Children and Adolescents with Neurodevelopmental Disabilities: Ecological Assessment Tools and Cognitive Analysis

Children and Adolescents with Neurodevelopmental Disabilities: Ecological Assessment Tools and Cognitive Analysis

Guest Editors

Yael Fogel
Naomi Josman

MDPI

Basel • Beijing • Wuhan • Barcelona • Belgrade • Novi Sad • Cluj • Manchester

Guest Editors
Yael Fogel
Department of Occupational Therapy
University of Ariel
Ariel
Israel

Naomi Josman
Department of Occupational Therapy
University of Haifa
Haifa
Israel

Editorial Office
MDPI AG
Grosspeteranlage 5
4052 Basel, Switzerland

This is a reprint of the Special Issue, published open access by the journal *Children* (ISSN 2227-9067), freely accessible at: https://www.mdpi.com/journal/children/special_issues/6N3300V02H.

For citation purposes, cite each article independently as indicated on the article page online and as indicated below:

Lastname, A.A.; Lastname, B.B. Article Title. *Journal Name* **Year**, *Volume Number*, Page Range.

ISBN 978-3-7258-6974-9 (Hbk)
ISBN 978-3-7258-6975-6 (PDF)
https://doi.org/10.3390/books978-3-7258-6975-6

Contents

About the Editors

Yael Fogel

Yael Fogel is a senior lecturer in the Department of Occupational Therapy, Faculty of Health Sciences, Ariel University, Israel, and the head of the Promoting Daily Executive Function Laboratory. Her research focuses on functional cognition, executive functions, and metacognitive processes, with an emphasis on how these higher-level cognitive mechanisms shape everyday functioning, participation, and independence. Her work primarily addresses children, adolescents, and young adults with neurodevelopmental difficulties, including attention, learning, and motor disorders, using ecological, performance-based assessment tools and strategy-based interventions. She completed her PhD at the University of Haifa and conducted a postdoctoral fellowship at Oxford Brookes University, UK. Dr. Fogel has published numerous peer-reviewed articles, serves as a guest editor and reviewer for international journals, and leads funded research projects aimed at developing innovative, ecologically valid tools for assessing and promoting daily executive functioning.

Naomi Josman

Naomi Josman is Professor Emerita of Occupational Therapy at the University of Haifa, Israel, and currently serves as an academic advisor for Horizon Europe at the Research Authority. She previously served as Associate Dean of Research at the Faculty of Social Welfare and Health Sciences at the University of Haifa between 2017 and 2021. Her research interests focus on cognition, metacognition, and executive functions and their impact on everyday functioning among individuals with central nervous system conditions, including stroke, Parkinson's disease, multiple sclerosis, schizophrenia, depression, and post-traumatic stress disorder. Her work spans diverse clinical populations, aiming to identify common and distinct functional profiles across disorders. She served as a member of the NATO scientific research initiative on virtual reality and rehabilitation for post-traumatic stress disorder and was invited to deliver keynote lectures at two NATO workshops. She has published more than 110 peer-reviewed articles and 14 book chapters and has presented her research at numerous national and international conferences.

Preface

This Reprint focuses on ecological assessment tools and cognitive analysis in children and adolescents with neurodevelopmental disabilities, emphasizing functional cognition and real-life performance. It presents performance-based, context-sensitive approaches that move beyond traditional decontextualized cognitive testing.

This Reprint is intended for researchers, clinicians, educators, and developers interested in ecologically valid assessment frameworks that capture authentic everyday functioning.

Yael Fogel and Naomi Josman
Guest Editors

children

MDPI

Editorial

Children and Adolescents with Neurodevelopmental Disabilities: Ecological Assessment Tools and Cognitive Analysis

Yael Fogel [1,*] and Naomi Josman [2]

1 Department of Occupational Therapy, Ariel University, Ariel 4070000, Israel
2 Department of Occupational Therapy, Faculty of Social Welfare and Health Sciences, University of Haifa, Haifa 3498838, Israel; njosman@univ.haifa.ac.il
* Correspondence: yaelfo@ariel.ac.il; Tel.: +972-52-616-2455

The Special Issue, "Children and Adolescents with Neurodevelopmental Disabilities: Ecological Assessment Tools and Cognitive Analysis," brings together a diverse collection of articles that highlight the rapidly evolving landscape of assessment, participation, and cognitive analysis in children and adolescents with neurodevelopmental disabilities (NDDs). As guest editors, we are grateful to the authors, the reviewers, and the *Children* journal for contributing to the success of this Special Issue, which now includes a rich set of 11 high-quality papers.

Functional cognition has emerged as one of the most critical domains in understanding children's and adolescents' participation in meaningful daily activities [1]. *Functional cognition* reflects the dynamic interplay of cognitive abilities, performance skills, environmental demands, and task requirements—elements that traditional, decontextualized cognitive tests cannot fully capture [2,3]. Over the past decade, the field has seen a conceptual shift: from focusing primarily on isolated cognitive components (bottom-up) toward emphasizing real-world functional performance (top-down) [4]. This shift aligns with broader occupational therapy and neuropsychological frameworks that emphasize ecological validity, contextual performance, and strategy use as essential indicators of meaningful cognitive functioning [5].

In our conceptual review on digitizing functional cognitive assessments, we found that although technology offers major opportunities, such as precise measurement, accessibility, and scalability, most performance-based assessment tools with the strongest ecological validity remain unavailable in digital formats.

The review demonstrates a persistent gap: Tools that best capture real-life functioning (e.g., complex cooking tasks, calendar planning, and naturalistic assessments) are precisely those most challenging to translate into digital platforms without compromising the richness of observation or strategy identification. At the same time, emerging technologies, such as virtual reality (VR), mobile platforms, and algorithm-driven adaptive assessments, show promise in bridging this gap by offering controlled yet naturalistic environments that can simulate real-life complexity. This technological evolution underscores the need for advanced digital tools that maintain representativeness, contextual fidelity, and the ability to capture strategy use—all hallmarks of ecologically valid functional cognitive assessment [6].

Collectively, the contributions to this Special Issue highlight a movement toward integrated assessment approaches that view cognitive abilities not as isolated mechanisms but as embedded within daily participation, emotional regulation, social interaction, and task demands. The articles span a wide range of populations (attention-deficit/hyperactivity

 https://doi.org/10.3390/children13010073

disorder [ADHD], autism spectrum disorder, traumatic brain injury, genetic syndromes, learning disabilities, and typically developing youth). They present tools that assess executive functions, memory, attention, problem-solving, and self-regulation using real-world or simulated tasks. Many contributions also integrate intervention perspectives, reflecting the growing understanding that assessment and treatment are interdependent—particularly within dynamic, context-sensitive frameworks.

A clear conceptual thread emerges across the Special Issue: the transition from bottom-up assessments, which assess cognitive components in isolation, toward top-down models, which evaluate performance within meaningful occupations. This transition is evident in the tools that examine participation, naturalistic behavior, everyday task complexity, and functional problem-solving. The studies collectively emphasize that understanding performance in real contexts is indispensable for accurately identifying strengths, challenges, learning potential, and intervention needs among children and adolescents with NDDs [7].

1. Future-Oriented Research Directions Across the Contributions

The collective body of work in this Special Issue highlights important opportunities for advancing the field of functional cognition. First, there is a clear need to continue developing ecologically valid digital assessment tools that preserve the richness of real-world observation while leveraging technological precision and scalability. Future studies should explore hybrid models that integrate naturalistic tasks with digital data capture, including VR-based simulations, sensor-supported monitoring, and adaptive mobile assessments. Second, there is a growing call for longitudinal research examining how functional cognition evolves across developmental stages and contexts, particularly in relation to participation, autonomy, and learning potential. Third, the contributions underscore the importance of cross-cultural validation and normative data for performance-based assessments, ensuring that assessment tools are sensitive to diverse environments and populations. Finally, future research should deepen the connection between assessment and treatment by investigating how performance-based measures can directly inform individualized strategy training, classroom accommodations, and family-centered support. Together, these directions point toward a dynamic, interdisciplinary future that seamlessly integrates ecological assessment, technological innovation, and participation-focused intervention.

2. An Overview of the Published Articles

2.1. *Diagnosis Identity Perception in Adolescents with ADHD and Its Relationship to Executive Functions, Self-Management, and Quality of Life (C1)*

This article explores how adolescents perceive their ADHD diagnosis and how this identity relates to executive functioning, self-management, and quality of life. The findings reveal that negative diagnosis identity predicts poorer executive function performance and reduced participation, highlighting the interplay between emotional experience, metacognition, and real-life functioning. This study contributes a unique psychosocial dimension to functional cognition, showing that identity and daily participation are intertwined. The study bridges assessment and intervention by pointing to the need for holistic, context-sensitive support.

2.2. *Occupation-Based Tele-Intervention for Children with Neurodevelopmental Disorders: A Pilot Study (C2)*

This pilot study adapts the cognitive orientation to daily occupational performance model for telehealth delivery, demonstrating meaningful functional gains in daily occupations. By focusing on self-selected goals and metacognitive strategies, the intervention aligns with top-down, participation-based assessment and treatment. Parents

 https://doi.org/10.3390/children13010073

and therapists reported that working in the child's natural home environment enhanced generalization—emphasizing the ecological strengths of tele-intervention. The study illustrates how assessment and intervention are interdependent processes shaped by real-life contexts.

2.3. Assessment of Fine Motor Abilities Among Children with Spinal Conditions (C3)

The authors evaluate fine-motor performance in children with spinal disorders using functional, activity-focused tools that capture real-life task execution (e.g., handling objects, manipulating materials). The results highlight significant gaps between impairment-level findings and actual performance in daily occupations, demonstrating the limits of bottom-up motor assessments. This article reinforces the need for ecologically valid, occupation-centered tools to understand how motor deficits influence participation and independence. Its focus on naturalistic performance connects directly to the Special Issue's emphasis on functional cognition.

2.4. Effects of Medical Cannabis Treatment for Autistic Children on Family Accommodation: An Open-Label Mixed-Methods Study (C4)

This mixed-methods study shows that cannabidiol-rich cannabis treatment reduced family accommodation behaviors and parental distress while improving family routines and participation. Although medical treatment is not a cognitive intervention per se, the findings demonstrate how reductions in behavioral rigidity can enhance functional participation within daily occupations. The study emphasizes the family context as a critical ecological layer influencing a child's functional cognition. It reinforces the relevance of participation-based outcomes as essential indicators of meaningful change.

2.5. Independence in Activities of Daily Living Among Autistic Toddlers: A Pilot Study Using Ecological Momentary Assessment (C5)

Using ecological momentary assessment, this study captures toddlers' daily living skills across real-time contexts. Results show that autistic toddlers demonstrate greater independence at home than indicated by one-time clinic assessments, highlighting the limitations of decontextualized evaluations. Ecological momentary assessment provides a rich, ecologically grounded picture of functional cognition, capturing variability, environment–task interactions, and natural performance. This article strongly supports the Special Issue's emphasis on real-world assessment and the top-down perspective.

2.6. ADHD Reporting in Developmental Age: The Role of the Informants (C6)

This article examines patterns of ADHD-symptom reporting across developmental stages using multi-informant perspectives. The study highlights the importance of contextualized behavioral observations, showing discrepancies among teachers, parents, and clinicians that reflect setting-dependent executive function performance. The findings align with functional cognition principles, illustrating that ADHD-related behaviors cannot be fully understood through isolated, component-based assessments. The paper underscores the need for ecologically grounded evaluations that consider context, participation demands, and daily routines.

2.7. Developmental Patterns in Autism and Other Neurodevelopmental Disorders in Preschool Children (C7)

This study analyzes developmental and adaptive profiles across autism spectrum disorder, language disorder, and mixed developmental disorder using multiple standardized tools and caregiver reports. Results confirm highly heterogeneous trajectories, demonstrating that diagnostic labels poorly generalize to functional performance in daily life.

https://doi.org/10.3390/children13010073

The authors show that caregiver-based ecological assessments add essential insight beyond clinic-based testing—especially regarding communication, motor skills, and adaptive functioning. This aligns strongly with the Special Issue's goal of understanding cognition within natural environments and across diverse NDD populations.

2.8. A Virtual Reality Platform for Evaluating Deficits in Executive Functions in Deaf and Hard of Hearing Children: Relation to Daily Function and to Quality of Life (C8)

This study introduces a VR-based assessment (supermarket) designed to simulate everyday executive-function challenges in a controlled yet ecologically valid environment. Findings show that VR tasks successfully capture real-world behaviors, such as planning, flexibility, and inhibition, beyond what traditional paper-and-pencil tests can measure. The virtual supermarket reflects the field's movement toward digital, performance-based assessments that preserve contextual demands. By replicating complex tasks in a safe virtual environment, the study demonstrates how technology can bridge the gap between top-down functional evaluation and quantifiable cognitive metrics.

2.9. Can Functional Cognitive Assessments for Children/Adolescents Be Transformed into Digital Platforms? A Conceptual Review (C9)

This conceptual review examines the feasibility and implications of digitizing performance-based functional cognitive assessments for children and adolescents. Reviewing 13 assessment tools, the authors show that most high-ecologically valid assessments remain nondigital, whereas existing digital tools often sacrifice contextual realism. The article highlights a major gap between clinical need and technological development and emphasizes that digital platforms must preserve real-world context, strategy observation, and process-oriented evaluation. It proposes a guiding conceptual framework to support future development of ecologically valid digital assessments. The review concludes with recommendations for leveraging VR, mobile devices, and advanced analytics to enhance the precision, accessibility, and scalability of functional cognitive evaluation.

2.10. Sleep Disorders in Children with Rett Syndrome (C10)

This review synthesizes evidence on sleep disturbances among children with Rett syndrome, a population in which approximately 80% experience significant sleep difficulties. The article details common issues, such as insomnia, abnormal nocturnal breathing, parasomnias, bruxism, and seizures, and examines genotype–phenotype associations. Objective findings from polysomnography reveal reduced sleep efficiency, elevated arousals, disrupted REM/NREM patterns, and both central and obstructive sleep apnea. Recommendations for management emphasize behavioral sleep interventions, careful pharmacological consideration due to autonomic and cardiac vulnerabilities, and the importance of individualized multimodal care. The authors call for more rigorous research and registry-based studies to advance evidence-based treatment strategies.

2.11. XR Technologies in Inclusive Education for Neurodivergent Children: A Systematic Review 2020–2024 (C11)

This systematic review synthesizes evidence on extended reality tools used to support neurodivergent students in inclusive education. The findings emphasize improvements in engagement, social communication, and cognitive participation within simulated learning environments. Extended reality emerges as a promising pathway for creating controlled yet realistic contexts that mirror daily classroom demands. The review highlights the potential of extended reality to bridge digital assessment with real-world participation, supporting the Special Issue's theme of emerging technologies in functional cognition.

https://doi.org/10.3390/children13010073

3. Authentic, Integrated, and Person-Centered Approaches

Collectively, the articles in this Special Issue advance the field toward more authentic, integrated, and person-centered approaches. They reinforce the importance of aligning assessments with real-world contexts and of acknowledging the rich diversity of children's experiences, abilities, and environments. It is our hope that this Special Issue will inspire continued innovation and collaboration across clinical, educational, community, and research settings.

We extend our sincere appreciation to all authors whose work contributed to this Special Issue and to the *Children* editorial team for their support and professionalism. We look forward to seeing how the ideas presented here will influence future research, shape practice, and expand our collective understanding of children and adolescents with neurodevelopmental disabilities.

Conflicts of Interest: The authors declare no conflicts of interest.

List of Contributions:

1. Zabar-Cahanovich, Y.; Stern, A.; Lamash, L. Diagnosis identity perception in adolescents with ADHD and its relationship to executive functions, self-management, and quality of life. *Children* **2025**, 12, 1532.
2. Ben Zagmi-Averbuch, S.; Rozen, D.; Aharon-Felsen, B.; Siman Tov, R.; Lowengrub, J.; Tal-Saban, M.; Gilboa, Y. Occupation-based tele-intervention for children with neurodevelopmental disorders: A pilot study. *Children* **2025**, *12*, 1521.
3. Klemm, I.; Danial-Saad, A.; Karlin, A.R.; Nassar-Yassien, R.; Eshel, I.; Levine, H.; Steinberg, T.; Aharoni, S. Assessment of fine motor abilities among children with spinal muscular atrophy treated with Nusinersen using a new touchscreen application: A pilot study. *Children* **2025**, *12*, 1378.
4. David, A.; Gal, E.; Ben-Sasson, A.; Kohn, E.; Berkovitch, M.; Stolar, O. Effects of medical cannabis treatment for autistic children on family accommodation: An open-label mixed-methods study. *Children* **2025**, *12*, 1373.
5. Hillel, S.; Aaronson, B.; Gilboa, Y. Independence in activities of daily living among autistic toddlers: A pilot study using ecological momentary assessment. *Children* **2025**, *12*, 1316.
6. Esposito, D.; Gigliotti, F.; Colotti, B.; Di Brina, C.; Pisani, F.; Romani, M. ADHD reporting in developmental age: The role of the informants. *Children* **2025**, *12*, 914.
7. Martelli, M.E.; Gigliotti, F.; Giovannone, F.; Lentini, G.; Manti, F.; Sogos, C. Developmental patterns in autism and other neurodevelopmental disorders in preschool children. *Children* **2025**, *12*, 125.
8. Hamed-Daher, S.; Josman, N.; Klinger, E.; Engel-Yeger, B. A virtual reality platform for evaluating deficits in executive functions in deaf and hard of hearing children—relation to daily function and to quality of life. *Children* **2024**, *11*, 1123.
9. Fogel, Y.; Josman, N.; Cohen Elimelech, O.; Zlotnik, S. Can functional cognitive assessments for children/adolescents be transformed into digital platforms? A conceptual review. *Children* **2025**, *12*, 1384.
10. Harner, C.; Gaffey, T.A.; Sullivan, S.S.; Witmans, M.; DelRosso, L.M.; Tablizo, M.A. Sleep disorders in children with Rett syndrome. *Children* **2025**, *12*, 869.
11. Valverde Olivares, B.; Muñoz Araya, L.; Valín, J.L.; Jarpa Azagra, M.; Hidalgo Escobar, R.; Cuevas Quezada, I.; Galleguillos Ketterer, C. XR technologies in inclusive education for neurodivergent children: A systematic review 2020–2024. *Children* **2025**, *12*, 1474.

References

1. Lee, Y.; Randolph, S.B.; Kim, M.Y.; Foster, E.R.; Kersey, J.; Baum, C.; Connor, L.T. Performance-based assessments of functional cognition in adults, part 1—Assessment characteristics: A systematic review. *Am. J. Occup. Ther.* **2025**, *79*, 7904205130. [CrossRef] [PubMed]

https://doi.org/10.3390/children13010073

2. Giles, G.M.; Edwards, D.F.; Morrison, M.T.; Baum, C.; Wolf, T.J. Screening for functional cognition in postacute care and the Improving Medicare Post-Acute Care Transformation (IMPACT) Act of 2014. *Am. J. Occup. Ther.* **2017**, *71*, 7105090010p1–7105090010p6. [CrossRef] [PubMed]
3. Wolf, T.J.; Edwards, D.F.; Giles, G.M. *Functional Cognition and Occupational Therapy: A Practical Approach to Treating Individuals with Cognitive Loss*; AOTA Press: Bethesda, MD, USA, 2019.
4. Weinstock-Zlotnick, G.; Hinojosa, J. Bottom-up or top-down evaluation: Is one better than the other? *Am. J. Occup. Ther.* **2004**, *58*, 594–599. [CrossRef] [PubMed]
5. Toglia, J.; Foster, E. *The Multicontext Approach: A Metacognitive Strategy-Based Intervention for Functional Cognition*; MC CogRehab Resources: New York, NY, USA, 2021.
6. Wallisch, A.; Little, L.M.; Dean, E.; Dunn, W. Executive function measures for children: A scoping review of ecological validity. *OTJR* **2017**, *38*, 6–14. [CrossRef] [PubMed]
7. Josman, N.; Rosenblum, S. A metacognitive model for children with atypical brain development. In *Cognition, Occupation, and Participation Across the Life Span: Neuroscience, Neurorehabilitation and Models for Intervention in Occupational Therapy*; Katz, N., Ed.; AOTA Press: Bethesda, MD, USA, 2018; pp. 223–248.

https://doi.org/10.3390/children13010073

children

MDPI

Article

Diagnosis Identity Perception in Adolescents with ADHD and Its Relationship to Executive Functions, Self-Management, and Quality of Life

Yael Zabar-Cahanovich [1], Adi Stern [2] and Liron Lamash [1,*]

[1] Department of Occupational Therapy, Faculty of Social Welfare & Health Sciences, University of Haifa, Haifa 3498838, Israel; yaelcahanovich@gmail.com

[2] Department of Occupational Therapy, Faculty of Health Sciences, Ben-Gurion University of the Negev, Beer Sheva 8410501, Israel; adister@bgu.ac.il

* Correspondence: llamash1@staff.haifa.ac.il

Highlights:

What are the main findings?

- Adolescents with ADHD reported significantly higher identity Acceptance scores compared to Rejection, Engulfment, and Enrichment, F (2.38, 149.89) = 32.41, $p < 0.001$.
- The total diagnosis identity score was strongly associated with self-management (r = 0.61, $p < 0.001$).
- The Engulfment dimension showed strong and consistent associations with both executive dysfunction and lower quality of life, despite the absence of correlations at the total score level.
- Regression analyses indicated that self-monitoring, social QoL, and self-evaluation together explained 45% of the variance in ADHD diagnosis identity. The Engulfment dimension of identity was a significant negative predictor of executive functioning (R^2 = 0.15), self-management (R^2 = 0.35), and QoL (R^2 = 0.17).

What are the implications of the main findings?

- The findings underscore the complex relationship between diagnosis identity and emotional as well as functional outcomes in adolescents with ADHD.
- Negative perceptions of one's diagnosis identity predict poorer executive functioning, self-management, and QoL, while core aspects of self-management and social well-being also significantly shape how adolescents with ADHD perceive their diagnosis.
- The results highlight the need for holistic, individualized interventions that address both the development of positive diagnosis identity and the strengthening of executive and self-management skills of adolescents with ADHD.
- Promoting a positive diagnosis identity may improve functional and emotional outcomes, which in turn may reinforce a more adaptive and accepting view of the diagnosis itself.

Abstract: Background/Objectives: This study aimed to describe how adolescents with attention-deficit/hyperactivity disorder (ADHD) perceive their diagnosis identity and examine its correlation with executive functions (EFs), self-management abilities, and quality of life (QoL). Methods: A total of 66 adolescents with ADHD, aged 12 to 18 years (M = 15.21, SD = 1.84), completed self-report questionnaires, including the Illness Identity Questionnaire, Behavior Rating Inventory of Executive Function, Self-Control and Self-Management Scale, and Pediatric QoL Inventory. We used ANOVA with Bonferroni post hoc tests to assess differences in diagnosis identity domains and Pearson correlations to examine correlations between diagnosis identity, EFs, self-management, and QoL. **Results**: Adolescents reported significantly higher ADHD *Acceptance* feelings compared to *Rejection*, *Engulfment*, and *Enrichment*, F (2.38, 149.89) = 32.41, $p < 0.001$. Total diagnosis identity score was strongly associated with self-management ($r = 0.61$, $p < 0.001$). While no significant correlations were found with overall EF or QoL, significant associations did emerge with their sub-scores. Regression analyses indicated that self-monitoring, social QoL, and self-evaluation together explained 45% of the variance in diagnosis identity. The *Engulfment* dimension of identity was a significant negative predictor of executive functioning ($R^2 = 0.15$), self-management ($R^2 = 0.35$), and QoL ($R^2 = 0.17$). **Conclusions**: Promoting a positive diagnosis identity may improve functional and emotional outcomes in adolescents with ADHD. In turn, better functional and emotional outcomes may help them embrace a diagnosis identity that is more positive.

Keywords: diagnosis identity; attention-deficit/hyperactivity disorder; adolescence; executive function; self-management; quality of life

1. Introduction

The neurodevelopmental condition, attention-deficit/hyperactivity disorder (ADHD), is characterized by difficulties with sustaining attention and/or hyperactivity-impulsivity that interfere with functioning and development [1]. As one of the most common neurodevelopmental disorders, the prevalence of ADHD among children and adolescents is estimated to be around 8% globally [2]. Although ADHD was traditionally considered a childhood disorder, it is currently recognized as a lifelong condition [3,4].

The World Health Organization [5] defines adolescence as the transitional stage between childhood and adulthood, occurring between the ages of 10 and 19. This period is marked by significant growth and development across all areas of life. In addition to physical changes, adolescents undergo substantial cognitive, emotional, and social transformations. Additionally, it is a time characterized by identity formation, development of social roles and interactions, self-exploration, and cultivation of autonomy and self-reliance [6].

For adolescents with ADHD, this stage can present particularly profound challenges. Increased academic and social demands make this period especially vulnerable because adolescents with ADHD often face higher rates of social rejection, isolation, and educational difficulties [7,8]. These challenges are compounded by low self-esteem, reduced motivation to achieve, social-skills deficits, and social withdrawal [9]. Studies also indicate that these deficits in social, physical, and emotional domains negatively affect quality of life (QoL), particularly during adolescence. Adolescents with ADHD often have a significantly lower QoL compared to their peers without an ADHD diagnosis [6,10].

One central deficit commonly associated with ADHD is impairments in executive functions (EFs) [11,12]. Approximately 67% of adolescents with ADHD exhibit clinically significant EF deficits, particularly in planning, organization, and working memory domains [13]. EFs are high-level cognitive processes involving complex, goal-directed behaviors such as planning, control, problem-solving, working memory, and inhibition which are necessary to perform tasks in diverse situations and environments [14]. They enable individuals to make informed decisions and use strategies to enhance performance, learning, and daily functioning [14]. Thus, EF deficits can have long-term implications for daily life and significantly affect planning, organization, decision-making, academic achievement, and social skills, potentially leading to maladaptive behaviors [15,16].

Adolescence is a period of significant EFs development [17]. Adolescents with ADHD often exhibit more deficits in tasks requiring EFs than their typically developing peers [18–20]. They frequently struggle with maintaining attention, inhibiting responses, and sustaining perseverance [11,18–20]. These difficulties may hinder them in developing various aspects of self-perception and identity, which are critical developmental tasks during this stage of life. Additionally, the challenges associated with EF deficits may impair daily functioning, academic performance, self-regulation, and self-management [16].

Self-management is a lifelong task that requires EFs, such as problem-solving and decision-making [21,22]. It involves managing time and adapting as circumstances change, with an acute awareness of experiences and their impact on one's physical and mental state [23]. These skills are designed to improve EFs, reduce core symptoms, and enhance QoL and self-identity perception. For youth with chronic health conditions, self-management skill development is a long, complex process shaped by psychological factors, social networks, and health system involvement [24–28]. Ultimately, this development can lead to positive changes in health and social outcomes [19].

Identity refers to internal self-awareness, encompassing an individual's direction in life and future goals [29]. Self-identity is a composite of skills, knowledge, and beliefs shaped by personal traits, characteristics, life roles, physical appearance, values, goals, past experiences, and ongoing interactions with significant others [29,30]. It enables individuals to work toward achieving their goals while recognizing their strengths and limitations and fosters a sense of capability and efficacy. This recognition is essential for self-definition and functioning as a successful societal adult. Adolescents with chronic illnesses tend to integrate their diagnosis into their identity [31], which may include their knowledge and goals related to their condition, guiding their actions, values, and behaviors in various situations [30]. Forming a well-integrated and consolidated identity by, for example, committing to plans and actively participating in life decisions can protect young people living with chronic illnesses against distress and depressive symptoms [32].

The term *illness identity* has recently been used to describe how a person integrates a chronic illness into their identity [33]. It refers to the attitudes and roles a person develops about their self, their health condition, and their integration of the condition into their daily life [34,35]. Using this concept, Oris et al. [34] described the degree to which a person integrates their chronic illness with their sense of self. They described four dimensions of illness identity: (a) *Acceptance*, how much a person accepts their illness and its challenges as part of their identity without being overwhelmed by it; (b) *Enrichment*, how much the person feels the illness allowed them to develop and discern advantages for their identity in it; (c) *Rejection*, how much the person rejects the illness and does not perceive it as part of their identity; and (d) *Engulfment*, how much the person's illness engulfs their identity and permeates all areas of their life. Whereas *Acceptance* and *Enrichment* are considered positive dimensions of identity perception, *Rejection* and *Engulfment* are considered negative [36].

Several studies have examined illness identity perception among adolescents and adults with chronic health conditions, such as type 1 diabetes, epilepsy, and celiac disease, and how these illnesses integrate into their sense of self [34,36–38]. These studies demonstrated that illness identity plays a central role in adapting to chronic illnesses. Adolescents who felt *Engulfment* were more likely to experience symptoms of depression and anxiety. On the other hand, *Acceptance* of the diagnosis was linked to better social abilities, improved coping skills, and increased social participation. Other studies have explored illness identity (herein renamed *diagnosis identity*) within neurodevelopmental conditions such as autism spectrum disorder and ADHD. A positive diagnosis identity in autistic individuals was associated with greater psychological well-being, higher QoL, and broader social participation [39–41]. Similarly, recent studies have examined diagnosis identity and its psychosocial implications among adolescents with ADHD, emphasizing how the interpretation of one's diagnosis shapes self-concept, social relationships, and adjustment [42–44]. These findings indicate that illness identity is not limited to the experience of chronic health conditions but reflects broader identity processes common to neurodevelopmental conditions.

In sum, adolescence is a critical period for development, which may be more complex for individuals with ADHD. Adolescents with ADHD often face various emotional and functional impairments, which further contribute to low self-esteem and QoL. Hence, developing a positive self-image, self-esteem, and identity perception can be particularly challenging for them [45]. The self-identity of adolescents with ADHD often incorporates aspects related to their diagnosis, challenges, and goals, influencing their behavior in various contexts. The absence of a stable identity may lead to difficulties in EFs, impair self-management abilities, and negatively impact QoL. These emotional and functional deficits may, in turn, further hinder identity formation. Despite the importance of this issue, it has yet to be thoroughly explored. Therefore, the aims of this study were to examine how adolescents with ADHD perceive their diagnosis identity and how it relates to their EFs, self-management abilities, and QoL.

2. Materials and Methods

2.1. Study Design

This was a cross-sectional study using an anonymous online survey. The sample was recruited using convenience sampling, and eligibility was confirmed through a brief parental screening process before data collection.

2.2. Participants

A sample size of approximately 70 participants was determined using the G-Power test based on a one-tailed correlation with an effect size of 0.03, alpha level of 0.05, and power of 80%. The final sample included 66 adolescents aged 12 to 18 years (M = 15.21 years, SD = 1.84) with a formal diagnosis of ADHD. Of these, 50 (75.8%) participants were male, 15 (22.7%) were female, and one (1.5%) did not want to specify gender. Other comorbid neurodevelopmental or chronic health conditions (e.g., autism spectrum disorder, intellectual disability, or chronic medical illnesses) served as exclusion criteria to minimize the influence of additional conditions on the experience related to having ADHD. Due to the anonymous nature of the online survey, verification of ADHD diagnosis provided by a qualified authority, and the absence of comorbidities, were confirmed at the parental screening stage. Table 1 presents additional participant demographic characteristics.

Table 1. Participants' demographic characteristics.

Characteristic	Range	*M (SD)*
Age of diagnosis (years)	4–17	10.11 (3.27)
Age of exposure to diagnosis (years)	3–17	10.20 (3.06)
	n (%)	
Educational setting		
Public school	62 (93.9)	
Anthroposophical/democratic	3 (4.5)	
External school/home school	1 (1.5)	
Class type		
Mainstream class/full matriculation	58 (87.9)	
Special education	3 (4.5)	
Gifted/sport	5 (7.6)	
Stimulant medication		
Yes	24 (36.4)	
No	42 (63.6)	

2.3. Measures

2.3.1. Demographic Questionnaire

Items in the demographic questionnaire developed for this study included parental confirmation of the child's ADHD and additional chronic or neurodevelopmental diagnoses. Other items collected general sociodemographic data, such as gender, age, and education settings.

2.3.2. Illness Identity Questionnaire

The Illness Identity Questionnaire (IIQ) [34] is a self-report questionnaire designed to measure the extent to which a chronic health or developmental condition integrates into the respondent's daily life and identity. For this study, the IIQ was explicitly adapted for ADHD following the authors' guidelines and with their permission. The questionnaire consists of 25 statements rated on a 5-point Likert scale from 1 (strongly disagree) to 5 (strongly agree). The IIQ assesses four dimensions of diagnosis identity: (a) *Rejection*, including five items; (b) *Engulfment*, including eight items; (c) *Acceptance*, including five items; and (d) *Enrichment*, including seven items. Each dimension's score is calculated as the average of its related items; a higher score indicates a greater expression of that dimension. Items from the negative dimensions (*Rejection* and *Engulfment*) are reverse-scored; mean scores are calculated across all items to achieve an overall score; higher overall scores reflect more positive identity perception. The IIQ has demonstrated high discriminant validity and internal consistency; reliability coefficients ranged from 0.75 to 0.95 among adolescents with chronic conditions [34,46]. In the current study, internal reliability was good for all IIQ items ($\alpha = 0.81$) and adequate for each component ($\alpha = 0.71 - 0.84$).

2.3.3. Behavior Rating Inventory of Executive Function-Self-Report

The Behavior Rating Inventory of Executive Function (BRIEF-SR) [47] is a self-report questionnaire designed to assess EFs in adolescents aged 11 to 18 years. The questionnaire comprises 80 statements in which participants are asked to rate the frequency of specific behaviors on a 3-point scale: 1 (never), 2 (sometimes), and 3 (often or always). The items are divided into eight categories that assess different aspects of executive functioning. Three categories, inhibition, shifting, and emotional regulation, form the behavioral regulation index (BRI); five categories, initiation, working memory, planning/organization, environmental organization, and monitoring, form the metacognition index (MI). Raw scores are computed for each category by summing the item ratings. Additionally, composite scores are calculated for the BRI, MI, and the global executive composite (GEC), which reflects overall executive functioning. Using gender- and age-specific norms to convert these raw scores provides a standardized score for executive functioning; a lower score reflects better executive functioning. Scores below 60 represent normal functioning, scores from 60 to 65 indicate at-risk functioning, and scores greater than 65 signify impaired functioning. The BRIEF-SR has demonstrated strong content validity, construct validity, and high internal reliability across its scales, with reported reliabilities of Cronbach's alphas of 0.93 (BRI), 0.94 (MI), and 0.96 (GEC) [47]. In the current study, internal reliability was similarly high, with $\alpha = 0.96$ for all items and $\alpha = 0.95$ to 0.96 across the categories.

2.3.4. Self-Control and Self-Management Scale

The Self-Control and Self-Management Scale (SCMS) [48] is a self-report questionnaire to assess self-management abilities in daily life. The questionnaire consists of 16 statements rated on a scale from 0 (does not describe me at all) to 5 (describes me very well). These items are divided into three subscales: self-monitoring (six statements), self-evaluating (five statements), and self-reinforcing (five statements) scales. Together, they produce an overall score reflecting self-management skills. Scores are calculated by summing the ratings of all relevant items; higher scores indicate better self-management abilities [49]. The SCMS has demonstrated construct and discriminant validity, along with high internal reliability for all items ($\alpha = 0.85$) and adequate to good reliability for the subscales ($\alpha = 0.72 - 0.80$). The current study found reliability acceptable, with a Cronbach's alpha of 0.75 for all items and subscale reliability ranging from 0.59 to 0.87.

2.3.5. Pediatric Quality of Life Inventory

The self-reported Pediatric Quality of Life Inventory (PedsQL), designed for adolescents aged 13 to 18 years [50], assesses health-related QoL. It applies to healthy adolescents and those with chronic health conditions. The questionnaire includes 23 items that evaluate four dimensions of QoL: eight physical-functioning items, five emotional-functioning items, five social-functioning items, and five school-functioning items. Adolescents are asked to indicate the extent to which each statement represents a difficulty or problem on a scale from 0 (never a problem) to 4 (almost always a problem). These ratings are converted to a linear score ranging from 0 to 100 (0 = 100, 1 = 75, 2 = 50, 3 = 25, 4 = 0), with higher scores indicating better QoL. In addition to an overall score, mean scores for the four dimensions are calculated. The PedsQL has demonstrated high internal reliability for self-reports ($\alpha = 0.88$) and possesses strong construct and discriminant validity between groups with varying morbidity levels [50]. In the current study, the PedsQL demonstrated acceptable internal reliability for all items ($\alpha = 0.72$) and good reliability across the categories ($\alpha = 0.79 - 0.84$).

2.4. *Procedure*

The University of Haifa Institutional Ethics Committee approved this study (No. 274/19-1). We recruited participants by directing advertisements to parents of adolescents with ADHD via relevant interest groups, forums, and social media. The advertisements included a link to an explanatory letter about the study and several screening questions designed to confirm eligibility. Parents who expressed interest in their child's participation were asked to complete an informed consent form. Subsequently, they forwarded the survey link to their adolescents, who independently completed the questionnaire on Google Forms. Because the online form required a response for every item, no forms were submitted with missing data. Completion time was approximately 25 min. Responses were transmitted automatically and anonymously to a secure database only the research team could access. Data collection took place between February and April 2024.

2.5. *Data Analyses*

We analyzed the data using IBM SPSS (Version 27). Descriptive statistics summarized the sample characteristics, including the variables' ranges, means, and standard deviations. An analysis of variance with Bonferroni post hoc analysis for repeated measures was performed to assess differences in diagnosis identity perception measures. Additionally, we conducted Pearson correlation analyses to explore the correlation between dimensions of diagnosis identity perception (IIQ) and EFs (BRIEF-SR), self-management (SCMS), and QoL (PedsQL).

3. Results

3.1. *Diagnosis Identity Perception of Adolescents with ADHD*

A repeated measures ANOVA was conducted to examine differences between the four dimensions of diagnosis identity (*Rejection*, *Acceptance*, *Engulfment*, and *Enrichment*), as measured by the IIQ. Mauchly's test indicated a violation of the sphericity assumption, $\chi^2(5) = 22.67$, $p < 0.001$; therefore, we applied the Greenhouse–Geisser correction ($\varepsilon = 0.795$).

The results showed a statistically significant effect of identity dimension on IIQ scores, $F\ (2.38, 149.89) = 32.41$, $p < 0.001$, partial $\eta^2 = 0.607$, indicating a large effect size. Multivariate tests (Wilks' Lambda = 0.393, $p < 0.001$) also confirmed a significant overall difference across the four dimensions. Post hoc comparisons using Bonferroni-adjusted pairwise tests showed that *Acceptance* scores ($M = 3.74$, $SD = 0.88$) were significantly higher than *Rejection* ($M = 2.54$, $SD = 0.91$), *Engulfment* ($M = 2.38$, $SD = 0.81$), and *Enrichment* ($M = 2.75$, $SD = 0.93$) scores ($p < 0.001$ for all comparisons). *Engulfment* scores were significantly lower than all other dimensions ($p < 0.001$), while *Enrichment* did not significantly differ from *Rejection* ($p > 0.05$). No significant gender differences were observed in IIQ scores, nor were there significant differences between adolescents who reported taking ADHD medication and those who did not.

3.1.1. Relationship Between Diagnosis Identity Perception and EFs, Self-Management, and QoL

We conducted correlational analyses to explore the relationships among adolescents' diagnosis identity perceptions (as measured by the IIQ) and their reported EFs, self-management, and QoL.

3.1.2. Relationship Between Diagnosis Identity and EFs

No significant correlations were found between the IIQ total score and the BRIEF-SR total (GEC), behavioral regulation (BRI), or metacognitive abilities (MI) scores. Further analysis explored the correlation between the IIQ dimensions and the specific BRIEF-SR scales. Most of the significant correlations were associated with the *Engulfment* dimension, suggesting that the participants who felt their ADHD diagnosis was more central or overwhelming tend to experience greater executive dysfunctions, and conversely, greater difficulties in executive functioning may reinforce a more engulfed or consuming sense of diagnosis identity. Table 2 presents these results, including detailed correlations between the IIQ dimensions and the BRIEF-SR scales.

Table 2. Correlations between the IIQ and the BRIEF-SR, SCMS, and PedsQL.

	IIQ				
	Rejection	***Acceptance***	***Engulfment***	***Enrichment***	***Total IIQ***
BRIEF-SR					
Inhibition	−0.25 *	0.20	0.38 **	0.26 *	0.11
Shift	−0.15	0.10	0.42 **	0.20	0.00
Emotional control	−0.16	0.13	0.32 **	0.26 *	0.08
BRI Score	−0.21	0.21	0.42 ***	0.24	0.05
Organization of material	−0.10	0.07	0.27 *	0.03	−0.04
Task completion	0.05	−0.05	0.37 **	−0.03	−0.19
Working memory	−0.12	0.13	0.40 ***	0.16	0.00
Plan/organize	−0.01	0.00	0.38 **	0.04	−0.18
Monitor	−0.14	−0.03	0.26 *	−0.03	−0.10
MI Score	0.05	0.13	0.43 ***	0.09	−0.12
GEC Score	−0.13	0.11	0.46 ***	0.17	−0.04
SCMS					
Self-monitoring	−0.30 *	0.47 ***	−0.29 *	0.46 **	0.58 **
Self-evaluation	−0.17	0.14	−0.02	0.23	0.20
Self-reinforcing	−0.22	0.28 *	−0.11	0.31 **	0.36 **
SCMS Total	−0.37 **	0.45 ***	−0.35 **	0.39 ***	0.61 ***
PedsQL					
Physical	−0.02	0.20	−0.42 **	0.03	0.30 *
Emotional	0.03	−0.15	−0.31 *	−0.14	0.05
Social	−0.27 *	−0.09	−0.28 *	−0.08	0.19
School	0.25 *	−0.13	−0.24	−0.11	−0.05
PedsQL Total	0.00	0.00	−0.41 ***	−0.07	0.17

Note. IIQ = Illness Identity Questionnaire; BRIEF-SR = Behavior Rating Inventory of Executive Function–Self-Report; SCMS = Self-Control and Self-Management; PedsQL = Pediatric Quality of Life Inventory; * $p < 0.05$, ** $p < 0.01$, *** $p < 0.001$.

3.1.3. Relationship Between Diagnosis Identity and Self-Management

A strong positive correlation was found between the IIQ total score and the SCMS total score ($r = 0.61$, $p < 0.001$), suggesting that adolescents with a more integrated diagnosis identity tend to report better self-regulation. Likewise, adolescents with stronger self-regulation tend to perceive their diagnosis identity more positively. Among the IIQ dimensions, *Acceptance* and *Enrichment* were most positively associated with SCMS subscales, while *Rejection* and *Engulfment* showed negative correlations. Detailed correlations between IIQ dimensions and SCMS subscales are presented in Table 2.

3.1.4. Relationship Between Diagnosis Identity and QoL

No significant correlation was found between the IIQ total score and overall PedsQL scores, suggesting that general diagnosis identity integration is not directly linked to perceived QoL. However, we observed significant negative correlations for the *Engulfment* dimension with the physical ($r = -0.42$, $p < 0.01$), emotional ($r = -0.31$, $p \leq 0.05$), and social ($r = -0.28$, $p = 0.05$) domains of QoL. These findings suggest that adolescents who feel more engulfed by their ADHD diagnosis tend to report lower well-being, and those experiencing reduced QoL may be more likely to perceive their diagnosis as overwhelming. Table 2 presents the full correlation results.

3.2. *Diagnosis Identity Perception: Bidirectional Prediction*

3.2.1. Predicting Diagnosis Identity by EFs, Self-Management, and QoL

A stepwise multiple regression analysis was conducted to examine predictors of diagnosis identity perception (IIQ total score). Three variables were entered sequentially as significant predictors: self-monitoring (SCMS), social QoL (PedsQL), and self-evaluation (SCMS). The final model accounted for 45.3% of the variance in diagnosis identity perception. No evidence of multicollinearity was observed, as all VIF values were close to 1. Table 3 presents a summary of the regression models.

Table 3. Summary of the model: predictors of diagnosis identity perception in stepwise multiple regressions.

Model	Predictor	B	*SE* B	β	*t*	*p*
1	Self-Monitoring (SCMS)	0.049	0.008	0.592	5.88	<0.001
			$F\ (1{,}64) = 34.57$, $p < 0.001$			
			$R = 0.592$, $R^2 = 0.351$, $Adj.\ R^2 = 0.341$			
2	Self-Monitoring (SCMS)	0.048	0.008	0.582	5.98	<0.001
	Social QoL (PedsQL)	0.007	0.003	0.231	2.37	0.021
			$F\ (2{,}63) = 21.35$, $p < 0.001$			
			$R = 0.636$, $R^2 = 0.404$, $Adj.\ R^2 = 0.385$			
3	Self-Monitoring (SCMS)	0.049	0.008	0.595	6.32	<0.001
	Social QoL (PedsQL)	0.007	0.003	0.226	2.40	0.019
	Self-Evaluation (SCMS)	0.029	0.012	0.221	2.35	0.022
			$F\ (3{,}62) = 17.09$, $p < 0.001$			
			$R = 0.673$, $R^2 = 0.453$, $Adj.\ R^2 = 0.426$			

3.2.2. Predicting EFs, Self-Management, and QoL by Diagnosis Identity Dimensions

A series of stepwise multiple regression analyses was conducted to examine the predictive value of diagnosis identity perception dimensions (IIQ) for executive functioning, self-monitoring, and QoL. *Engulfment* emerged as a significant negative predictor of both executive functioning and QoL; specifically, adolescents who reported greater identification with their diagnosis showed poorer cognitive and well-being outcomes. In contrast, *Enrichment* was a positive predictor of self-management skills, reflecting that perceiving one's diagnosis as meaningful and growth-promoting was associated with better self-regulatory abilities. Together, these models explained approximately 15% to 35% of the variance across the outcome measures. No evidence of multicollinearity was observed in any model (all VIFs < 1.05). The results are summarized in Table 4.

Table 4. Summary of the model: Predicting EF, self-management, and QoL by IIQ dimensions in stepwise multiple regressions.

Outcome Variable	Predicator (IIQ Dimension)	B	*SE* B	β	*t*	*p*
Executive functions (BRIEF-SR GEC)	Engulfment	6.50	1.94	0.386	3.35	0.001
			F (1,64) = 11.20, p = 0.001			
			R = 0.386, R^2 = 0.149, *Adj.* R^2 = 0.136			
Self-management-Step 1	Enrichment	6.24	1.30	0.514	4.80	<0.001
			F (2,63) = 23.01, p < 0.001			
			R = 0.514, R^2 = 0.264, *Adj.* R^2 = 0.253			
Self-Management-Step 2	Enrichment	6.75	1.25	0.557	5.42	<0.001
	Engulfment	−4.05	1.43	−0.292	−2.84	0.006
			F (2,63) = 16.80, p < 0.001			
			R = 0.590, R^2 = 0.348, *Adj.* R^2 = 0.327			
Quality of life (PedsQL)	Engulfment	−6.52	1.83	−0.407	−3.56	0.001
			F (3,62) = 12.69, p < 0.001			
			R = 0.407, R^2 = 0.165, *Adj.* R^2 = 0.152			

4. Discussion

The present study reveals that adolescents with ADHD are more likely to perceive their diagnosis identity in positive terms, with *Acceptance* emerging as the most prominent dimension compared to *Rejection* and *Engulfment*. This tendency aligns with prior research on other neurodevelopmental and chronic conditions, such as celiac disease [38] and autism [51], where a positive component of diagnosis identity has also been observed. Moreover, our results complement prior work with adolescents with ADHD, who often characterize their experience in terms of openness, honesty, empathy, high energy and motivation, creativity, agreeableness, hyperfocus, and strong willingness to help others [52]. Recognizing and validating these strengths can foster greater acceptance, more adaptive coping strategies, and, in some cases, even a sense of pride in one's diagnosis [53]. The positive aspects of ADHD have also been emphasized in the growing influence of the Neurodiversity Movement [54], which highlights individuals' strengths, talents, and unique contributions and views neurological differences as natural and valuable expressions of human variation [55].

However, our findings also reveal that the diagnosis identity perceptions of adolescents with ADHD are not exclusively positive or negative. Instead, most participants demonstrated a nuanced and multidimensional profile, experiencing both *Acceptance* and *Enrichment* alongside feelings of *Rejection* and *Engulfment*. This internal complexity echoes recent qualitative research showing that adolescents with ADHD often navigate a dynamic mix of pride, self-acceptance, and meaning, while simultaneously contending with stigma, self-doubt, or a sense of difference [44,56,57]. Such findings highlight that diagnosis identity in ADHD is shaped by ongoing negotiation between positive self-concepts and the psychological or social challenges associated with the diagnosis.

The present study found that feelings of *Engulfment*, meaning the sense that ADHD becomes central and overwhelming to one's identity, were significantly associated with EF deficits among adolescents. This finding supports the conceptualization of ADHD diagnosis identity as closely intertwined with self-regulation processes. Qualitative and quantitative research has suggested that when adolescents experience their diagnosis as engulfing, they may also struggle more with inhibitory control and emotional regulation, core components of EF [13,56,58]. Our results further indicate that better inhibition and emotional regulation are linked to more positive perceptions of the ADHD diagnosis, echoing previous studies emphasizing the centrality of these EFs for developing a coherent and adaptive self-concept [58–60]. Together, these findings highlight the value of considering both the cognitive and diagnosis identity dimensions of ADHD in intervention planning. Specifically, addressing feelings of *Engulfment* and fostering executive functioning skills, particularly inhibition and emotional regulation, may help adolescents with ADHD develop a more positive and balanced identity.

Our study demonstrates that adolescents with ADHD who report higher levels of *Acceptance* and *Enrichment* also tend to exhibit better self-management abilities, particularly in self-monitoring and self-reinforcement. Conversely, greater feelings of *Rejection* and *Engulfment* are linked to poorer self-management. These findings align with previous research in other chronic conditions, where a positive illness or diagnosis identity has been associated with improved self-management and a more adaptive self-concept [61–63]. Self-monitoring, a key aspect highlighted in the current study, is crucial to behavior change and self-regulation among youth with ADHD [64,65]. Recent qualitative research further supports that when adolescents constructively internalize their diagnosis, they develop a stronger sense of agency and are better able to adopt effective coping strategies [44]. Additionally, the positive association between diagnosis identity and self-reinforcement underscores the importance of fostering not only knowledge and skills but also a healthy, empowered self-perception as part of interventions for adolescents with ADHD. Given the limited research on self-reinforcement in neurodevelopmental populations, future studies should investigate how enhancing positive diagnosis identity can strengthen core self-management processes and contribute to better outcomes for this group.

A growing body of research on chronic and neurodevelopmental conditions demonstrates that negative diagnosis identity, particularly the sense of *Engulfment*, can have substantial adverse effects on QoL, including greater psychosocial distress and lower functioning in physical, social, and emotional domains [34,37,66]. The current study extends these findings to adolescents with ADHD, revealing that negative dimensions of diagnosis identity are strongly linked to reduced physical, social, and emotional QoL. Importantly, these associations emerged even though positive perceptions were more prevalent overall among participants. Similarly to reports in other conditions (e.g., [67]), adolescents with ADHD who exhibit higher acceptance of their diagnosis tend to report better QoL. Conversely, those experiencing greater *Engulfment* and *Rejection* face a heightened risk for poor psychosocial outcomes. These results highlight the importance of developing targeted interventions that not only cultivate strengths and talents but also address and reduce negative diagnosis identity, as these negative emotions are closely related to adolescents' daily functioning and well-being [34,37,51].

The decision to also examine bidirectional predictive associations between ADHD diagnosis identity and functional outcomes reflects the view that these domains influence one another dynamically. A coherent and positively integrated sense of diagnosis identity can enhance self-awareness, motivation, and coping, contributing to improved executive functioning and overall well-being (e.g., [44]). At the same time, well-developed executive abilities and psychosocial adjustment provide the cognitive and emotional resources necessary to reflect on one's diagnosis and develop a stable, adaptive identity (e.g., [68]). The results of the regression analyses highlight this bidirectional relationship between diagnosis identity perception and functional and emotional outcomes in adolescents with ADHD. On one hand, dimensions of diagnosis identity, particularly *Engulfment* and *Enrichment*, were significant predictors of executive functioning, self-management, and QoL. A more positive diagnosis identity predicted better daily functioning, while a negative diagnosis identity predicted greater impairment. On the other hand, self-monitoring and self-evaluation, as well as social QoL, predicted overall diagnosis identity perception, jointly accounting for nearly half the variance. These findings indicate that adolescents' day-to-day skills and well-being not only reflect their sense of diagnosis identity but also actively shape it. This relationship aligns with recent theoretical frameworks suggesting that identity development in chronic and neurodevelopmental conditions is a dynamic process, continually influenced by both internal capacities and external experiences [34,37,44].

Practically, these findings highlight the importance of holistic and differentiated interventions across clinical, educational, and family contexts. For clinicians and educators, the results emphasize the need to assess adolescents with ADHD in terms of not only their clinical symptoms and functional abilities but also their diagnosis identity—how they perceive and internalize their diagnosis. Therefore, interventions should aim to reduce negative meanings associated with ADHD, foster interpretations that are more positive and empowering, and strengthen self-efficacy. Such approaches can enhance daily functioning, social experiences, and overall QoL. Promoting executive and self-management skills may further support adaptive development of diagnosis identity. For families, addressing adolescents' diagnosis identities can guide parents and caregivers in providing emotional and practical support that reinforces self-regulation, confidence, and inclusion. Collaboration among teachers, counselors, and family members around this shared understanding may foster a more adaptive and positive identity formation process, ultimately improving the well-being and daily functioning of adolescents with ADHD. It is important for future research to explore the mechanisms underlying these correlations, including the role of environmental factors (e.g., family support, school climate) and the potential for targeted interventions to disrupt maladaptive feedback loops between diagnosis identity perception and daily functioning.

This study's limitations should be acknowledged. The ADHD diagnoses were based solely on parental confirmation of a formal clinical diagnosis, without independent verification. The relatively small sample size ($N = 66$) and use of convenience sampling may have reduced the statistical power to detect subtle effects and limited the generalizability of the findings to the broader population of adolescents with ADHD. Participants with parent-reported neurodevelopmental or chronic comorbidities were excluded to focus specifically on illness identity related to ADHD. This deliberate decision enhanced conceptual clarity but limited the generalizability of the findings to adolescents with ADHD who present additional conditions. Moreover, participants who voluntarily chose to participate might differ in motivation, awareness, or coping strategies from those who did not, potentially introducing selection bias. The requirement for adolescents to independently complete a relatively long online questionnaire (approximately 25 min) may have further excluded those with more severe attentional or behavioral difficulties. Although symptom severity was assessed, it was not significantly related to diagnosis identity or outcome measures. Therefore, we did not include it in the main analyses. Additionally, the study did not distinguish between ADHD subtypes (inattentive, hyperactive-impulsive, or combined). These subtypes may differ in behavioral and emotional characteristics and could potentially mediate or moderate the relationships observed in this study.

The gender distribution (76% male) is higher than typically reported in epidemiological studies (e.g., [69]) but consistent with clinical samples where boys are typically overrepresented; this may limit generalizability, particularly to girls with ADHD who are often underdiagnosed [70]. While no gender differences were observed in diagnosis identity (IIQ), some independent variables (e.g., self-regulation, executive functioning) did show differences, suggesting gender may act as a confounding or moderating factor. Similarly, although stimulant medication use was not associated with any of the study variables, the modest sample size limited examination of dosage or duration effects, and thus, medication influences cannot be entirely ruled out. Additional limitations include the study's use of self-report measures, which could introduce response bias, and its cross-sectional design, which precludes causal inference regarding the directionality of relationships.

Future studies should recruit larger and more diverse samples through randomized or stratified procedures across multiple settings to enhance external validity and enable subgroup analyses (e.g., gender or medication status). They should also consider ADHD subtype distinctions to better understand their possible influence on the study variables. Incorporating longitudinal or experimental designs and developing parallel tools for other diagnosis groups to enable cross-condition comparisons. Finally, qualitative approaches could further enrich understanding of how adolescents with ADHD experience and integrate their diagnoses into daily life.

5. Conclusions

This study's findings underscore the complex relationship between diagnosis identity and emotional and functional outcomes in adolescents with ADHD. Not only do negative perceptions of diagnosis identity, such as *Engulfment* and *Rejection*, predict poorer executive functioning, self-management, and QoL, but core aspects of self-management and social well-being also significantly shape how adolescents perceive their diagnosis. These results spotlight the importance of and need for holistic, individualized interventions that address both the development of positive diagnosis identity and the strengthening of executive and self-management skills. Clinicians, educators, and families should be aware of the ongoing interplay between diagnosis identity and daily functioning, supporting adolescents in embracing their diagnosis and building practical coping strategies to improve QoL.

Author Contributions: Conceptualization, Y.Z.-C., A.S. and L.L.; methodology, Y.Z.-C., A.S. and L.L.; formal analysis, Y.Z.-C., A.S. and L.L.; investigation, Y.Z.-C., A.S. and L.L.; data curation, Y.Z.-C.; writing—original draft preparation, Y.Z.-C.; writing—review and editing, A.S. and L.L.; supervision, A.S. and L.L. All authors have read and agreed to the published version of the manuscript.

Funding: This research received no external funding.

Institutional Review Board Statement: The study was approved by the Institutional Review Board of the University of Haifa (approval number 274/19-1, 20 January 2024).

Informed Consent Statement: Informed consent was obtained from all subjects involved in the study.

Data Availability Statement: The data that support the findings of this study are available from the corresponding author upon reasonable request. Due to ethical considerations and the involvement of minors, the data are not publicly available to protect participant confidentiality.

Conflicts of Interest: The authors declare no conflicts of interest.

Abbreviations

The following abbreviations are used in this manuscript:

ADHD	Attention-deficit/hyperactivity disorder
BRI	Behavioral regulation index (BRIEF)
BRIEF	Behavior Rating Inventory of Executive Function
EF	Executive function
GEC	Global executive composite (BRIEF)
IIQ	Illness Identity Questionnaire
MI	Metacognition index (BRIEF)

PedsQL	Pediatric Quality of Life Inventory
QoL	Quality of life
SCMS	Self-Control and Self-Management Scale

References

1. American Psychiatric Association. *Diagnostic and Statistical Manual of Mental Disorders*, 5th ed.; text rev.; American Psychiatric Association Publishing: Washington, DC, USA, 2022.
2. Ayano, G.; Demelash, S.; Gizachew, Y.; Tsegay, L.; Alati, R. The global prevalence of attention deficit hyperactivity disorder in children and adolescents: An umbrella review of meta-analyses. *J. Affect. Disord.* **2023**, *339*, 860–866. [CrossRef]
3. Fayyad, J.; Sampson, N.A.; Hwang, I.; Adamowski, T.; Aguilar-Gaxiola, S.; Al-Hamzawi, A.; Andrade, L.H.S.G.; Borges, G.; de Girolamo, G.; Florescu, S.; et al. The descriptive epidemiology of DSM-IV adult ADHD in the World Health Organization World Mental Health Surveys. *Atten. Deficit Hyperact. Disord.* **2017**, *9*, 47–65. [CrossRef]
4. Kooij, J.; Bijlenga, D.; Salerno, L.; Jaeschke, R.; Bitter, I.; Balázs, J.; Thome, J.; Dom, G.; Kasper, S.; Filipe, C.N.; et al. Updated European consensus statement on diagnosis and treatment of adult ADHD. *Eur. Psychiatry* **2019**, *56*, 14–34. [CrossRef] [PubMed]
5. World Health Organization. *Basic Documents*, 49th ed.; World Health Organization: Geneva, Switzerland, 2020.
6. Mitic, M.; Woodcock, K.A.; Amering, M.; Krammer, I.; Stiehl, K.A.M.; Zehetmayer, S.; Schrank, B. Toward an integrated model of supportive peer relationships in early adolescence: A systematic review and exploratory meta-analysis. *Front. Psychol.* **2021**, *12*, 589403. [CrossRef] [PubMed]
7. Gardner, D.; Gerdes, A. A review of peer relationships and friendships in youth with ADHD. *J. Atten. Disord.* **2015**, *19*, 844–855. [PubMed]
8. Grygiel, P.; Humenny, G.; Rębisz, S.; Bajcar, E.; Świtaj, P. Peer rejection and perceived quality of relations with schoolmates among children with ADHD. *J. Atten. Disord.* **2018**, *22*, 738–751. [CrossRef]
9. Abecassis, M.; Isquith, P.K.; Roth, R.M. Characteristics of ADHD in the emerging adult: An overview. *Psychol. Inj. Law* **2017**, *10*, 197–208. [CrossRef]
10. Krauss, A.; Schellenberg, C. ADHD symptoms and health-related quality of life of adolescents and young adults. *Eur. J. Health Psychol.* **2022**, *29*, 165–174. [CrossRef]
11. Adler, L.A.; Dirks, B.; Deas, P.; Raychaudhuri, A.; Dauphin, M.; Saylor, K.; Weisler, R. Self-reported quality of life in adults with attention-deficit/hyperactivity disorder and executive function impairment treated with lisdexamfetamine dimesylate: A randomized, double-blind, multicenter, placebo-controlled, parallel-group study. *BMC Psychiatry* **2013**, *13*, 253. [CrossRef]
12. Barkley, R.A. *Attention-Deficit Hyperactivity Disorder: A Handbook for Diagnosis and Treatment*, 4th ed.; Guilford Press: New York, NY, USA, 2015.
13. Molitor, S.J.; Oddo, L.E.; Eadeh, H.-M.; Langberg, J.M. Executive function deficits in adolescents with ADHD: Untangling possible sources of heterogeneity. *J. Emot. Behav. Disord.* **2019**, *27*, 165–177. [CrossRef]
14. Toglia, J.; Foster, E.R. *The Multi Context Approach to Cognitive Rehabilitation: A Metacognitive Strategy Intervention to Optimize Functional Cognition*; Gatekeeper Press: Citrus Park, FL, USA, 2021.
15. Shimoni, M.; Engel-Yeger, B.; Tirosh, E. Executive dysfunctions among boys with attention deficit hyperactivity disorder (ADHD): Performance-based test and parents report. *Res. Dev. Disabil.* **2012**, *33*, 858–865. [CrossRef]
16. Tonks, J.; Williams, W.H.; Slater, A.M.; Frampton, I.J. Is damage to the pre-frontal cortex dormant until adolescence, or difficult to detect? Looking for keys that unlock executive functions in children in the wrong place. *Med. Hypotheses* **2017**, *108*, 24–30. [CrossRef]
17. Blakemore, S.J.; Choudhury, S. Development of the adolescent brain: Implications for executive function and social cognition. *J. Child Psychol. Psychiatry* **2006**, *47*, 296–312. [CrossRef]
18. Al-Yagon, M.; Borenstein, T. Adolescents' executive functions: Links to inattention, hyperactivity-impulsivity, trait mindfulness, and academic performance. *J. Adolesc.* **2022**, *95*, 30–42.
19. Barkley, R.A. *Executive Functions: What They Are, How They Work, and Why They Evolved*; Guilford Press: New York, NY, USA, 2012.
20. Weyandt, L.L.; Willis, W.G.; Swentosky, A.; Wilson, K.; Janusis, G.M.; Chung, H.J.; Turcotte, K.; Marshall, S. A review of the use of executive function tasks in externalizing and internalizing disorders. In *Handbook of Executive Functioning*; Goldstein, S., Naglieri, J.A., Eds.; Springer: London, UK, 2014; pp. 69–87.
21. Munsell, E.G.S.; Orsmond, G.I.; Fulford, D.; Coster, W.J. Self-management of daily life tasks in diploma-track youth with disabilities. *Disabil. Rehabil.* **2022**, *44*, 8011–8021. [CrossRef]
22. Lorig, K.R.; Holman, H. Self-management education: History, definition, outcomes, and mechanisms. *Ann. Behav. Med.* **2003**, *26*, 1–7. [CrossRef] [PubMed]
23. Van de Velde, D.; De Zutter, F.; Satink, T.; Costa, U.; Janquart, S.; Senn, D.; De Vriendt, P. Delineating the concept of self-management in chronic conditions: A concept analysis. *BMJ Open* **2019**, *9*, e027775. [CrossRef]

24. Araújo-Soares, V.; Hankonen, N.; Presseau, J.; Rodrigues, A.; Sniehotta, F.F. Developing behavior change interventions for self-management in chronic illness: An integrative overview. *Eur. Psychol.* **2019**, *24*, 7–25. [CrossRef] [PubMed]
25. Audulv, Å. The overtime development of chronic illness self-management patterns: A longitudinal qualitative study. *BMC Public Health* **2013**, *13*, 452. [CrossRef] [PubMed]
26. Cronly, J.A.; Savage, E. Developing agency in the transition to self-management of cystic fibrosis in young people. *J. Adolesc.* **2019**, *75*, 130–137. [CrossRef]
27. Lozano, P.; Houtrow, A. Supporting self-management in children and adolescents with complex chronic conditions. *Pediatrics* **2018**, *141* (Suppl. S3), S233–S241. [CrossRef]
28. Sawyer, S.M.; Aroni, R.A. Self-management in adolescents with chronic illness: What does it mean and how can it be achieved? *Med. J. Aust.* **2005**, *138*, 405–409.
29. Erikson, E. *Identity: Youth and Crisis*; W.W. Norton: New York, NY, USA, 1968.
30. Dunn, D.S.; Burcaw, S. Disability identity: Exploring narrative accounts of disability. *Rehabil. Psychol.* **2013**, *58*, 148–157. [CrossRef] [PubMed]
31. Raymaekers, K.; Prikken, S.; Vanhalst, J.; Moons, P.; Goossens, E.; Oris, L.; Weets, I.; Luyckx, K. The social context and illness identity in youth with type 1 diabetes: A three-wave longitudinal study. *J. Youth Adolesc.* **2020**, *49*, 449–466.
32. Luyckx, K.; Seiffge-Krenke, I.; Schwartz, S.J.; Goossens, L.; Weets, I.; Hendrieckx, C.; Groven, C. Identity development, coping, and adjustment in emerging adults with a chronic illness: The sample case of type 1 diabetes. *J. Adolesc. Health* **2008**, *43*, 451–458.
33. Charmaz, K. Struggling for a self: Identity levels of the chronically ill. *Res. Sociol. Health Care* **1987**, *6*, 283–321.
34. Oris, L.; Seiffge-Krenke, I.; Moons, P.; Goubert, L.; Rassart, J.; Luyckx, K. Illness identity in adolescents and emerging adults with type 1 diabetes: Introducing the Illness Identity Questionnaire. *Diabetes Res. Clinical Pract.* **2016**, *112*, 148–155. [CrossRef]
35. Yanos, P.T.; Roe, D.; Lysaker, P.H. The impact of illness identity on recovery from severe mental illness. *Am. J. Psychiatr. Rehabil.* **2010**, *13*, 73–93.
36. Van Bulck, L.; Goossens, E.; Luyckx, K.; Oris, L.; Apers, S.; Moons, P. Illness identity: A novel predictor for healthcare use in adults with congenital heart disease. *J. Am. Heart Assoc.* **2018**, *7*, e008723.
37. Luyckx, K.; Oris, L.; Raymaekers, K.; Rassart, J.; Moons, P.; Verdyck, L.; Mijnster, T.; Mark, R.E. Illness identity in young adults with refractory epilepsy. *Epilepsy Behav.* **2018**, *80*, 48–55. [CrossRef]
38. Meyer, S.; Lamash, L. Illness identity in adolescents with celiac disease. *J. Pediatr. Gastroenterol. Nutr.* **2021**, *72*, e42–e47. [CrossRef]
39. Gray, S.M.; McMorris, C.A.; Mudry, T.E.; McCrimmon, A.W. An exploration of diagnostic identity for autistic individuals: A systematic review of existing literature. *Res. Autism Spectr. Disord.* **2024**, *114*, 102394. [CrossRef]
40. Lamash, L.; Sagie, D.; Selanikyo, E.; Meyer, S.; Gal, E. Autism identity in young adults and the relationships with participation, quality of life, and well-being. *Res. Autism Spectr. Disord.* **2024**, *111*, 102311. [CrossRef]
41. Lamash, L.; Meyer, S. Confirmatory factor analysis of an identity questionnaire among autistic adolescents and young adults. *Autism Dev. Lang. Impair.* **2025**, *10*, 23969415251325337. [CrossRef]
42. Abu Raya-Ghanayem, N.; Stern, A.; Lamash, L. Diagnosis identity perception of adolescents with ADHD and its relationship to social participation and quality of life. *Res. Dev. Disabil.* **2025**, *165*, 105102. [CrossRef] [PubMed]
43. Grimell, J. Identity work among girls with ADHD: Struggling with Me and I, impression management and social camouflaging in school. *Front. Psychol.* **2025**, *16*, 1591135. [CrossRef]
44. Frick, K.; Skoglund, C.; Wästfelt, E. ADHD and identity formation: Adolescents' experiences from the healthcare system and peer relationships. *BMC Psychol.* **2024**, *12*, 152. [CrossRef]
45. Jones, S.; Hesse, M. Adolescents with ADHD: Experiences of having an ADHD diagnosis and negotiations of self-image and identity. *J. Atten. Disord.* **2018**, *22*, 92–102. [CrossRef]
46. Oris, L.; Luyckx, K.; Rassart, J.; Goubert, L.; Goossens, E.; Apers, S.; Arat, S.; Vandenberghe, J.; Westhovens, R.; Moons, P. Illness identity in adults with a chronic illness. *J. Clin. Psychol. Med. Settings* **2018**, *25*, 429–440. [CrossRef] [PubMed]
47. Guy, S.C.; Isquith, P.K.; Gioia, G.A. *Behavior Rating Inventory of Executive Function–Self-Report Version (BRIEF-SR)*; Psychological Assessment Resources: Lutz, FL, USA, 2004.
48. Mezo, P.G. The Self-Control and Self-Management Scale (SCMS): Development of an adaptive self-regulatory coping skills instrument. *J. Psychopathol. Behav. Assess.* **2009**, *31*, 83–93. [CrossRef]
49. Mezo, P.G.; Short, M. Construct validity and confirmatory factor analysis of the Self-Control and Self-Management Scale. *Can. J. Behav. Sci.* **2012**, *44*, 1. [CrossRef]
50. Varni, J.W.; Seid, M.; Kurtin, P.S. PedsQL™ 4.0: Reliability and validity of the Pediatric Quality of Life Inventory™ Version 4.0 Generic Core Scales in healthy and patient populations. *Med. Care* **2001**, *39*, 800–812. [CrossRef]
51. Lamash, L.; Gutman, Y.; Meyer, S.; Gal, E. Self & parent-reported autism identity perception among adolescents with ASD. *Am. J. Occup. Ther.* **2024**, *78* (Suppl. S2), 7811500005p1. [CrossRef]

52. Mahdi, S.; Viljoen, M.; Massuti, R.; Selb, M.; Almodayfer, O.; Karande, S.; de Vries, P.J.; Rohde, L.; Bölte, S. An international qualitative study of ability and disability in ADHD using the WHO-ICF framework. *Eur. Child Adolesc. Psychiatry* **2017**, *26*, 1219–1231. [CrossRef]
53. Schippers, L.M.; Horstman, L.I.; Velde, H.V.D.; Pereira, R.R.; Zinkstok, J.; Mostert, J.C.; Greven, C.U.; Hoogman, M. A qualitative and quantitative study of self-reported positive characteristics of individuals with ADHD. *Front. Psychiatry* **2022**, *13*, 922788. [CrossRef]
54. Kapp, S.K.; Gillespie-Lynch, K.; Sherman, L.E.; Hutman, T. Deficit, difference, or both? Autism and neurodiversity. *Dev. Psychol.* **2013**, *49*, 59–71. [CrossRef] [PubMed]
55. Singh, A. Neurodiversity in education: Celebrating differences and embracing strengths. *Int. J. Res. Publ. Semin.* **2022**, *13*, 271–276.
56. Rasmussen, L.A.; Almvik, A. "A bit lost"—Living with attention deficit hyperactivity disorder: A qualitative longitudinal study. *BMC Psychol.* **2024**, *12*, 152.
57. Rasmussen, L.A.; Almvik, A.; Nortvedt, P. Just being a kid, or an ADHD kid? A qualitative study of children's experiences of attention deficit hyperactivity disorder. *J. Atten. Disord.* **2018**, *26*, 985–993.
58. Barkley, R.A. Behavioral inhibition sustained attention, and executive functions: Constructing a unifying theory of ADHD. *Psychol. Bull.* **1997**, *121*, 65–94. [CrossRef]
59. Diamond, A. Executive functions. *Ann. Rev. Psychol.* **2013**, *64*, 135–168. [CrossRef]
60. Hirsch, O.; Chavanon, M.; Riechmann, E.; Christiansen, H. Emotional dysregulation is a primary symptom in adult attention-deficit/hyperactivity disorder (ADHD). *J. Affect. Disord.* **2018**, *232*, 41–47. [CrossRef]
61. Hosseinzadeh, H.; Downie, S.; Shnaigat, M. Effectiveness of health literacy- and patient activation-targeted interventions on chronic disease self-management outcomes in outpatient settings: A systematic review. *Aust. J. Prim. Health* **2022**, *28*, 83–96. [CrossRef]
62. Kralik, D.; Koch, T.; Price, K.; Howard, N. Chronic illness self-management: Taking action to create order. *J. Clin. Nurs.* **2004**, *13*, 259–267. [CrossRef]
63. Peters, L.; Brown, E. The relationship between illness identity and the self-management of inflammatory bowel disease. *Br. J. Health Psychol.* **2022**, *27*, 956–970. [CrossRef] [PubMed]
64. Falkenberg, C.A.; Barbetta, P.M. The effects of a self-monitoring package on homework completion and accuracy of students with disabilities in an inclusive general education classroom. *J. Behav. Educ.* **2013**, *22*, 190–210. [CrossRef]
65. Hoekstra, T.; Dam, M.; Klaassen, G.; Bos, W.J.W.; van der Boog, P.J.M.; Vogt, L.; van Jaarsveld, B.; van Dijk, S.; Navis, G.; Meuleman, Y. Self-monitoring and self-efficacy in patients with chronic kidney disease during low-sodium diet self-management interventions: Secondary analysis of the ESMO and SUBLIME trials. *Int. J. Behav. Med.* **2025**, *32*, 34–44.
66. Knödler, L.L.; Thomann, P.A.; Ebert, M.P. The concept of illness identity in inflammatory bowel disease. *J. Crohn's Colitis* **2020**, *14* (Suppl. S1), S414–S415. [CrossRef]
67. Karademas, E.C.; Karamvakalis, N.; Zarogiannos, A. Life context and the experience of chronic illness: Is the stress of life associated with illness perceptions and coping? *Stress Health* **2009**, *25*, 405–412. [CrossRef]
68. Korfmacher, A.-K.; Hirsch, O.; Chavanon, M.-L.; Albrecht, B.; Christiansen, H. Self-management training vs. neurofeedback interventions for attention deficit hyperactivity disorder: Results of a randomized controlled treatment study. *Front. Psychiatry* **2022**, *13*, 969351. [CrossRef]
69. Danielson, M.L.; Claussen, A.H.; Bitsko, R.H.; Katz, S.M.; Newsome, K.; Blumberg, S.J.; Ghandour, R. ADHD prevalence among U.S. children and adolescents in 2022: Diagnosis, severity, co-occurring disorders, and treatment. *J. Clin. Child Adolesc. Psychol.* **2024**, *53*, 343–360. [CrossRef] [PubMed]
70. Mowlem, F.D.; Rosenqvist, M.A.; Martin, J.; Lichtenstein, P.; Asherson, P.; Larsson, H. Sex differences in predicting ADHD clinical diagnosis and pharmacological treatment. *Eur. Child Adolesc. Psychiatry* **2019**, *28*, 481–489. [CrossRef]

children

MDPI

Article

Occupation-Based Tele-Intervention for Children with Neurodevelopmental Disorders: A Pilot Study

Stav Ben Zagmi-Averbuch [1,2,*], Deena Rozen [1], Bathia Aharon-Felsen [1], Revital Siman Tov [1], Jeffrey Lowengrub [1], Miri Tal-Saban [2,†] and Yafit Gilboa [2,†]

1 Meuhedet Health Maintenance Organization (HMO), Ashdod 9108601, Israel; deena_rozen@meuhedet.co.il (D.R.); batia.a@meuhedet.co.il (B.A.-F.); simantov_revital@meuhedet.co.il (R.S.T.); lowengrub_j@meuhedet.co.il (J.L.)

2 School of Occupational Therapy, Faculty of Medicine, The Hebrew University of Jerusalem, Jerusalem 9124001, Israel; miri.tal-saban@mail.huji.ac.il (M.T.-S.); yafit.gilboa@mail.huji.ac.il (Y.G.)

* Correspondence: stav.benzagmi@mail.huji.ac.il

† These authors contributed equally to this work.

Highlights:

What are the main findings?

- Tele-CO-OP enables meaningful functional gains in children with NDDs through telehealth.

What are the implications of the main findings?

- Home-based delivery enhances the generalization of treatment to the child's natural environment.
- Key facilitators and barriers identified can inform sustainable teleintervention.

Abstract: Background: There is a growing gap between the increasing prevalence of children with neurodevelopmental disorders (NDDs) and the limited availability of developmental services. This raises an urgent need for effective and accessible intervention models. Hybrid intervention offers an innovative and practical solution, yet evidence regarding its feasibility and efficacy for children remains limited. This study aimed to adapt an evidence-based occupational therapy (OT) intervention model for remote delivery and to examine its feasibility and preliminary efficacy among children with NDDs. **Methods**: Using a quasi-experimental pre–post, mixed-methods design, children aged 5–8 years with NDDs were recruited from child development units in southern Israel. The intervention comprised 12–15 weekly video-conference sessions utilizing the Cognitive Orientation to (daily) Occupational Performance (CO-OP) approach. Standardized outcome measures assessed feasibility and preliminary efficacy. Focus groups with parents and therapists explored facilitators and barriers to implementation. **Results**: Of the 26 participants enrolled, 14 children (71% boys) completed the intervention and reported high satisfaction. Clinically significant improvements were observed in personal goal training, reported by both children (80%) and parents (73.68%). Content analysis identified three key themes: parents' engagement, ecological intervention, and technological literacy. **Conclusions:** Tele-CO-OP intervention was found to be feasible for children with NDDs and showed potential to improve occupational performance in personal goals. Findings provide a practical foundation for developing hybrid OT services as a valuable complement to in-person care for this growing population.

Keywords: child development; occupational therapy; cognitive orientation to (daily) occupational performance (CO-OP); Tele-CO-OP; tele-intervention

1. Introduction

Neurodevelopmental disorders (NDDs) are a group of developmental conditions, including attention deficit hyperactivity disorder (ADHD), autistic spectrum disorders (ASD), and developmental coordination disorder (DCD), characterized by developmental deficits that can be detected during early childhood [1]. They affect 5–20% of the general population and are more frequent in males than females [1]. NDDs are among the most prevalent conditions associated with disability and participation restrictions during childhood. NDDs are also associated with disrupted brain development that affects different aspects of daily life functions [2]. Recent evidence demonstrates, for example, altered resting-state functional connectivity in children with ADHD, reflecting atypical brain network organization [3].

Children with NDDs face significant delays in at least one developmental skill, such as motor, language, behavioral, social, and cognitive development [4]. They also struggle in performing activities, including self-care tasks (e.g., dressing, feeding, and toileting), academic and pre-academic activities (e.g., handwriting, reading, and following classroom routines), and play and leisure activities that require social interaction, motor coordination, or sustained attention [5]. These difficulties lead to functional limitations in daily participation, raising the need for appropriate support and developmental services, sometimes even before the child enters school [6].

NDDs usually continue into adolescence and adulthood, characterized by problems in many areas of function (e.g., work and education), increasing the risks of unemployment, social isolation, injuries, gambling addictions, and delinquency [7]. Lack of early and appropriate intervention can lead to deterioration in overall health and functioning, as well as increase the risk for the emergence of comorbid mental health disorders. Therefore, early intervention among children with NDDs is essential for their long-term health [8].

An intervention approach with strong evidence for improving functioning in children with NDDs is the task-oriented approach [9]. This intervention focuses on a client's personal goals, empowering them to acquire functional skills and increase participation in their natural environments [10,11]. One example of task-oriented intervention is The Cognitive Orientation to (daily) Occupational Performance [CO-OP; [12]].

The CO-OP approach is a performance-based use of metacognitive strategies and problem-solving principles to improve daily functions [12]. Its aims are to accomplish the following: (a) meet the client's functional goals through task acquisition; (b) facilitate self-generated cognitive strategy acquisition; and (c) promote generalization and transfer to other occupations and contexts [13]. The key elements of this approach include setting personal functional goals according to the child's preference; dynamic performance analysis (DPA), using global and specific strategies; and a guided discovery process with enabling principles. The process known as "Goal-Plan-Do-Check" is a global problem-solving strategy that outlines four steps toward achieving goals: setting a functional goal, designing a plan to achieve it, implementing the plan, and checking that it was implemented and that it succeeded. If the plan does not succeed, new plans are generated, and the cycle is repeated [14].

The CO-OP was originally developed to improve functioning and participation in daily activities for children with DCD [13]. Recent evidence has demonstrated the successful application of this approach among children with additional NDDs such as learning disability [LD], ASD, and ADHD [15]. Improvements in goal attainment, activity performance, and transfer to untrained tasks were reported in studies involving children following acquired brain injury (ABI), and in a systematic review of CO-OP interventions with children aged 0–18 years diagnosed with conditions such as DCD and ADHD, it showed evidence for the intervention's effectiveness [15,16]. Furthermore, evidence from a recent systematic review reinforces the added value of the CO-OP approach compared to other interventions. The review emphasized that the transfer of learned skills is a realistic and attainable outcome across different ages and populations following CO-OP training, with consistently higher levels of transfer observed relative to control interventions. This focus on metacognitive learning, client-driven goal setting, and generalization represents CO-OP's added value in comparison with traditional top-down or bottom-up interventions, making it particularly relevant for pediatric populations with neurodevelopmental challenges [17,18].

The CO-OP approach is widely used in an in-person format in clinics with children with NDDs [15]. However, access to in-person interventions is often limited due to barriers such as geographical distance, shortage of trained professionals, and long waiting lists, making it difficult for many families to receive timely services using this approach [19]. A possible solution is to provide service through telemedicine platforms to address these issues [20].

Telemedicine is defined as accessibility to health services and clinical information through the use of a variety of technologies [21]. Occupational therapy (OT) tele-intervention is one of the services included in the American Telemedicine Association [ATA] definition [22]. The use of telemedicine services is rapidly increasing in developed countries because it appears to be cost-effective compared to traditional treatment methods, and it offers additional benefits for patients, caregivers, and organizations [23,24]. Key benefits for patients include improved access to services, especially for those living in peripheral areas; the ability to perform intervention in a patient's natural environment; increased client service availability; and interaction between patients' home-based caregivers [25,26]. In addition, tele-intervention may improve the caregiver's sense of confidence and facilitate the application of the clinician's primary therapy goals [27].

Previous studies have indicated the utility of tele-intervention among children with NDDs, as well as the responsiveness and satisfaction of their families [28], alongside its complexity and barriers [29]. In addition, a few preliminary studies support the effectiveness of tele-interventions for child development, but the evidence is insufficient due to the small sample sizes, very short interventions, and low sensitivity of outcome measures [30]. Furthermore, the value of remote health services for child development has not been sufficiently assimilated among the health professions, including OT [31,32].

Previous researchers have demonstrated the feasibility and effectiveness of the remote CO-OP approach (tele-CO-OP) among diverse populations with chronic health conditions and functional impairments, such as adolescents with spina bifida [33], cancer survivors [34], and adults with acquired brain injuries [35]. However, to the best of our knowledge, the feasibility and efficacy of tele-CO-OP for children with NDDs have not yet been tested.

The rise in pediatric tele-intervention has created new opportunities to deliver occupation-based interventions in children's natural environments, increasing access and enabling parent-mediated practice [25,36]. Despite growing evidence for tele-intervention feasibility, there remains limited rigorous data on how cognitive-strategy-based approaches, such as CO-OP, function when delivered remotely, and on the roles of family engagement and digital literacy as mediators of outcome [16,37] The tele-CO-OP model adapts CO-OP principles for remote delivery by incorporating simplified, developmentally appropriate mnemonic supports, visual aids, and explicit parent scaffolding to enhance comprehension and strategy application.

Therefore, the goal of this study was to investigate the feasibility, acceptability, and preliminary efficacy of the tele-CO-OP approach among children aged 5–8 years with NDDs. The specific research hypotheses were as follows:

(1) Feasibility: The tele-CO-OP will be found to be applicable in terms of adherence (the number of participants who complete the intervention program, and the number of sessions completed).

(2) Acceptability: The tele-CO-OP will be found to be acceptable to the patients and therapists, as indicated by questionnaires and insights from focus groups.

(3) Preliminary Efficacy: The tele-CO-OP will be found to be measurably effective in improving the function and participation of children with NDDs.

2. Materials and Methods

2.1. Design

This pilot study employed a mixed-methods, quasi-experimental pre–post design that integrated quantitative and qualitative approaches. The intervention phase served as a preliminary step in preparation for a full-scale study and was complemented by post-intervention focus groups. Mixed-methods designs are commonly used in pilot research to inform the development of larger and more complex studies [38].

2.2. Participants

Using a convenience sampling, 26 children and their parents underwent baseline assessments; out of this group, 14 children (71% boys) aged 5–8 (M = 6 years, 5 months, SD = 1.1) and their parents completed the entire intervention. The recruitment was conducted across child development centers in the southern region of Israel. The participants were children who either had a confirmed diagnosis of NDD or were suspected to have an NDD based on professional recommendation. The latter group included children referred by parents or educational staff who had received a developmental evaluation by an occupational therapist, indicating the need for further intervention. Inclusion criteria were as follows: (a) Hebrew at a mother-tongue level; (b) child's ability to identify at least three functional difficulties, in order to set personal goals; and (c) availability of a computer/iPad with a web camera and wireless connectivity in the child's home. Exclusion criteria were as follows: (a) children diagnosed with autistic spectrum disorder (ASD) or brain injury; and (b) children with a primary diagnosis of a mental health disorder. These exclusion criteria were defined due to the heterogeneity of functional profiles in these populations and the cognitive–linguistic abilities required for meaningful participation in the CO-OP approach.

Following the pilot study, all the parents and OTs who took part in the study were invited to participate in separate focus groups. Eventually, two focus groups of mothers were conducted (n = 7) and a third focus group that included OTs (n = 5). The OTs were all females, aged between 28 and 50 years, with professional experience ranging from 2 to 24 years.

2.3. Measures

2.3.1. Socio-Demographic Questionnaire and Clinical Data

Parents completed a brief sociodemographic questionnaire, providing information about their child's age, gender, family composition, and educational setting.

2.3.2. Therapist Feasibility Log

The OTs who conducted the intervention documented field notes following each session, regarding the number and duration of the meetings performed. They also reported the use of the key elements in the CO-OP approach to ensure the implementation of its critical components as described in fidelity checklists [39].

2.3.3. Parents as Partners in Intervention—Satisfaction Questionnaire [PAPI-Q; [40]]

This structured questionnaire, developed originally in Hebrew, was designed to assess parental involvement with OT service, such as therapy procedures, session attendance, and general parental satisfaction. In the current study, the parents as well as the OTs were asked to fill out the questionnaire following the intervention to assess the acceptability of the tele-CO-OP. The questionnaire includes 17 items ranked on a 1–5 Likert scale, with a higher score indicating a higher level of satisfaction.

Cronbach's alpha was good ($\alpha = 0.80$), suggesting high internal reliability. Content validity was established by a group of 12 OTs. Moreover, the PAPI-Q and the Canadian Occupational Performance Measure (COPM) have been found to have a strong relationship, with a significant positive correlation between parent satisfaction scores, which suggests that both tools are measuring related aspects of the intervention experience [41,42].

2.3.4. Canadian Occupational Performance Measure (COPM), 5th Edition [41]

The COPM is a widely used, valid outcome measure in OT and specifically in developmental services, designed to measure the clients' self-perceptions of their activity performance, satisfaction with their performance, and changes over time. Participants, in collaboration with their parents, were asked to identify personal and functional goals. Thereafter, they were asked to rate their performance and their satisfaction on a scale of 1 to 10, where 10 indicates optimal performance and/or satisfaction. A clinically significant difference is a minimum of a 2-point change in the COPM performance ratings [41]. Each child completed the COPM performance and satisfaction ratings on an individual form while their parent was present in the same room. The therapist facilitated the process to ensure that children understood the questions and responded independently. Parents completed a separate COPM form reflecting their own perceptions of their child's performance and satisfaction. Psychometric properties include good predictive validity, which improves therapists' understanding of clients' goals and enhances predictive outcome accuracy [43]. Furthermore, it demonstrates good test–retest reliability (0.80 on the performance scale for 1–2 weeks), sensitivity to change in many studies, and usefulness as an outcome measure among various populations, including children [44].

2.3.5. Performance Quality Rating Scale [PQRS; [45]]

The PQRS is an observational measure of performance quality in client-selected, personally meaningful activities that complements the COPM by assessing actual, rather than perceived, performance of the identified goals. The PQRS was originally developed for children with NDDs. The therapist scores each activity pre- and post-intervention, using a 10-point performance rating scale between 1 ("unable to perform") and 10 ("performs well"). The instrument is commonly used in studies involving intervention according to the CO-OP approach [11]. It has good inter-rater reliability (0.71–0.77) and good test–retest reliability (>0.80). However, convergent validity with the COPM is inconsistent, and further validation is required [46].

2.4. Focus Groups

Focus groups were conducted post-intervention to gather in-depth feedback on the tele-CO-OP intervention. Two researchers with experience in facilitating focus groups and qualitative data collection conducted the group sessions. Both were independent of the intervention process to ensure objectivity. Using structured, open-ended questions, parents and therapists were invited to reflect on their overall experience, including factors that facilitated or hindered the process. This approach aimed to evaluate the acceptability of the intervention while also capturing participants' perspectives to inform future refinement and implementation of the tele-CO-OP model.

Example questions included the following: "Which component of the intervention was most helpful in supporting the process?" (therapists' focus group protocol) and "If you were aware that two service delivery modes had equal effectiveness, which would you prefer and why?" (parents' focus group protocol).

2.5. Procedure

The research was conducted at the child development centers of Israel's "Meuhedet" HMO. Ethical authorization was obtained from the Israeli HMO—Meuhedet Health Services (Israel) in 2017 (Ethical code: HMO #05-02-09-20).

Children who applied for OT service were screened for eligibility. Parents provided written informed consent for their child's participation, and children gave verbal assent in accordance with ethical procedures. Baseline and post-intervention assessment sessions (around 1 h each) were conducted in-person in the clinics by the same OT who provided the intervention. In addition, focus groups were conducted post-intervention with parents and therapists to obtain feedback regarding the tele-CO-OP intervention. They were facilitated by researchers who did not conduct the intervention themselves and were conducted via videoconferencing, recorded, and transcribed.

At the baseline assessment, each participant (with the parent) identified three to five functional goals and rated the importance of each goal using the COPM. Three out of these goals were practiced directly during the intervention (trained goals), while the two remaining goals were untrained in order to allow an examination of the generalization transfer of the strategies learned during the intervention to the other stated goals (untrained goals).

2.6. Intervention

The intervention protocol (Appendix A) was based on an adapted remote version of the CO-OP approach [33,35], along with findings from a survey among OTs regarding occupation-based tele-intervention [47]. The protocol included 12–15 weekly videoconference sessions and was based on the CO-OP principles, without any changes in the key elements of the approach [12]. The adjustments mainly involved the therapy setting and environment organization (e.g., choosing the room, gathering required tools, and reducing external stimuli). In addition, electronic tools (such as whiteboards and computerized games) were made available using the Poppins platform (https://femi.com/technology/poppins-3/, accessed on 8 November 2025.), a secure software licensed for use in Meuhedet HMO child development clinics.

The intervention was carried out by eight OTs who were trained by two senior occupational therapists certified by the International Cognitive Approaches Network (ICAN) and who served as study supervisors.

All OTs worked in child development clinics in Israel's southern district and had at least two years of experience. The OTs were further trained in the use of the research instruments, as well as in the delivery of the treatment protocol. In addition to experience in using the CO-OP approach, OTs underwent additional training that taught them the adjustments needed for remote access.

As part of the first intervention session, the OT and participant reviewed the goals and discussed them; then, the global problem-solving strategy (Goal-Plan-Do-Check) was taught. In subsequent sessions, the OTs guided the participants in using this strategy to discover their performance problems and develop specific strategies in order to improve their performance and accomplish their goals. Examples of domain-specific strategies used during the adapted version of the tele-CO-OP intervention are summarized in Table 1.

Rather than providing solutions, the OTs facilitated this process by asking questions and providing feedback.

Table 1. Domain-specific strategies (DSS) used to promote goal achievement.

Goal	CO-OP Strategy Use	Example
Organizing the required equipment for school according to the class schedule	Attention to doing	Therapist: How will you remember the required equipment for each day? Client: I will write the schedule on my board inside my room.
	Task specification\modification	Therapist: Where should you place your books? Client: I can reach the lower shelf above the desk by myself.
	Verbal-motor mnemonic	Therapist: How can we call the required stages of this activity? Client: Take out, choose, put in and checking.
Complete writing assignment independently	Body position	Therapist: (demonstrate sitting bent over and away from the table) What do you think about my sitting posture? Client: Your back will hurt. Therapist: What should I do? Client: Approach the table and straighten your back.
	Task specification\modification	Therapist: Which place will allow you enough space to study with no other distractions? Client: My brother and my room, near the desk with my study equipment, while my brother is in the playroom.
	Verbal-motor mnemonic	Therapist: (displays a group of letters) What do all these letters have in common? Client: They are all written in the same direction. A balanced line from above and going straight down. Therapist: Great. What do you think will be a proper name for this group? Client: The ceiling and the wall.
Eating a meal independently using a spoon without dropping the food	Attention to doing	Therapist: Demonstrate eating while standing and watching television. Client: You are spilling the food everywhere Therapist: I didn't notice, what should I do differently? Client: Your mouth is very far from the plate. Maybe you should sit down and watch the food instead the TV.
	Task specification\modification	An observation on mealtime was performed and recommendations were given by the occupational therapist, such as the following: replace the chair (higher one), and use a shorter spoon and a bowl instead of a flat plate.
	Verbal–rote script	Therapist: How can we remember the sequence of all the steps we need to do? Client: Sit, closer, pick a little, and directly into the mouth.

At the beginning of the intervention, the therapist emphasized the crucial nature of the caregiver's involvement during the process: according to the CO-OP principles [14], their role is to facilitate the execution of plans and generalizing strategies and skills in daily routines. The parents' expected involvement was further explained in two categories. First was their role as an agent of change, to encourage their child to acquire problem-solving abilities in various functions and relationships. Second was parental presence during the technical aspects of the treatment, which included assisting with accessibility as needed. Examples included helping the child use technological devices, changing the camera angle when needed, making and sending videos, and organizing the home environment. Occasionally, their supervision was necessary for safety reasons (e.g., cutting food in the kitchen).

Since the CO-OP is a performance-based approach, some of the activities were performed by the participants during the sessions. Whenever possible, the therapist observed those activities performed in the participant's natural environment via video conferencing. Certain activities could not be performed online, because they required either another setting (e.g., a playground) or privacy (e.g., dressing themselves); the performance strategies and plans for these activities were discussed during online sessions.

In addition, participants received a folder with pictorial aids for use in the sessions. The visual symbols represented the "Goal-Plan-Do-Check" process, in order to make the global strategy more accessible and easier to practice. The visual aids were divided into boys' and girls' versions. In some cases, changes were made in the visual aids for cultural adaptation, such as adhering to religious dress codes.

2.7. Data Analysis

The data analysis was performed using the SPSS software (Version 25; IBM Corp, Armonk, NY, USA). Descriptions of sample characteristics were analyzed using descriptive statistics. A nonparametric statistical (Wilcoxon) analysis for paired samples was used to assess differences pre- and post-intervention (goals accomplished and changes in quality of activity performance). The significance level for confirming the research hypothesis was $p < 0.05$. Qualitative data were analyzed using a conventional content analysis method [48]. Researchers conducted a reflective process throughout the entire analysis regarding their ideas, perspectives, and thoughts to ensure trustworthy findings. The process included three researchers, all of whom had expertise in child development and remote intervention, and two of them had prior experience in qualitative research, to strengthen the reliability of the findings. One researcher performed the initial open coding of the focus-group transcripts, after which two additional researchers independently reviewed and commented on the emerging codes. The three researchers then met to discuss the coding, refine the categories, and reach full agreement on the final themes.

3. Results

Of the 26 children who initially enrolled in the study, 14 completed the full tele-CO-OP intervention (retention rate = 54%), aged 5–8 years (M = 6 years, 5 months; SD = 1.1); the male–female ratio was 10:4. All fourteen children were born in Israel, and their family size ranged from two to eight children (M = 3.86, SD = 1.91). All 14 children studied at regular education programs, and half of them (n = 7) had participated in OT sessions before the current study. The socio-demographic and clinical characteristics of the participants are presented in Table 2.

Table 2. Socio-demographic and clinical characteristics of the participants (N = 14).

Characteristics	N (%)	Median (IQR)
Age		6.66 (6.04–7.81)
Gender		
Girls	10 (71.43)	
Boys	4 (28.57)	
Fathers		
Age (years:months)		38:6 (32–42)
Education (years)		15 (12–16)
Mothers (years)		
Age (years:months)		39:6 (35–45)
Education (years)		16 (15–16)
Number of children in the family		3 (2.75–5.25)
Native language		
Hebrew	10 (71.43)	
Bilingual	4 (28.57)	

3.1. Feasibility

A flow diagram provides details regarding the process of recruitment and intervention (see Figure 1). All the children had been referred to one of three child development centers;

they were screened for eligibility during a recruitment period of six months. A total of 62 children and their families were found to be suitable and were invited to participate in the study. Of these, 42% (26/62) agreed to participate and started the procedure. Fourteen of the 26 participants completed the 3-month tele-CO-OP program (A retention rate of 54%). Dropouts occurred after 1–6 sessions. The main reasons for discontinuing were as follows: (a) child's lack of motivation to participate in the intervention (e.g., preference for playing with other toys in the room, limited interest in the treatment activities or conversations, or preference for in-person sessions among children with previous face-to-face therapy experience); (b) parent's lack of involvement during sessions and training (e.g., being occupied with household tasks or other siblings, or having difficulty practicing and integrating the strategies at home between sessions); and (c) technological issues (e.g., difficulties logging into the platform, unstable internet connection, or poor audio quality).

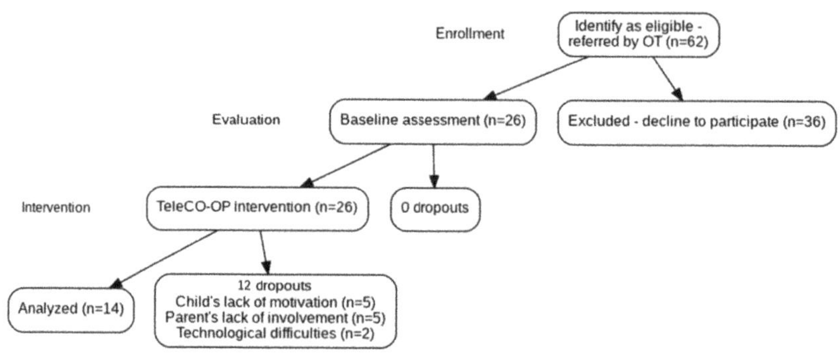

Figure 1. Flow diagram of the study enrollment, evaluation, intervention, and analysis.

Participants altogether defined, using the COPM, 64 basic activities from which were derived participation goals (trained and untrained). They covered three main life domains: (a) self-care (n = 16; 25%), for example: eating a meal independently, using a spoon without dropping the food, or getting dressed independently in the morning; (b) productivity in education (n = 40; 62.5%), for example, organizing the required equipment for school, according to the class schedule; and (c) leisure (n = 8; 12.5%), for example, playing chess with a brother, or riding a bicycle independently at the playground. It should be noted that all participants chose at least one education productivity goal.

3.2. Acceptability

Acceptability of the intervention was based on a post-intervention satisfaction questionnaire (PAPI-Q). Overall, both parents and OTs expressed high satisfaction with tele-intervention, although the parents reported higher satisfaction. On a scale of 1–5, the average PAPI-Q score was 4.34 $\pm$ 0.47 for parents and 4.17 $\pm$ 0.53 for occupational therapists (Table 3). Eleven parents (84.6%) and seven therapists (50%) expressed high to very high satisfaction (4–5) with the intervention in general (item 17).

Beyond quantitative satisfaction ratings, a qualitative content analysis was performed to reflect the perspectives of both parents and therapists and to gain insight into their subjective experiences with the intervention process. Three primary themes emerged from the combined analysis of all focus groups. The first theme was *Parents' engagement*. Participants in all groups indicated that the presence and active participation of parents were necessary conditions for the intervention to succeed. Several parents reported that they learned about their child's needs this way and felt obligated to remain involved during and between meetings. For example: "Parental involvement was crucial. They need to be involved in every aspect of the session, including documenting, photographing, and listening to what the therapist says." (Parent 2). A similar perspective was echoed by the occupational therapists in their focus groups, who emphasized that parental presence and trust were essential for both the therapeutic process and its continuation at home. As OT 3 noted, "Relationship with parents was highly meaningful because, without their presence, therapy would not have been possible. In my opinion, the trust of the parent in us, in the therapeutic process, and in its significance in the room to conduct the session and continue the practice at home was fundamental."

Table 3. Descriptive statistics of parents' and therapists' satisfaction with the tele-CO-OP.

PAPI-Q Statements	Parents M (SD)	Occupational Therapists M (SD)
Did the number of sessions match the child's needs?	4.38 (0.65)	4.43 (0.51)
Did you feel like a partner in the process?	4.54 (0.66)	4.82 (0.40)
Did the child participate in most of the sessions?	4.77 (0.60)	4.64 (0.74)
Did you/the child and his parent practice at home according to the guidance?	4 (0.58)	3.69 (1.18)
In your opinion, did you/the parent acquire tools to implement with other difficulties?	4 (1.00)	3.89 (0.60)
General satisfaction with the therapeutic process.	4.38 (0.77)	3.71 (0.99)
Satisfaction with the topics the therapy dealt with.	4.36 (0.46)	4.08 (0.76)
Total	4.34 (0.47)	4.17 (0.53)

The second theme was ecological intervention. Developmental treatments are often performed in clinics, which simulate "laboratory conditions". Thus, remote treatment in the participants' homes provided a new therapeutic environment. It was noted positively by many therapists that the tele-intervention enables working on goals that are relevant to daily activities using tools and methods the child is familiar with. As OT 2 described, "I strongly believe in it (therapy in the natural environment) because, in the clinic, there are controlled conditions. However, being in their home, it allowed us to see the family in their own space. We could understand their living conditions, explain and adapt the environment based on their changing needs." At the same time, therapists described difficulties in delivering the intervention in the home environment, such as coping with distractions and having no control over the treatment conditions. OT 3 explained that, "for some, distractions occur, such as siblings entering and leaving the room, wanting to show things, or being in different parts of the house. Thus, therapy becomes dynamic and unpredictable. As a therapist, you become limited beyond the screen, posing a significant challenge." Parents, however, also described the home environment as an opportunity for meaningful preparation and adaptation. For instance, Parent 2 noted that "As part of our preparation, we organized our environment. Our therapist asked us to see our home first, explaining how adjustments could be made. She helped us understand how to create the optimal environment for our child. Additionally, we were asked to prepare specific materials before each session. It wasn't complicated, and we came prepared."

The third theme was technological literacy. Infrastructure and technological platforms were mentioned by participants with differing opinions. Some reported that the platform served the therapist and the patient's needs. Parent 4 noted that, "It (the software) was very user-friendly, and we did not encounter many issues. There were games and interesting tools included in the software that my child eagerly looked forward to". While others found it difficult to learn, use, and operate the technology. Apart from platform type, many OTs mentioned the need to gain more in-depth knowledge, understanding, and proficiency with technological tools. For example, one person said that, "It was challenging to conduct the session many times because the technology didn't work as it should. Even a slight interruption in the internet made it challenging. I found it to be extremely challenging." (OT 4).

3.3. Preliminary Efficacy

Changes before and after the intervention were measured by the COPM and were analyzed using the Wilcoxon signed-rank test, including effect sizes. The results are shown in Table 4. Significant improvement was found in performance and satisfaction ratings reported by the child and the parent, for both trained and untrained goals. Further analysis of the results demonstrated a clinically significant improvement (≥2 points) in the COPM performance scale relating to 80% and 73.68% of the individual goals practiced during treatment, as reported by children and parents, respectively.

Table 4. Changes over time from baseline to post-intervention in the COPM and PQRS.

Measures	Pre Median (IQR)	Post Median (IQR)	Z	P	r (ES)
COPM—performance					
Child (trained goals)	5 (3.29–6.08)	9 (8.1–9.75)	−3.279	0.001	−0.881
Child (untrained goals) [a]	5 (4–6)	8.5 (7.5–10)	−2.937	0.003	−0.885
Parent (trained goals)	4.83 (3.83–5.67)	(7.17–8.69)	−3.062	0.002	−0.818
Parent (untrained goals) [a]	6.5 (5.5–7)	8.5 (6.5–9)	−2.392	0.017	−0.721
COPM—satisfaction					
Parent (trained goals)	5 (3.08–5.81)	9.17 (8.1–10)	−3.185	0.001	−0.851
Parent (untrained goals) [a]	6.5 (4.5–6.5)	9 (8–10)	−2.606	0.009	−0.786
PQRS (trained goals)	4.58 (3.25–5.5)	8 (7.67–8.54)	−3.298	0.001	0.881

Notes. An effect size (r) was calculated from the z value of the Wilcoxon signed-rank test ($r = z/\sqrt{n}$) and can be interpreted as a small ($r \leq 0.10$), medium ($r = 0.30$), or large ($r \geq 0.50$) effect size. [a] n = 11.

Similar results were also found on the COPM satisfaction scale, which showed clinically significant improvement in 85% of the goals practiced, according to the parents' reports. Children's responses on the satisfaction scale were not analyzed due to their consistent difficulty in distinguishing between the scales of the COPM. In addition, another clinically significant improvement (≥2 points) was found on the PQRS scale between pre- and post-intervention, with large effect sizes (see Table 4).

The sample size required for a future study was calculated based on the results of the current (pilot) study we recently conducted. In order to estimate sample size, we relied on the largest conservative effect size found in our primary outcome results (COPM; ES = 0.88) with a two-sided significance level of 0.05 and power of 80% with equal allocation to two arms. According to this calculation, a minimum sample size of 22 participants in each group is required. Following the results of the pilot study, we expect a dropout rate of about 20%; therefore, we decided to recruit 27 participants for each study group.

4. Discussion

The current study assessed the feasibility, acceptability, preliminary efficacy, and implementation barriers and facilitators of the CO-OP approach in a tele-intervention format for children with NDDs. Our findings indicated that tele-CO-OP was feasible and acceptable among parents and OTs. In addition, the study provided preliminary evidence for the intervention's efficacy, as demonstrated by significant clinical improvements in both trained and untrained functional goals. Furthermore, the qualitative analyses of the focus groups revealed three overarching themes that informed meaningful refinements and adaptations to the intervention.

4.1. Feasibility

In terms of adherence, 54% of the participants completed all sessions of the tele-CO-OP as required by the research protocol. The retention rate in the current study compares favorably to those reported in a systematic review of 23 tele-intervention studies conducted by healthcare providers among children with disabilities, where the highest reported retention rate was 40% [49]. Despite being consistent with previous reports, these findings highlight the ongoing need for future research to better understand and improve adherence in pediatric tele-interventions.

4.2. Acceptability

High levels of satisfaction were reported by the parents, demonstrating the acceptability of the protocol. These findings are consistent with previous studies. For example, a survey found that the majority (80.5%) of parents or caregivers of children with NDDs were satisfied with tele-interventions conducted by health professionals during the COVID-19 pandemic [50]. Even though therapists were generally satisfied with tele-interventions, their satisfaction levels were slightly lower than those of parents. Previous studies have found that the major factor affecting therapists' satisfaction and confidence with remote services is their previous experience [51,52]. Therefore, the small gap in our study can be explained by the fact that they were first-time users of a tele-intervention [53]. In addition, the lack of a therapist's previous experience with tele-interventions in the present study might also influence the dropout rate. These findings highlight the need for future research to further explore the relationship between therapists' prior experience, confidence, and engagement in tele-intervention, as well as the types of support or training that may enhance their satisfaction and sustain participation over time.

The implementation of the tele-CO-OP protocol revealed several key facilitators and barriers that emerged from the focus groups, many of which align with findings from the recent literature [12,29,54,55]. One notable facilitator was active parental engagement, which was identified in our focus groups as a critical component for successful intervention. As mentioned in other studies, pediatric tele-interventions are most effective when clients and their primary caregivers (usually parents) are empowered and guided remotely by OTs [54]. Implementing tele-intervention, as was performed in this study, includes parental and child involvement (a key recommendation in the CO-OP approach) [12]. Similar findings were reported by Steinberg et al. [29], who found that parents who embraced a more central role in remote sessions contributed significantly to reconstructing therapeutic conditions at home. Furthermore, low parental involvement emerged as a barrier, which is consistent with a systematic review by Jimenez-Arberas et al. [55], who found that reduced caregiver availability was associated with lower fidelity and completion rates in tele-intervention.

Another strong facilitator identified in our study was the ecological validity of conducting therapy in the child's natural environment. Therapists emphasized that delivering sessions at home enabled them to address authentic, everyday challenges using familiar materials and routines. This finding is consistent with Steinberg et al. [29], who, in their qualitative study of telehealth in pediatric rehabilitation, described "home as a new therapeutic opportunity," highlighting how the home environment can expand the relevance and meaningfulness of intervention. At the same time, therapists in our study also noted practical challenges, including limited physical space, background noise, and competing household stimuli, all of which disrupted the traditional structure of therapy and occasionally hindered session flow. Similar limitations were reported by Buitrago et al. [56], who found that household distractions and privacy concerns require careful planning and adaptation in order to optimize remote intervention.

A third influential factor was technological literacy. While some participants adapted easily to digital platforms, others, especially therapists new to tele-intervention, expressed discomfort or a lack of confidence. Similar concerns were widely reported in the literature, with therapists frequently describing technology-related stress as limiting their ability to focus on therapeutic content [29]. These insights support calls for formal training and digital competence development as a prerequisite for effective implementation.

Taken together, these findings underscore the importance of thorough pre-intervention preparation. This includes providing parents or primary caregivers with an initial orientation, clear guidance, and setting their expectations regarding their role during and between sessions. In addition, technical training on the tele-intervention platform should be offered to both parents and therapists, accompanied by ongoing technical support throughout the intervention process. Regarding the home environment, preparatory steps should focus on organizing the physical space, anticipating and managing potential distractions, and ensuring the availability of appropriate equipment and environmental adaptations.

Integrating these elements may enhance a future implementation's fidelity and sustainability of tele-intervention services in pediatric rehabilitation.

4.3. Preliminary Efficacy

Improving daily activity performance and participation is a highly desired outcome in pediatric OT intervention [57]. Accordingly, the primary outcome in our study was perceived performance change and satisfaction relating to participant-chosen functional goals. Despite the small sample, significant statistical and clinical improvements were found in individual functional goals post-intervention. These results are in line with previous systematic reviews and studies that evaluated the efficacy of tele-interventions among children with a variety of disabilities [32,37,58–60]. Our results are also in line with previous studies that evaluated the efficacy of the traditional in-person CO-OP approach among children with NDDs, as well as the use of tele-CO-OP among other populations [34,35]. Capistran and Martini's study [61], for instance, found similar percentages of goals in which children reported a significant improvement according to the COPM.

In the current study, gains were found in untrained goals, as reported by both parents and children. Our results were similar to those in previous CO-OP studies among children, showing significant improvements not only in trained goals but also suggesting transfer to untrained activities and everyday contexts [62,63]. This confirms that the principles of the CO-OP were designed to allow generalization of the results and transfer to other performance challenges, specifically the metacognitive nature of the approach and the emphasis on generalization and transfer to the child's natural environment during the sessions. Consequently, participants will be able to use global and domain-specific strategies on their own in a broad range of situations [64].

4.4. Limitations and Future Study

Study limitations should be taken into account when interpreting the results. First, these analyses were exploratory, and the sample size was small and relatively homogeneous, as participants were recruited from a specific region in the country. Furthermore, this was a pilot study without a control group, so we cannot necessarily attribute the improvements exclusively to the intervention. Nonetheless, since no other OT service was provided during the intervention period, we can assume that the improvement in activity performance was caused at least in part by the intervention being evaluated. In future studies, we recommend including a larger and more diverse sample, as well as a control group, to strengthen the validity of the findings and confirm this assumption.

Additionally, we included a heterogeneous group of participants with NDDs who had different functional difficulties, while excluding children with ASD, brain injury, and a primary diagnosis of mental health disorders. However, we recommend that future studies change the inclusion criteria to be based on functional profile rather than on etiology.

A further limitation of this study relates to the research measures employed. All outcome measures were subjective in nature, relying on the perspectives and self-reports of the children and their parents. Moreover, these evaluations were administered by the same therapists who delivered the intervention, which may have introduced potential bias. To address these limitations, future studies should incorporate objective assessment tools capable of capturing specific changes in body functions (e.g., executive functions) as a result of the intervention. In addition, outcome evaluations should be conducted by independent therapists, separate from those delivering the intervention, to minimize the risk of bias and strengthen the validity of the findings.

5. Conclusions

Based on the findings gleaned from the pilot study, tele-CO-OP for children with NDDs appears to be feasible and has potential efficacy in improving occupational performance to attain participants' functional goals. Our study contributes to the growing body of evidence supporting the use of tele-intervention as a valuable supplement to in-person interventions, overcoming accessibility barriers and the limited availability of services in remote areas. However, issues have arisen during the focus groups that require attention and adjustment for applicability and scalability. Consequently, a specialized panel was convened for expert discourse, leading to modifications to the protocol, such as the following: (1) The necessity for promoting parental involvement in the therapeutic process; (2) the incorporation of occupational performance coaching [OPC; [65]] as the foundation of the intervention; and (3) adding the parenting sense of competence [PSOC; [66]] as an outcome measure.

In the long run, it can be assumed that integration of accessible and effective services in child development centers will help reduce the burden on families and promote their functioning. Building on these findings, future research can now be conducted through randomized controlled trials with adequately powered sample sizes to rigorously establish the effectiveness of the tele-CO-OP approach.

Author Contributions: Y.G. and M.T.-S. are equal primary investigators (co-PIs). Conceptualization, methodology, formal analysis and investigation, resources, data curation, writing—original draft preparation, and writing—review and editing: Y.G., M.T.-S., and S.B.Z.-A. Resources: D.R., B.A.-F., R.S.T., and J.L. Supervision, project administration, and funding acquisition: Y.G. and M.T.-S. M.T.-S. and Y.G. should be considered senior authors, based on their equal and significant contributions to this paper. All authors have read and agreed to the published version of the manuscript.

Funding: This research was funded by the Ministry of Health of Israel, grant number 3011005798.

Institutional Review Board Statement: The study was conducted in accordance with the Declaration of Helsinki and approved by the Ethics Committee of Meuhedet Health Services, Israel (protocol code #05-02-09-20 in 12 September 2022).

Informed Consent Statement: Informed consent was obtained from all subjects involved in the study.

Data Availability Statement: Data is contained within the article.

Acknowledgments: The authors thank all study participants and their families for taking part in this study, as well as the occupational therapy staff who supported the enrollment process of the study in the child developmental clinics of Meuhedet HMO.

Conflicts of Interest: The authors declare that there is no conflict of interest concerning the authorship and/or publication of this article.

Appendix A. Tele CO-OP Intervention Process

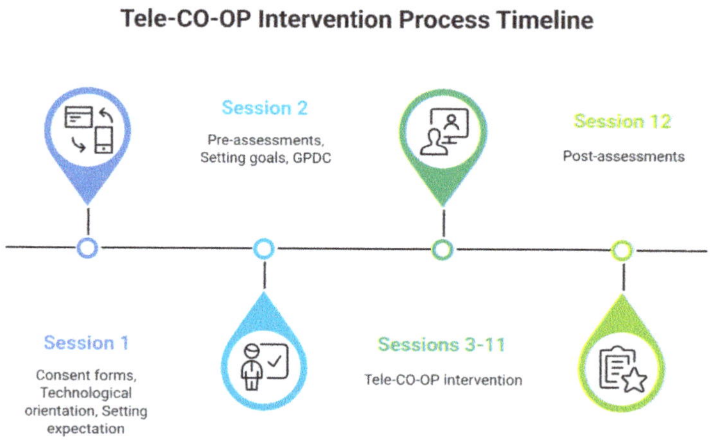

References

1. Patel, D.R.; Merrick, J. Neurodevelopmental and neurobehavioral disorders. *Transl. Pediatr.* **2020**, *9* (Suppl. S1), S1. [CrossRef]
2. Nair, K.S.; George, R.L.; Remya, V.R.; A, R.P.; Saji, C.V.; Mullasseril, R.R.; AShenoi, R.; Nair, J.; Krishna, R.; N, K.K.; et al. Prevalence Estimates of Neurodevelopmental Disorders (NDDs) in a South Indian Population. *Ann. Neurosci.* **2025**, 09727531251348188. [CrossRef] [PubMed]
3. Misra, R.; Gandhi, T.K. Functional connectivity dynamics show resting-state instability and rightward parietal dysfunction in ADHD. In Proceedings of the 2023 45th Annual International Conference of the IEEE Engineering in Medicine & Biology Society (EMBC), Sydney, Australia, 24–27 July 2023; pp. 1–4. [CrossRef]
4. Chauhan, R.; Kakkar, S.; Singhal, R.; Negi, A. Neurodevelopmental Disabilities: Current Perspectives on Burden of Care and Stigma—A Comprehensive Review. In *Health Psychology in Integrative Health Care*; Routledge: Abingdon, UK, 2024; pp. 129–135.
5. Blanco-Martínez, N.; Delgado-Lobete, L.; Montes-Montes, R.; Ruiz-Pérez, N.; Ruiz-Pérez, M.; Santos-del-Riego, S. Participation in everyday activities of children with and without neurodevelopmental disorders: A cross-sectional study in Spain. *Children* **2020**, *7*, 157. [CrossRef] [PubMed]
6. American Psychiatric Association. *Neurodevelopmental Disorders: DSM-5® Selections*; American Psychiatric Pub: Washington, DC, USA, 2015.
7. Faraone, S.V.; Banaschewski, T.; Coghill, D.; Zheng, Y.; Biederman, J.; Bellgrove, M.A.; Newcorn, J.H.; Gignac, M.; Al Saud, N.M.; Manor, I.; et al. The world federation of ADHD international consensus statement: 208 evidence-based conclusions about the disorder. *Neurosci. Biobehav. Rev.* **2021**, *128*, 789–818. [CrossRef] [PubMed]
8. Ministry of Health. Child Development Services. Available online: https://www.health.gov.il/Subjects/KidsAndMatures/child_development/Pages/default.aspx (accessed on 27 October 2025). (In Hebrew)
9. Lucas, B.R.; Elliott, E.J.; Coggan, S.; Pinto, R.Z.; Jirikowic, T.; McCoy, S.W.; Latimer, J. Interventions to improve gross motor performance in children with neurodevelopmental disorders: A meta-analysis. *BMC Pediatr.* **2016**, *16*, 1–16. [CrossRef]
10. Novak, I.; Honan, I. Effectiveness of pediatric occupational therapy for children with disabilities: A systematic review. *Aust. Occup. Ther. J.* **2019**, *66*, 258–273. [CrossRef]
11. Smits-Engelsman, B.; Vincon, S.; Blank, R.; Quadrado, V.H.; Polatajko, H.; Wilson, P.H. Evaluating the evidence for motor-based interventions in developmental coordination disorder: A systematic review and meta-analysis. *Res. Dev. Disabil.* **2018**, *74*, 72–102. [CrossRef]
12. Polatajko, H.J. Cognitive orientation to daily occupational performance (CO-OP) approach. *Perspect. Hum. Occup. Theor. Underlying Practice. Phila. FA Davis* **2017**, 183–206.
13. Polatajko, H.J.; Mandich, A.D.; Missiuna, C.; Miller, L.T.; Macnab, J.J.; Malloy-Miller, T.; Kinsella, E.A. Cognitive orientation to daily occupational performance (CO-OP) part III-the protocol in brief. *Phys. Occup. Ther. Pediatr.* **2001**, *20*, 107–123. [CrossRef]

14. McEwen, S.E.; Polatajko, H.J. *Cognitive Orientation to Daily Occupational Performance in Occupational Therapy: Using the CO-OP Approach to Enable Participation Across the Lifespan*; Dawson, D.R., McEwen, S.E., Polatajko, H.J., Eds.; AOTA Press, The American Occupational Therapy Association, Incorporated: Bethesda, MD, USA, 2017. Available online: https://lccn.loc.gov/2017950778 (accessed on 1 November 2025).
15. Madieu, E.; Gagné-Trudel, S.; Therriault, P.Y.; Cantin, N. Effectiveness of CO-OP approach for children with neurodevelopmental disorders: A systematic review. *Arch. Rehabil. Res. Clin. Transl.* **2023**, *5*, 100260. [CrossRef]
16. Vezinat, C.; Lebrault, H.; Câmara-Costa, H.; Martini, R.; Chevignard, M. Transfer of skills acquired through Cognitive Orientation to daily Occupational Performance (CO-OP) approach in children with executive functions deficits following acquired brain injury. *Aust. Occup. Ther. J.* **2025**, *72*, e70040. [CrossRef]
17. Araujo, C.R.S.; Cardoso, A.A.; Polatajko, H.J.; de Castro Magalhães, L. Efficacy of the Cognitive Orientation to daily Occupational Performance (CO-OP) approach with and without parental coaching on activity and participation for children with developmental coordination disorder: A randomized clinical trial. *Res. Dev. Disabil.* **2021**, *110*, 103862. [CrossRef] [PubMed]
18. Shiozu, H.; Kurasawa, S. Cognitive orientation to daily occupational performance (CO-OP) approach as telehealth for a child with developmental coordination disorder: A case report. *Front. Rehabil. Sci.* **2023**, *4*, 1241981. [CrossRef]
19. Sapiets, S.J.; Hastings, R.P.; Stanford, C.; Totsika, V. Families' access to early intervention and supports for children with developmental disabilities. *J. Early Interv.* **2023**, *45*, 103–121. [CrossRef]
20. Tanner, K.; Bican, R.; Boster, J.; Christensen, C.; Coffman, C.; Fallieras, K.; Long, R.; Mansfield, C.; O'Rourke, S.; Pauline, L.; et al. Feasibility and acceptability of clinical pediatric telerehabilitation services. *Int. J. Telerehabilitation* **2020**, *12*, 43–52. [CrossRef]
21. American Telemedicine Association (ATA). American Telemedicine Association—ATA. Available online: https://www.americantelemed.org/ (accessed on 27 October 2025).
22. Boccalandro, E.A.; Dallari, G.; Mannucci, P.M. Telemedicine and telerehabilitation: Current and forthcoming applications in haemophilia. *Blood Transfus.* **2019**, *17*, 385. [CrossRef]
23. Medvedeva, E.I.; Aleksandrova, O.A.; Kroshilin, S.V. Telemedicine in modern conditions: The attitude of society and the vector of development. *Ekon. I Sotsialnye Peremeny* **2022**, *15*, 200–222. [CrossRef]
24. Peretti, A.; Amenta, F.; Tayebati, S.K.; Nittari, G.; Mahdi, S.S. Telerehabilitation: Review of the state-of-the-art and areas of application. *JMIR Rehabil. Assist. Technol.* **2017**, *4*, e7. [CrossRef] [PubMed]
25. Baker, A.R.; Barents, E.R.; Cole, A.G.; Klaver, A.L.; Van Kampen, K.; Webb, L.M.; Wolfer, K.A. Use and perceptions of telehealth by pediatric occupational therapists post COVID-19 pandemic: A mixed-methods survey. *Am. J. Occup. Ther.* **2025**, *16*, e6655. [CrossRef]
26. Suso-Martí, L.; La Touche, R.; Herranz-Gómez, A.; Angulo-Díaz-Parreño, S.; Paris-Alemany, A.; Cuenca-Martínez, F. Effectiveness of telerehabilitation in physical therapist practice: An umbrella and mapping review with meta–meta-Analysis. *Phys. Ther.* **2021**, *101*, pzab075. [CrossRef]
27. American Occupational Therapy Association (AOTA). *Telehealth Guidelines in Occupational Therapy Practice*; AOTA Press: Bethesda, MD, USA, 2025.
28. Thompson, L.A.; Rasmussen, S.A. Potentials of telerehabilitation for families of children with special health care needs during the coronavirus disease 2019 emergency—Reply. *JAMA Pediatr.* **2021**, *175*, 105–106. [CrossRef]
29. Steinberg, P.; Gefen, N.; Weiss, P.L.; Beeri, M.; Landa, J.; Krasovsky, T. What does "tele" do to rehabilitation? Thematic analysis of therapists' and families' experiences of pediatric telerehabilitation. *Disabil. Rehabil.* **2025**, 1–9. [CrossRef]
30. Pratte, G.; Couture, M.; Morin, M.; Berbari, J.; Tousignant, M.; Camden, C. Evaluation of a web platform aiming to support parents having a child with developmental coordination disorder: Brief report. *Dev. Neurorehabilit.* **2020**, *23*, 64–67. [CrossRef] [PubMed]
31. Almog, T.; Gilboa, Y. Remote delivery of service: A survey of occupational therapists' perceptions. *Rehabil. Process Outcome* **2022**, *11*, 11795727221117503. [CrossRef]
32. Sarsak, H.I. Telerehabilitation services: A successful paradigm for occupational therapy clinical services. *Int. Phys. Med. Rehabil. J.* **2020**, *5*, 62–65. [CrossRef]
33. Steinhart, S.; Raz-Silbiger, S.; Beeri, M.; Gilboa, Y. Occupation Based Telerehabilitation Intervention for Adolescents with Myelomeningocele: A Pilot Study. *Phys. Occup. Ther. Pediatr.* **2020**, *41*, 1–16. [CrossRef] [PubMed]
34. Maeir, T.; Makranz, C.; Peretz, T.; Odem, E.; Tsabari, S.; Nahum, M.; Gilboa, Y. Cognitive Retraining and Functional Treatment (CRAFT) for adults with cancer related cognitive impairment: A preliminary efficacy study. *Support. Care Cancer* **2023**, *31*, 152. [CrossRef]
35. Beit Yosef, A.; Jacobs, J.M.; Shames, J.; Schwartz, I.; Gilboa, Y. A performance-based teleintervention for adults in the chronic stage after acquired brain injury: An exploratory pilot randomized controlled crossover study. *Brain Sci.* **2022**, *12*, 213. [CrossRef]
36. Dehghani, S.; Mirzakhany, N.; Dehghani, S.; Pashmdarfard, M. The use of tele-occupational therapy for children and adolescents with different disabilities: Systematic review of RCT articles. *Med. J. Islam. Repub. Iran* **2023**, *37*, 17. [CrossRef]

37. Oprandi, M.C.; Bardoni, A.; Corno, L.; Guerrini, A.M.; Molatore, L.; Negri, L.; Beretta, E.; Locatelli, F.; Strazzer, S.; Poggi, G. Feasibility and Acceptability of a Real-Time Telerehabilitation Intervention for Children and Young Adults with Acquired Brain Injury During the COVID-19 Pandemic: An Experience Report. *Int. J. Telerehabilitation* **2021**, *13*, e6423. [CrossRef]
38. Aschbrenner, K.A.; Kruse, G.; Gallo, J.J.; Plano Clark, V.L. Applying mixed methods to pilot feasibility studies to inform intervention trials. *Pilot Feasibility Stud.* **2022**, *8*, 217. [CrossRef]
39. International Cognitive Approaches Network (ICAN). (n.d.). CO-OP: An Evidence-Based Approach. Available online: https://www.icancoop.org/pages/copy-of-co-op-an-evidence-based-approach (accessed on day month year).
40. Hirsch, A.; Waldman-Levi, A.; Porush, S. Questionnaires to evaluate the effectiveness of the intervention given to children in occupational therapy: Questionnaires for expectations and satisfaction of parents and questionnaires for a teacher. *Isr. J. Occup. Ther.* **2005**, *14*, H232–H235. (In Hebrew)
41. Law, M.; Baptiste, S.; Carswell, A.; McColl, M.A.; Polatajko, H.; Pollock, N. *Canadian Occupational Performance Measure*, 5th ed.; CAOT Publications: Ottawa, Canada, 2017. Available online: https://www.thecopm.ca/learn/ (accessed on 1 November 2025).
42. Waldman-Levi, A.; Hirsch, I.; Gutwillig, G.; Parush, S. Psychometric properties of the Parents as Partners in Intervention (PAPI) Questionnaires. *Am. J. Occup. Ther.* **2017**, *71*, 7102220020p1–7102220020p8. [CrossRef]
43. Carswell, A.; McColl, M.A.; Baptiste, S.; Law, M.; Polatajko, H.; Pollock, N. The Canadian Occupational Performance Measure: A research and clinical literature review. *Can. J. Occup. Ther.* **2004**, *71*, 210–222. [CrossRef]
44. Canadian Occupational Performance Measure (COPM). The COPM is in Use. 2018. Available online: http://www.thecopm.ca/advanced/using-the-copm-with-children (accessed on day month year).
45. Miller, L.; Polatajko, H.J.; Missiuna, C.; Mandich, A.D.; Macnab, J.J. A pilot trial of a cognitive treatment for children with developmental coordination disorder. *Hum. Mov. Sci.* **2001**, *20*, 183–210. [CrossRef]
46. Martini, R.; Rios, J.; Polatajko, H.; Wolf, T.; McEwen, S. The performance quality rating scale (PQRS): Reliability, convergent validity, and internal responsiveness for two scoring systems. *Disabil. Rehabil.* **2015**, *37*, 231–238. [CrossRef]
47. Ben Zagmis Rozen, D.; Amar, E.; Hershkowitz, F.; Gilboa, Y. Occupational therapists' perspective on remote service after initial experience trail during the COVID-19 pandemic. *Isr. J. Occup. Ther.* **2021**, *30*. Available online: https://www.researchgate.net/publication/356459254_Occupational_Therapists%E2%80%99_Perspective_on_Remote_Service_after_Initial_Experience_Trail_During_the_COVID-19_Pandemic (accessed on 27 October 2025). (In Hebrew)
48. Hsieh, H.F.; Shannon, S.E. Three approaches to qualitative content analysis. *Qual. Health Res.* **2005**, *15*, 1277–1288. [CrossRef]
49. Camden, C.; Couture, M.; Pratte, G.; Morin, M.; Roberge, P.; Poder, T.; Maltais, D.B.; Jasmin, E.; Hurtubise, K.; Ducreux, E.; et al. Recruitment, use, and satisfaction with a web platform supporting families of children with suspected or diagnosed developmental coordination disorder: A randomized feasibility trial. *Dev. Neurorehabilit.* **2019**, *22*, 470–478. [CrossRef] [PubMed]
50. Frigerio, P.; Del Monte, L.; Sotgiu, A.; De Giacomo, C.; Vignoli, A. Parents' satisfaction of tele-rehabilitation for children with neurodevelopmental disabilities during the Covid-19 Pandemic. *BMC Prim. Care* **2022**, *23*, 146. [CrossRef] [PubMed]
51. Buckingham, S.A.; Anil, K.; Demain, S.; Gunn, H.; Jones, R.B.; Kent, B.; Logan, A.; Marsden, J.; Playford, E.D.; Freeman, J. Telerehabilitation for people with physical disabilities and movement impairment: A survey of United Kingdom practitioners. *JMIRx Med.* **2022**, *3*, e30516. [CrossRef] [PubMed]
52. Corey, T. Perspectives of Occupational Therapy Practitioners on Benefits and Barriers on Providing Occupational Therapy Services via Telehealth. Ph.D. Thesis, Nova Southeastern University, Fort Lauderdale, FL, USA, 2019. [CrossRef]
53. Ullah, S.; Maghazil, A.M.; Qureshi, A.Z.; Tantawy, S.; Moukais, I.S.; Aldajani, A.A. Knowledge and attitudes of rehabilitation professional toward telerehabilitation in Saudi Arabia: A cross-sectional survey. *Telemed. e-Health* **2021**, *27*, 587–591. [CrossRef]
54. Leochico, C.F.D.; Tyagi, N. Teleoccupational Therapy. In *Telerehabilitation, E-Book: Principles and Practice*; Elsevier: Amsterdam, The Netherlands, 2022; p. 297.
55. Jimenez-Arberas, E.; Casais-Suarez, Y.; Fernandez-Mendez, A.; Menendez-Espina, S.; Rodriguez-Menendez, S.; Llosa, J.A.; Prieto-Saborit, J.A. Evidence-based implementation of the family-centered model and the use of tele-intervention in early childhood services: A systematic review. *Healthcare* **2024**, *12*, 112. [CrossRef]
56. Buitrago, D.C.C.; Rattner, M.; James, L.E.; García, J.F.B. Barriers and facilitators to implementing a community-based psychosocial support intervention conducted in-person and remotely: A qualitative study in Quibdó, Colombia. *Glob. Health Sci. Pract.* **2024**, *12*, e2300032. [CrossRef] [PubMed]
57. Houtrow, A.; Murphy, N.; Council on Children with Disabilities. Prescribing physical, occupational, and speech therapy services for children with disabilities. *Pediatrics* **2019**, *143*, e20190285. [CrossRef]
58. Camden, C.; Silva, M. Pediatric telehealth: Opportunities created by the COVID-19 and suggestions to sustain its use to support families of children with disabilities. *Phys. Occup. Ther. Pediatr.* **2021**, *41*, 1–17. [CrossRef]
59. Hung, K.N.G.; Fong, K.N. Effects of telerehabilitation in occupational therapy practice: A systematic review. *Hong Kong J. Occup. Ther.* **2019**, *32*, 3–21. [CrossRef] [PubMed]
60. Ogourtsova, T.; Boychuck, Z.; O'Donnell, M.; Ahmed, S.; Osman, G.; Majnemer, A. Telerehabilitation for children and youth with developmental disabilities and their families: A systematic review. *Phys. Occup. Ther. Pediatr.* **2022**, *43*, 129–175. [CrossRef]

61. Capistran, J.; Martini, R. Exploring inter-task transfer following a CO-OP approach with four children with DCD: A single subject multiple baseline design. *Hum. Mov. Sci.* **2016**, *49*, 277–290. [CrossRef] [PubMed]
62. Araújo, C.R.S.; Cardoso, A.A.; Magalhães, L.D.C. Efficacy of the cognitive orientation to daily occupational performance with Brazilian children with developmental coordination disorder. *Scand. J. Occup. Ther.* **2019**, *26*, 46–54. [CrossRef]
63. Houldin, A.; McEwen, S.E.; Howell, M.W.; Polatajko, H.J. The cognitive orientation to daily occupational performance approach and transfer: A scoping review. *Occup. Particip. Health* **2018**, *38*, 157–172. [CrossRef]
64. Pierpont, R.; Berman, E.; Hildebrand, M. Increasing Generalization and Caregiver Self-Efficacy Through Cognitive Orientation to Daily Occupational Performance (CO-OP) Training. *Am. J. Occup. Ther.* **2020**, *74*, 7411520499p1. [CrossRef]
65. Graham, F.; Kennedy-Behr, A.; Ziviani, J. *Occupational Performance Coaching: A Manual for Practitioners and Researchers*; Routledge: Oxfordshire, UK, 2020.
66. Gibaud-Wallston, J.; Wandersman, L.P. *Parenting Sense of Competence Scale (PSOC)*; APA PsycTests: Washington, DC, USA, 1978.

children

MDPI

Article

Assessment of Fine Motor Abilities Among Children with Spinal Muscular Atrophy Treated with Nusinersen Using a New Touchscreen Application: A Pilot Study

Inbal Klemm [1,†], Alexandra Danial-Saad [2,†], Alexis R. Karlin [3], Rya Nassar-Yassien [2], Iuliana Eshel [1], Hagit Levine [4,5], Tamar Steinberg [3,5] and Sharon Aharoni [3,5,*]

1 Department of Occupational Therapy, Schneider Children's Medical Center of Israel, Petach Tikva 4920235, Israel; inbalke2@clalit.org.il (I.K.)
2 Department of Occupational Therapy, Faculty of Social Welfare and Health Sciences, University of Haifa, Haifa 349002, Israel; asaad@univ.haifa.ac.il (A.D.-S.)
3 Institute of Pediatric Neurology, Schneider Children's Medical Center of Israel, Petach Tikva 4920235, Israel
4 Institute of Pulmonology, Schneider Children's Medical Center of Israel, Petach Tikva 4920235, Israel
5 Gray Faculty of Medical & Health Sciences, Tel Aviv University, Tel Aviv 6139001, Israel
* Correspondence: sharonah@clalit.org.il; Tel.: +972-3-9253132; Fax: +972-3-9253871
† These authors contributed equally to this work.

Abstract: Background/Objectives: Spinal Muscular Atrophy (SMA) is a genetic neurodegenerative disease characterized by severe muscle weakness and atrophy. Advances in disease-modifying therapies have dramatically changed the natural history of SMA and the outcome measures that are used to assess the clinical response to therapy. Standard assessment methods for SMA are limited in their ability to detect minor changes in fine motor abilities and in patients' daily functions. The aim of this pilot study was to evaluate the feasibility and preliminary use of the Touchscreen-Assessment Tool (TATOO) alongside standardized tools to detect changes in upper extremity motor function among individuals with SMA receiving nusinersen therapy. **Methods:** Thirteen individuals with genetically-confirmed SMA, aged 6–23 years, eight with SMA type 2, and five with SMA type 3, participated. The patients continued the maintenance dosing of nusinersen during the study period. They were evaluated at the onset of the study, then twice more at intervals at least six months apart. Upper extremity functional assessments were performed via the TATOO and standardized tools: the Hand Grip Dynamometer (HGD), Pinch Dynamometer (PD), Revised Upper Limb Module (RULM), and Nine-Hole Peg Test (NHPT). **Results:** Significant changes in fine motor function were detected using the TATOO together with other standardized tools. Participants demonstrated notable improvements in hand grip strength and fine motor performance, as measured by the NHPT. The RULM results were not statistically significant for the total study group, particularly in ambulatory patients with SMA type 3. TATOO provided detailed metrics, and revealed enhancements in accuracy and speed across various tasks. However, given the small sample size, the lack of a control group, and the lack of baseline assessment before receiving therapy, these findings should be considered preliminary and exploratory. **Conclusions:** The findings suggest that the TATOO, alongside traditional assessment tools, offers a sensitive measure of fine motor function changes in patients with SMA. This study highlights the potential of touchscreen-based assessments to address gaps in current outcome measures and emphasizes the need for larger, multicenter studies that will include pre-treatment, baseline, and control data.

Keywords: spinal muscular atrophy; hand function; upper extremity motor function; Touchscreen Assessment Tool

1. Introduction

Spinal muscular atrophy (SMA) is a rare autosomal recessive neuromuscular disease characterized by the progressive loss of motor neurons, and the subsequent atrophy of skeletal muscles and muscle weakness. The phenotypic spectrum is classically categorized into four subtypes according to the age of onset and the maximum motor milestone achieved. However, the classification has evolved to focus on milestone achievements (non-sitters, sitters, walkers) to better tailor interventions [1,2].

Prior to the development of gene- and RNA-based therapies, treatment for SMA largely consisted of supportive therapies including non-invasive ventilation and enteral feeding when the disease progressed. In recent years, disease-modifying therapies, including nusinersen, risdiplam, and onasemogene abeparvovec, have dramatically altered the course and outcomes of the disease. These advances have created a growing need for outcome measures that are sensitive to subtle motor changes and applicable across the SMA spectrum, in both adolescents and adults.

Clinical tools used to evaluate shifts in motor function in individuals with SMA focus on the physical examination of the range of motion of the musculoskeletal system and on related functional impairments. In addition, strength and timed tests are used to monitor aspects of function that reflect activities of daily living [1]. Assessment tools, such as the Revised Upper Limb Module (RULM) and Hand Grip Dynamometer (HGD) that were standardized before the emergence of current therapies, are still in use despite their limitations [3–9]. For example, the RULM is limited by a ceiling effect—meaning that, in patients with relatively preserved upper limb function, such as many with SMA type 3, changes in fine motor skills cannot be reliably detected [9,10]. Hand-held dynamometers provide quantitative measures of strength but do not reflect the complexity of fine motor skills [11]. The Nine-Hole Peg Test (NHPT) has been widely used as a standard tool for hand function assessment, including for various muscular atrophy conditions, whilst its revised version has been found to be more sensitive to upper extremity (UE) fatigue. Thus, it achieves better validation for assessing changes in dexterity in the SMA population [12,13]. Through the course of SMA treatment, individuals may undergo apparently minor changes in UE fine motor skills, which are undetected by traditional assessment methods, but may significantly impact daily functioning [10,14,15].

To address the gap in the functional assessment of fine motor skills for patients with neuromuscular disorders, a member of our team (A.D.S.) developed a Touchscreen Assessment Tool (TATOO) [16–18]. TATOO comprises multiple tasks, each designed to provide objective data on the performance of distinct functional components and motor skills necessary for touchscreen interaction [17]. Subsequent research has demonstrated the effectiveness of TATOO as an assessment tool for fine motor skills in diverse populations, including elderly individuals and children. Its applicability to individuals with type 2 diabetes mellitus is currently being investigated [15,18]. However, the tool has not been systematically studied among individuals with neuromuscular diseases like the SMA population.

The aim of this study was to evaluate the feasibility and preliminary use of TATOO alongside standard functional assessment tools to detect even subtle changes in UE motor function among individuals with SMA undergoing nusinersen therapy. We aimed to test three hypotheses. First, we hypothesized that the UE functional assessment via the TATOO application, along with standard assessment tools, including the HGD, the Pinch Dynamometer (PD), and the NHPT, would detect changes in functional motor skills. Second, we hypothesized that the RULM would not detect significant UE functional changes over the study period. Third, we hypothesized that correlations would be apparent between the standardized fine motor assessment tools (HGD, PD, and NHPT) and the TATOO assessment.

2. Methods

2.1. Study Design and Participants

This was a prospective pilot study conducted during the period 2020–2022 at the multidisciplinary neuromuscular clinic of Schneider Children's Medical Center of Israel. As an exploratory study, no formal power calculation was performed. We aimed to assess the feasibility and to generate preliminary data for larger studies. The inclusion criteria were (1) genetically confirmed 5q SMA; (2) SMA type 2 or 3; (3) age $\geq$ 3 years; and (4) the ability to participate in standardized assessments. All participants received nusinersen therapy prior to study initiation and continued maintenance dosing every four months during the study period as part of standard care in our clinic. The patients were both ambulatory and non-ambulatory. The study population reflected the demographics of our clinical population, including individuals speaking Hebrew, Arabic, and Russian as their native tongues. Patients with comorbidities that could influence motor, sensory, and cognitive functions were excluded.

Written informed consent was obtained from all participants. The study was approved by the hospital review board (RMC-0031-20). All patients were evaluated during regularly scheduled clinic visits. Demographic and clinical data recorded at every visit included age, gender, SMA type, functional level, and dominant hand. Hand dominance was determined by asking participants about their preferred hand for daily tasks such as eating and writing, rather than by performing a standardized assessment. Each participant completed the standard assessments of UE gross and fine motor functions and the TATOO assessments of UE fine motor function, as detailed below. The participants underwent a total of three evaluation sessions: at the initiation of the study, at eight months ($\pm$2 months), and at 17 months ($\pm$5 months).

2.2. Assessment Tools

2.2.1. Standard Assessment Tools for UE Function

The standard assessment tools included the HGD, PD, NHPT, and the RULM.

Two types of hand grip were assessed. Hand Grip Dynamometer (HGD) was assessed to measure hammer grip and lateral pinch strength using a calibrated JAMAR device, following the American Society of Hand Therapists protocol. These tasks were selected as they are reliable indicators of overall hand strength, and are feasible in individuals with SMA and variable abilities. Pinch Dynamometer (PD) was assessed to quantify precision pinch strength [3–5]. The NHPT was used to assess manual dexterity, defined as the ability to manipulate small objects via finger coordination in a timely manner. The test is scored by the number of seconds required to place nine pegs in a pegboard and then to remove them from the pegboard, first using the dominant then the non-dominant hand [6,7].

The RULM includes 19 items that correlate various proximal and distal UE functions. Each item is scored as 0 (unable), 1 (able, with modification), or 2 (able, no difficulty) [9,19]. All the assessments were conducted by an experienced occupational therapist and physical therapist.

2.2.2. The Touchscreen Assessment Tool

TATOO provides an objective measure of the abilities required to use a touchscreen tool [16,17].

In the current study, the participants performed each of the seven following tasks: (1) touch and tap the entire screen area; (2) touch and tap all the corners; (3) double tapping;

(4) tap on static and moving objects accurately; (5) drag objects in all directions; (6) drag objects along straight horizontal paths; and (7) pinching (Figure 1).

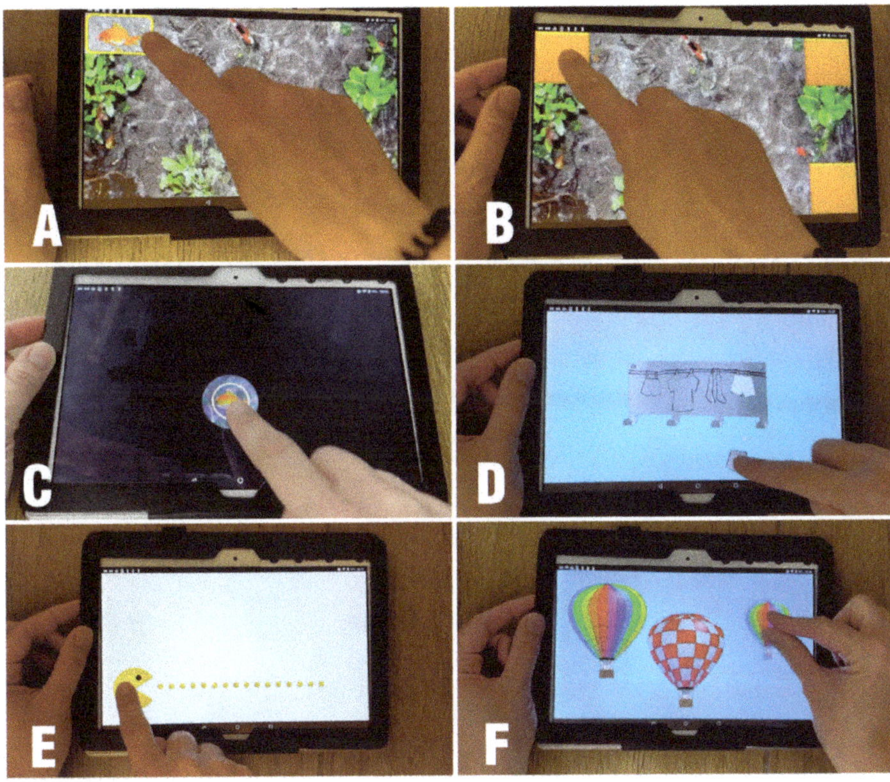

Figure 1. TATOO tasks. (**A**) touch and tap all corners; (**B**) double tapping; (**C**) tap on static and moving objects accurately; (**D**) drag objects in all directions; (**E**) drag objects along straight horizontal paths; and (**F**) pinching.

Performance on each task is summarized by numerical and graphical reports of the temporal metrics and accuracy metrics. The temporal metrics (in seconds) include reaction time, task duration, touch time (the total time in seconds during which the finger touches the screen surface), and flight time (the time in seconds during which the finger does not touch the screen surface). The accuracy metrics include the number of taps, drag attempts, drag completed successfully, and touch outside (the number of errors) [18]. As TATOO is a novel tool in SMA, this study focused on feasibility and sensitivity, and not on reliability and construct validity, which should be investigated in future studies.

2.3. Statistical Analysis

The data were analyzed using SPSS® version 27. Descriptive statistics were used to summarize demographic and clinical data. The normality of data distribution was assessed using the Shapiro–Wilk test. As most variables did not meet the assumption of normality, and due to the small sample size ($n = 13$), we employed non-parametric tests throughout the analysis.

First, we evaluated the differences in the performance of the participants' right and left hands during the first assessment to scrutinize whether hand dominance influences performance. Second, we assessed the changes between the first and last assessments for each outcome measure. Due to the exploratory nature of this pilot study, multiple comparisons were not corrected. Instead, emphasis was placed on the effect size, which was calculated as $r = Z/\sqrt{N}$ to quantify the magnitude of observed changes. Interpretations were based on Cohen's criteria (small: r = 0.1–0.3, moderate: r = 0.3–0.5, large: r > 0.5). We report both statistically significant findings ($p \leq 0.05$) and statistical trends ($0.05 < p < 0.10$). These are accompanied by moderate-to-large effect sizes, which may indicate clinically meaningful changes warranting investigation in further studies. Spearman's rank correlation coefficient test was used to examine the correlation between the parameters of standardized fine motor tools (HGD, PD, NHPT), assessed separately for each hand.

3. Results

A total of 16 individuals with SMA were recruited. After excluding three individuals due to missed evaluations, the participants included 13 individuals aged 6–23 years. Eight were diagnosed with SMA type 2 and five were diagnosed with SMA type 3. Their clinical and demographic characteristics are shown in Table 1.

Table 1. Clinical and demographic characteristics of the patients, $n = 13$.

Variable	Total Patients
Age, years	
Mean (SD)	14.1 (±5.81)
Median (p25–p75)	15 (7.9–19.15)
Gender, *n* (%)	
Male	6 (46.2)
Female	7 (53.8)
SMA type, *n* (%)	
Type 2	8 (61.5)
Type 3	5 (38.5)
SMN2 copy number, *n*	
3	10
4	3
Dominant hand, *n* (%)	
Right	11 (84.6)
Left	2 (15.4)
Ambulatory, *n* (%)	
No	8 (61.5)
Yes	5 (38.5)

SMA: spinal muscular atrophy.

3.1. Comparison of Right- and Left-Hand Performance

At the first assessment, no significant differences were found between right- and left-hand performance across all the standard assessment tools. Based on this finding, subsequent statistical analyses were conducted without stratification by hand dominance but only for right–left performance disparities.

3.2. Comparison Between First and Last Assessments—Standard Tools

Longitudinal analysis revealed significant improvements in several standardized measures of upper limb function. HGD increased significantly in both hands ($z = -2.76$, $p < 0.01$).

Manual dexterity, as measured by the NHPT, showed asymmetric improvement patterns. The left hand demonstrated statistically significant improvement with a reduced task completion time (median change from 28.35 to 23.03 s; $Z = -2.22$, $p = 0.026$, $r = 0.67$). The right hand paradoxically showed a slight increase in completion time, though this change was not statistically significant (Z = −1.69, p = 0.09, r = 0.51). Despite the lack of statistical significance, the large effect size suggests potential clinical relevance requiring further investigation.

Pinch strength measurements assessed by PD revealed minimal changes, with only the right hand showing a trend toward improvement (Z = −1.34, p = 0.18, r = 0.37). This represents a moderate effect size without reaching statistical significance (See Table 2).

Table 2. Comparison between participants' first and last assessments using standard tools.

Variable	Hand	First Assessment	Last Assessment	Z	Effect Size	Relative Size
		Mdn.	Mdn.			
HGD (kg)	R	4.65	6.05	−2.76 **	0.80	
	L	4.50	5.75	−2.76 **	0.80	
PD (kg)	R	1.7	1.9	−1.34 +	0.37	Moderate
	L	1.6	1.1	−0.42	0.12	
NHPT (sec.)	R	22.90	23.32	−1.69 +	−0.51	Large
	L	28.35	23.03	−2.22 *	0.67	

* $p < 0.05$, ** $p < 0.01$, + Clinical change without statistical significance. The relative effect size was added: small (r = 0.1–0.3), moderate (r = 0.3–0.5), large (r > 0.5). Mdn. = median score. HGD = Hand grip Dynamometer, PD = Pinch Dynamometer, NHPT = Nine-Hole Peg Test, R = Right Hand, L = Left Hand. Kg = kilograms, sec. = seconds.

3.3. Comparison Between First and Last Assessments Using TATOO

Using the TATOO application, significant improvements were observed primarily in right-hand performance for both temporal metrics and accuracy metrics across the various tasks. The temporal metrics improved markedly. The median reaction time decreased by 19% (from 3.14 to 2.54 s, z = −2.97, $p < 0.01$). The median flight time decreased by 18% (from 9.49 to 7.79 s, z = −3.11, $p < 0.01$). The median test duration decreased by 20% (from 14.24 to 11.44 s, z = −2.04, $p < 0.01$). The accuracy metrics also improved. The median number of errors of touch outside the desired area decreased by 78% (from 1.29 to 0.29, z = −1.43, $p < 0.05$). The total drag attempts decreased from 10 to 9 (z = −2.02, $p < 0.05$). Metrics such as touch time, the number of taps, and the number of drags completed successfully demonstrated moderate effect sizes despite not reaching statistical significance (Table 3). This suggests potential clinical relevance in a larger sample.

In contrast to the above, fewer significant improvements were observed with left hand performance. A significant reduction by 10% was observed only in reaction time, from 2.77 to 2.47 s (z = −2.27, $p < 0.05$). This asymmetric pattern may reflect differential use in daily activities or in hand-specific therapeutic responses. Other left-hand metrics—including flight time, task duration, and accuracy-related variables, demonstrated small to moderate effect sizes without statistical significance. This highlights consistent trends but requires confirmation in future studies (see Supplemental Table S1).

Table 3. Comparison between participants' first and last assessments using the TATOO application.

Variable	Hand	First Assessment	Last Assessment	Z	Effect Size	Relative Size
		Mdn (IQR)	Mdn (IQR)			
Reaction time (sec.)	R	3.14 (1.14)	2.54 (0.73)	−2.97 **	0.82	
Flight time (sec.)	R	9.49 (2.01)	7.79 (2.18)	−3.11 **	0.86	
Touch time (sec.)	R	4.14 (1.68)	4.00 (1.23)	−1.22 +	0.33	Moderate
Test duration (sec.)	R	14.24 (4.23)	11.44 (3.32)	−2.04 **	0.84	
Number taps (*n*)	R	138 (63.50)	132 (63.50)	−1.26 +	0.35	Moderate
Touch outside (*n*)	R	1.29 (2.36)	0.29 (0.64)	−1.43 *	0.67	
Drag completed successfully (*n*) #	R	8 (0)	8 (0)	−1.41 +	0.39	Moderate
Total drag attempts (*n*)	R	10 (2.50)	9 (0.50)	−2.02 *	0.56	

* $p < 0.05$, ** $p < 0.01$, + Clinical change without statistical significance. Relative effect size was added. Mdn = median score, IQR = interquartile range. R = right, L = left, sec. = seconds, *n* = number. # The median score range in the first assessment was 1 (7–8), and in the last assessment was 0 (8–8).

3.4. Comparison Between First and Last Assessments—RULM

The first and last RULM assessments showed contrasting patterns between the SMA total group and the SMA subtypes. Considering all the participants analyzed, the RULM results revealed no statistically significant differences (z = −1.44, p = 0.15) although a moderate effect size (r = 0.4) showed a trend of change. The first median score was 26 (interquartile range [IQR]: 13.5–36.5) compared with 24 (IQR: 14–37) at the last assessment. Subgroup analysis revealed important distinctions. Participants with SMA Type 2 demonstrated a statistically significant improvement, with median scores increasing from 16 to 18 points (Z = −2.39, p = 0.02), representing an 11% gain in upper limb function. This improvement is clinically meaningful in this population in which first-time function is limited.

In contrast, participants with SMA Type 3 showed no measurable change (first time median 36.5/37, final 37/37; Z = −1.07, p = 0.29).

These findings underscore the RULM's variable utility, namely its appropriateness for monitoring Type 2 patients with moderate impairment, and inadequacy for Type 3 patients who approached maximum scores.

3.5. Correlations Between Standardized Tools and TATOO

Finally, we examined the correlations between measurements of standardized fine motor tools and TATOO for both hands. In the right hand, the parameter "number of taps" of the first task ("Touch all screen areas") correlated significantly with HGD (r = 0.81, p = 0.01) and PD (r = 0.74, p = 0.02). This suggests that tap frequency reflects the underlying force generation capacity. As expected, tap frequency correlated negatively with NHPT (r = −0.63, p = 0.03), indicating that faster tapping corresponds to better manual dexterity.

For both hands, the "pinch ability" task duration showed strong correlations with NHPT performance. For the right hand, rs = 0.67, p = 0.02. For the left hand, rs = 0.90, p < 0.001. This particularly strong left-hand correlation suggests that TATOO's pinch task captures similar fine motor control demands as traditional pegboard tasks.

Taken together, these findings provide the preliminary evidence of convergent validity for TATOO, as the temporal and accuracy-based measures demonstrate consistent associations with the established fine motor performance tools. A comprehensive overview of all correlation analyses is provided in Supplemental Table S1.

4. Discussion

To date, only a few studies have evaluated innovative tools to assess fine motor skills or dexterity in the SMA population, particularly in individuals undergoing treatment [14]. This raises the need to establish standardized fine motor assessment tools that are sensitive to subtle changes in function, accessible to all individuals with SMA regardless of functional status or SMA type, and efficient and easy to administer. Our study demonstrated that TATOO, alongside standardized fine and gross motor assessment tools, was able to detect significant changes in motor function among individuals with SMA types 2 and 3 receiving nusinersen over a 12–18-month period.

Importantly, TATOO provided detailed temporal and accuracy-based metrics, including reaction time, task duration, and the accuracy of finger movements. These parameters are directly relevant to daily activities that rely on touchscreen technology, underscoring the ecological validity of this tool [16–18]. Taken together, our preliminary findings suggest that TATOO may serve as a complementary, sensitive assessment method for monitoring functional changes in the SMA population.

In contrast to the above, the RULM alone was insufficient to capture significant changes at the group level, which was consistent with prior studies [20,21]. Literature reviews and meta-analyses in recent years have indicated that the RULM is hampered by a ceiling effect. Accordingly, the assessment is more effective for detecting motor changes among SMA Type 2 and non-ambulatory Individuals; and less for individuals with SMA Type 3, ambulatory, and with higher baseline functional abilities [22–25]. The median score of our participants with SMA type 3 was 36.5/37 at the first test, which may explain the lack of significant findings. Compared to our other findings, our study suggests that the ceiling effect may be mitigated by a combination of assessments with TATOO, HGD and PD, and the NHPT.

We report significant improvements over time in the hand grip strength of both hands, as measured by the HGD. This is consistent with studies that found statistically significant improvements in hand grip strength among young and adult participants with SMA types 2, 3, and 4, compared to assessments before receiving therapy [10,20,21,26]. However, in our study, the participants had already initiated nusinersen therapy at the time of the first assessment, which may partly explain the differences with prior studies.

Regarding fine motor skills and dexterity, the results revealed significant improvements in performance time for the left hand, and a trend towards improvement for the right hand using the NHPT. These findings align with the study by Gu, Minsu, and Hyun-Ho Kong, published in 2021 [27]. They also reported significant improvements in dexterity for both hands among five participants with SMA type 2, following 18 months of novel therapy using a similar standard dexterity test, the PERDEU Pegboard. This improvement may be attributed to the practice learning effect, which leads to relatively permanent changes in the capability for skilled performance, and which is considered the most crucial factor for improvement in performing motor skills [28].

Finally, our study revealed a strong significant correlation between one of our parameters ("number of taps") in TATOO and all the standardized motor assessment tools. This provides evidence of convergent validity, indicating that TATOO captures dimensions of motor function comparable to established measures of speed, accuracy, stability, strength, precision, durability, and range of motion. In addition, the tool's other metrics offer further functional and pragmatic assessments. We also found a significant correlation between the NHPT (measured by performance time) and the test duration parameter of the Pinch Ability task in TATOO. In both tests, the participants are required to "pinch objects" as fast as they can in all areas of the screen or peg board. Therefore, the resemblance between these tasks likely explains the positive correlation. Other TATOO metrics inconsistently correlated with standardized tools, highlighting that the application may assess both overlapping and unique facets of fine motor performance. Gabyzon, M. et al. [15] examined correlations of TATOO with tests of hand strength and manual dexterity among independent community-living older individuals. They reported no significant correlations between most of the TATOO-measured parameters and the parameters of those assessment tools. However, they did note a moderately positive trend between the number of double taps and manual dexterity (r = 0.32, p = 0.07). Taken together, these diverse findings underscore the complexity of fine motor skill assessment and highlight the potential of TATOO to provide nuanced insights across various populations and conditions.

In the future, measurement tools like TATOO may prove to be a welcome alternative to standardized assessment tools. This is due both to their accurate and precise measuring of functional fine motor ability, and their distinct advantages over prior tools. Indeed, our study has revealed many potential advantages of this tool. A crucial advantage of TATOO is its ability to measure functional changes in individuals with SMA, regardless of age and functional limitations, including those limited by contractures, thus effectively eliminating both floor and ceiling effects. Furthermore, TATOO does not need to be modified or adapted according to functional ability, making the application a more accessible and standardized tool than the NHPT or HGD. Moreover, TATOO does not require the use of specialized equipment. Indeed, the test administrator only needs an electronic tablet with the application downloaded.

Finally, the now nearly universal use of touchscreen tools to perform daily tasks of living, including academic pursuits, social engagement and communication, and purchase of food and other essentials provides a clear opportunity for an innovative approach to ecological clinical assessments. During the present period, the primary advantage of TATOO is its ability to simulate nearly universal tasks of daily living, thereby providing meaningful and pragmatic functional evaluations.

The study had several limitations, which limit the real-world usability of TATOO as a stand-alone tool, yet provide opportunities for further investigation. Firstly, we were unable to test TATOO with a demographically similar control population. Though validation is in process, we do not currently have the norms for a healthy population nor the norms for individuals with SMA along various functional stratifications. This has limited our ability to provide standardized "scores" to summarize an individual's fine motor abilities. Rather, we measured motor abilities across an abundance of parameters. As our current quantification technique may well prove burdensome to providers in the future, it is critical to devise a simple scoring metric based on standardized measurements. Secondly, we recruited participants when they were already receiving nusinersen therapy. Therefore, we did not attain a pre-treatment assessment, and the treatment course itself varied among participants. Nevertheless, we did demonstrate the usability of the tool in conjunction with other tools to measure changes during treatment. Furthermore, given timeframe discrepancies between assessments, we were unable to compare baseline standardized assessments to the TATOO assessment. In addition, the time interval between assessments was not consistent among all participants due to scheduling disruptions related to the COVID pandemic at the time. This mostly impacted the timing of the second visit. Indeed, we also found that the time interval between first and second assessments was too short for our findings to be significant for most patients. For these two reasons, we used only the first and last assessments in the final analysis. Finally, our small sample size limited our statistical analysis, and we cannot exclude a potential learning effect with repeated exposure to TATOO tasks. No formal learning-effect analysis was conducted. Further studies may opt to split groups according to SMA type or functional status.

5. Conclusions

The results of this pilot study suggest that the skills necessary for the operation of touchscreen devices entail specific capabilities that are generally not captured by traditional assessment tools. The clinical implication is that the hand function assessment toolbox should be expanded. Tools such as TATOO can be used to capture the skills required for touchscreen manipulation in the context of the modern digital milieu. We hope that this pilot study may influence the development of new tools aimed to better detect subtle functional changes in individuals with SMA, particularly those receiving novel therapies. This may pave the way to tailor therapies and even contribute to the development of personalized functional technologies using similar touchscreen tools. Finally, the use of such tools may contribute to the developing knowledge about the influence of these gene- and RNA-based therapies on the motor functions of the upper extremity in the SMA population.

Supplementary Materials: The following supporting information can be downloaded at: https://www.mdpi.com/article/10.3390/children12101378/s1.

Author Contributions: I.K., A.D.-S., and S.A. conceptualized and designed the study. R.N.-Y. performed the statistical analysis. All authors wrote sections of the first draft of the manuscript, and critically reviewed and revised the manuscript for important intellectual content. All authors have read and agreed to the published version of the manuscript.

Funding: Funding was provided by the Research Authority at Schneider Children's Medical Center of Israel. Haifa University wishes to thank Prof. Chiari Lorenzo and Dr. Corzani Mattia from the University of Bologna, Italy, for developing the UNIBO TATOO software application.

Institutional Review Board Statement: The study was conducted according to the guidelines of the Declaration of Helsinki, and approved by the Institutional Review Board of Beilinson Hospital (RMC 0031-20, 17-06-2020).

Informed Consent Statement: Informed consent was obtained from all subjects involved in the study.

Data Availability Statement: The research data are not shared.

Conflicts of Interest: The authors declare no conflicts of interest. Disclosures: S.A. is a site principal investigator for clinical trials of Biogen, Novartis Gene Therapies, Inc., and Roche; has participated on advisory boards for Novartis Gene Therapies, Inc./Novartis, and Roche; received speaker's fees from Biogen, Novartis, and Roche; and received a research grant from Novartis Gene Therapies, Inc.

Abbreviations

UE:	Upper Extremity
HGD:	Hand Grip Dynamometer
NHPT:	Nine-Hole Peg Test
PD:	Pinch Dynamometer
RULM:	Revised Upper Limb Module
SMA:	Spinal Muscular Atrophy
TATOO:	Touchscreen-Assessment Tool

References

1. Mercuri, E.; Finkel, R.S.; Muntoni, F.; Wirth, B.; Montes, J.; Main, M.; Mazzone, E.S.; Vitale, M.; Snyder, B.; Quijano-Roy, S.; et al. Diagnosis and management of spinal muscular atrophy: Part 1: Recommendations for diagnosis, rehabilitation, orthopedic and nutritional care. *Neuromuscul. Disord.* **2018**, *28*, 103–115. [CrossRef]
2. Mercuri, E.; Bertini, E.; Iannaccone, S.T. Childhood spinal muscular atrophy: Controversies and challenges. *Lancet Neurol.* **2012**, *11*, 443–452. [CrossRef]

3. Gatt, I.; Smith-Moore, S.; Steggles, C.; Loosemore, M. The Takei handheld dynamometer: An effective clinical outcome measure tool for hand and wrist function in boxing. *Hand* **2018**, *13*, 319–324. [CrossRef]
4. Shaheen, A.A.M.; Omar, M.T.A.; Ali, O.I. Normative values of handgrip and pinch strengths in healthy female college students in Riyadh, Saudi Arabia: A cross-sectional study. *Bull. Fac. Phys. Ther.* **2021**, *26*, 1. [CrossRef]
5. Vargas-Pinilla, O.C.; Rodríguez-Grande, E.I. Reproducibility and agreement between three positions for handgrip assessment. *Sci. Rep.* **2021**, *11*, 12906. [CrossRef]
6. Wang, Y.C.; Magasi, S.R.; Bohannon, R.W.; Reuben, D.B.; McCreath, H.E.; Bubela, D.J.; Gershon, R.C.; Rymer, W.Z. Assessing dexterity function: A comparison of two alternatives for the NIH toolbox. *J. Hand Ther.* **2011**, *24*, 313–321. [CrossRef] [PubMed]
7. Smith, Y.; Hong, E.; Presson, C. Normative and validation studies of the Nine-Hole Peg Test with children. *Percept. Mot. Ski.* **2000**, *90*, 823–843. [CrossRef]
8. McGraw, S.; Qian, Y.; Henne, J.; Jarecki, J.; Hobby, K.; Yeh, W.S. A qualitative study of perceptions of meaningful change in spinal muscular atrophy. *BMC Neurol.* **2017**, *17*, 68. [CrossRef]
9. Pera, M.C.; Coratti, G.; Mazzone, E.S.; Montes, J.; Scoto, M.; De Sanctis, R.; Main, M.; Mayhew, A.; Muni Lofra, R.; Dunaway Young, S.; et al. Revised upper limb module for spinal muscular atrophy: 12-month changes. *Muscle Nerve* **2019**, *59*, 426–430. [CrossRef] [PubMed]
10. Milev, E.; Selby, V.; Wolfe, A.; Rohwer, A.; Tillmann, R.; Ramsey, D.; Iodice, M.; Hogrel, J.Y.; Baranello, G.; Scoto, M.; et al. Assessment of the upper limb function, strength, and mobility in treatment-naive children with spinal muscular atrophy types 2 and 3. *Muscle Nerve* **2024**, *69*, 340–348. [CrossRef] [PubMed]
11. Abd El-Samad, A.A.; El-Meniawy, G.H.; Nour El-Din, S.M.; El-Basatiny, H.M. Pinch grip strength and fine manual control in children with diplegic cerebral palsy: A cross-sectional study. *Bull. Fac. Phys. Ther.* **2021**, *26*, 28. [CrossRef]
12. Niu, H.X.; Wang, R.H.; Xu, H.L.; Song, B.; Yang, J.; Shi, C.H.; Li, Y.S.; Zhang, B.Q.; Wang, S.P.; Yong, Q.; et al. Nine-hole Peg Test and Ten-meter Walk Test for evaluating functional loss in Chinese Charcot-Marie-Tooth disease. *Chin. Med. J.* **2017**, *130*, 1773–1778. [CrossRef]
13. Czell, D.; Neuwirth, C.; Weber, M.; Sartoretti-Schefer, S.; Gutzeit, A.; Reischauer, C. Nine Hole Peg Test and transcranial magnetic stimulation: Useful to evaluate dexterity of the hand and disease progression in amyotrophic lateral sclerosis. *Neurol. Res. Int.* **2019**, 7397491. [CrossRef] [PubMed]
14. Cortés, P.L.; Poveda Verdú, D.; Férriz, A.A.; Ñungo-Garzón, N.C.; Domine, M.C.; Sevilla-Mantecón, T.; Pitarch-Castellano, I.; Vázquez-Costa, J.F. Validation of Neuromyotype: A smart keyboard for the evaluation of spinal muscular atrophy patients. *Neurología (Engl. Ed.)* **2024**, *39*, 733–742. [CrossRef] [PubMed]
15. Elboim-Gabyzon, M.; Danial-Saad, A. Correlation between the ability to manipulate a touchscreen device and hand strength and manual dexterity among community-living older individuals. *Int. J. Environ. Res. Public Health* **2021**, *18*, 9408. [CrossRef] [PubMed]
16. Danial-Saad, A.; Chiari, L. Developing an assessment tool for touch screen devices. *Stud. Health Technol. Inform.* **2017**, *242*, 755–761.
17. Danial-Saad, A.; Chiari, L. A multidisciplinary approach for developing an assessment tool for touch screen devices. *Disabil. Rehabil. Assist. Technol.* **2018**, *13*, 745–753. [CrossRef]
18. Danial-Saad, A.; Corzani, M.; Tacconi, C.; Chiari, L. Usability of a touchscreen assessment tool (TATOO) prototype for clinicians and typically developing children. *Disabil. Rehabil. Assist. Technol.* **2024**, *19*, 951–961. [CrossRef]
19. Mazzone, E.S.; Mayhew, A.; Montes, J.; Ramsey, D.; Fanelli, L.; Young, S.D.; Salazar, R.; De Sanctis, R.; Pasternak, A.; Glanzman, A.; et al. Revised upper limb module for spinal muscular atrophy: Development of a new module. *Muscle Nerve* **2017**, *55*, 869–874. [CrossRef]
20. Weber, C.; Schallner, J.; von der Hagen, M. Handgrip and finger flexion strength in children: A cross-sectional assessment of age-related normative data and application as a clinical functional marker in paediatric neuromuscular disorders. *Brain Dev.* **2023**, *45*, 26–38. [CrossRef]
21. De Wel, B.; Goosens, V.; Sobota, A.; Van Camp, E.; Geukens, E.; Van Kerschaver, G.; Jagut, M.; Claes, K.; Claeys, K.G. Nusinersen treatment significantly improves hand grip strength, hand motor function and MRC sum scores in adult patients with spinal muscular atrophy types 3 and 4. *J. Neurol.* **2021**, *268*, 923–935. [CrossRef] [PubMed]
22. Coratti, G.; Pane, M.; Lucibello, S.; Pera, M.C.; Pasternak, A.; Montes, J.; Sansone, V.A.; Duong, T.; Dunaway Young, S.; Messina, S.; et al. Age-related treatment effect in type II spinal muscular atrophy pediatric patients treated with nusinersen. *Neuromuscul. Disord.* **2021**, *31*, 596–602. [CrossRef]
23. Pane, M.; Coratti, G.; Pera, M.C.; Sansone, V.A.; Messina, S.; d'Amico, A.; Bruno, C.; Salmin, F.; Albamonte, E.; De Sanctis, R.; et al. Nusinersen efficacy data for 24-month in type 2 and 3 spinal muscular atrophy. *Ann. Clin. Transl. Neurol.* **2022**, *9*, 404–409. [CrossRef] [PubMed]

24. Coratti, G.; Cutrona, C.; Pera, M.C.; Bovis, F.; Ponzano, M.; Chieppa, F.; Antonaci, L.; Sansone, V.; Finkel, R.; Pane, M.; et al. Motor function in type 2 and 3 SMA patients treated with nusinersen: A critical review and meta-analysis. *Orphanet J. Rare Dis.* **2021**, *16*, 430. [CrossRef]
25. Pechmann, A.; Behrens, M.; Dörnbrack, K.; Tassoni, A.; Wenzel, F.; Stein, S.; Vogt, S.; Zöller, D.; Bernert, G.; Hagenacker, T.; et al. Improved upper limb function in non-ambulant children with SMA type 2 and 3 during nusinersen treatment: A prospective 3-years SMArtCARE registry study. *Orphanet J. Rare Dis.* **2022**, *17*, 384. [CrossRef]
26. Weber, C.; Müller, A.; Freigang, M.; von der Hagen, M.; Günther, R. 'Reading the palm'—A pilot study of grip and finger flexion strength as an outcome measure in 5q spinal muscular atrophy. *Brain Dev.* **2024**, *46*, 189–198. [CrossRef] [PubMed]
27. Gu, M.; Kong, H.H. Improvement in fine manual dexterity in children with spinal muscular atrophy type 2 after nusinersen injection: A case series. *Children* **2021**, *8*, 1039. [CrossRef]
28. Schmidt, R.A.; Lee, T.D.; Winston, C.; Wulf, G.; Zelaznik, H. *Motor Control and Learning: A Behavioral Emphasis*, 6th ed.; Human Kinetics: Champaign, IL, USA, 2018.

children

MDPI

Article

Effects of Medical Cannabis Treatment for Autistic Children on Family Accommodation: An Open-Label Mixed-Methods Study

Ayelet David [1,*], Eynat Gal [1], Ayelet Ben-Sasson [1], Elkana Kohn [2], Matitiahu Berkovitch [2,3] and Orit Stolar [2,4]

[1] Department of Occupational Therapy, Faculty of Social Welfare & Health Sciences, University of Haifa, Haifa 3490002, Israel
[2] Clinical Pharmacology and Toxicology, Shamir Medical Center (Assaf Harofeh), Zerifin 6093000, Israel
[3] Clinical Pharmacology and Toxicology, Tel-Aviv University, Tel-Aviv 69978, Israel
[4] Child Development Centers, Sharon District-Maccabi Healthcare Services, Kfar Saba 4465141, Israel
* Correspondence: adavid2@staff.haifa.ac.il

Highlights:

What are the main findings?

- CBD-rich cannabis treatment over 6 months was associated with reduced family accommodation (FA) and parental distress in families of autistic children.
- Qualitative findings showed improved family routines, parental well-being, and greater engagement in meaningful activities and social interactions.

Implications

- CBD-rich cannabis treatment may reduce FA and parental distress, while improving family routines and well-being.
- These results provide preliminary support for CBD-rich cannabis treatment in autistic children, though further controlled studies are needed.

Abstract: Background/Objectives: Parents of autistic children often face behavioral and participation challenges of their children, leading them to make accommodations to maintain a stable daily family routine. These family accommodations (FA) involve adapting family routines, actively engaging with the child's support needs and symptoms, and avoiding specific situations. Methods: This open-label, mixed-methods study investigated the impact of CBD-rich cannabis treatment on FA. In the quantitative phase, analyses included 44 parents (from 87 initially recruited) who had complete FAS-RRB data at baseline, 3 months, and 6 months. In the following qualitative phase, 15 parents from the full sample participated in semi-structured interviews. Results: Quantitative results showed reductions in FA frequency and parental distress at 3 and 6 months. Qualitative findings revealed positive changes in family routines, enhanced well-being, and improved parental engagement in meaningful activities and social interactions. Conclusions: This study provides preliminary evidence that CBD-rich cannabis treatment may reduce family accommodation (FA) and parental distress, while improving family routines and well-being. However, given the open-label design and observed adverse events and withdrawals, the findings should be interpreted with caution.

Keywords: autism; family accommodation; parental well-being; CBD-rich cannabis

1. Introduction

Autism spectrum disorder (ASD) is a pervasive clinically and etiologically heterogeneous neurodevelopmental condition. Its diagnostic criteria in the Diagnostic and Statistical

https://doi.org/10.3390/children12101373

Manual of Mental Disorders (5th ed.; DSM-5) include differences in social communication and restricted and repetitive behaviors (RRBI) [1]. Many autistic children have co-occurring maladaptive behaviors like aggression, tantrums, impulsiveness, sleep problems, and mealtime challenges [2] and diagnoses such as attention-deficit/hyperactivity disorder and anxiety [3].

These common behaviors and diagnoses have been associated with decreased daily functioning and participation of children with autism [4–6]. Consequently, they increase parental stress and adversely affect family participation and quality of life [7]. Despite various available interventions for autistic children, parents report that their children continue to experience serious challenges that influence the child and the entire family unit. Presentations vary widely across individuals and are influenced by context factors such as sleep, sensory environment, and daily routines.

Although the cannabis plant has been used medicinally since ancient times, only in the past decade has a more comprehensive understanding of its structure enabled extensive research into its potential health benefits [8]. Previous research distinguished two main phytocannabinoids: cannabidiol (CBD) and tetrahydrocannabinol (THC) [9,10]. The primary psychoactive substance in the plant, THC, is responsible for the "high" sensation, whereas CBD is an antioxidant, anti-inflammatory substance with antipsychotic and anti-anxiety properties [11,12]. By isolating these cannabinoids, medical cannabis can be tailored to treat specific medical needs. In the past decade, the FDA approved using CBD-rich cannabis to treat children with specific types of refractory epilepsy [13]. Interestingly, parents of autistic children treated for epilepsy with CBD-rich cannabis noticed improved ASD symptoms [14]. Recent studies showed the effectiveness of CBD-rich cannabis treatment for many conditions and symptoms common in ASD [15]. Nevertheless, previous studies also reported side effects and treatment withdrawals; these issues are discussed below.

These findings led to more research that found CBD-rich cannabis treatment effective and safe for autistic children [16–19]. Specifically, studies reported improved communication and socialization skills [16,18–20] and participation in daily activities like sleeping [18,21] and eating [22]. Furthermore, studies reported that cannabis consumption reduced co-occurring symptoms, including self-injury, tantrums, restlessness, and anxiety [16–18,20]. In our recently published study [23], we observed significant reductions in RRBI, particularly in compulsive, ritualistic, and sameness behaviors, alongside notable improvements in overall anxiety and specific subtypes, such as general, social, panic, and separation anxieties, following 6 months of CBD-rich cannabis treatment in autistic children. Our findings suggest that reductions in anxiety, especially in panic- and separation-related subtypes, predicted subsequent decreases in RRBI, specifically in sameness behaviors.

However, studies have also highlighted that CBD-rich cannabis treatment is not without limitations, including common side effects. These adverse effects include changes in appetite, gastrointestinal symptoms, irritability, somnolence, psychoactive effects, and sleep disturbances [16–19,21,23,24]. A recent study found that while 75% of parents reported only mild side effects and were able to adhere to the treatment, 9% of participants experienced severe side effects leading to treatment withdrawal. Additional reasons for withdrawal included challenges with the treatment regimen and, in some cases, unrealistic parental expectations, which complicated adherence for certain families [25].

These findings emphasize the need for professional guidance to help parents of autistic children understand both the benefits and potential challenges of CBD-rich cannabis treatment for their children and themselves. A recent study by Mazza et al. [26] further suggests that the benefits of CBD treatment extend beyond clinical and medical outcomes, positively impacting not only the child's quality of life but also that of their families.

Family accommodation (FA) is a collection of the family's responses or adjustments to the daily life demands of a child with a disability, intended to minimize the stress associated with the disorder and sustain the family's daily routine [27,28]. These responses may include modifying family routines, actively participating in the disorder symptoms, or avoiding situations that might trigger symptoms associated with the syndrome [28].

Studies indicated that FA is prevalent among families of children with obsessive-compulsive disorder (OCD) [29,30], anxiety [31,32], sensory modulation disorders [33–35], and ASD [27,36–38]. They also associated FA with adverse clinical presentations, including more severe symptoms, poorer treatment outcomes, increased parental burden, and more disrupted family functioning [28].

Increased interest motivated the development of several scales to measure FA associated with anxiety, OCD [39], and sensory over-responsivity [33]. Feldman et al. [27] adapted the Family Accommodation Scale to measure RRBI accommodation for the ASD population. They found that 80% of parents of autistic children engage in FA at least monthly, and 55% engage daily. Studies linked higher FA frequency in ASD to higher RRBI appearance [27,38], more disruptive behaviors [40], poorer communication and daily living skills [27], increased difficulty tolerating uncertainty [36], and increased child anxiety [31].

Although these studies emphasized how the high FA prevalence interferes with child presentation, they inevitably referred to the parents' role within this process. Beyond the child's behaviors, studies correlating FA with parenting stress [40] recently demonstrated that both the child's and the parents' anxiety contribute to increased FA [36].

While parents perform FA to relieve stress, most parents report feeling distress due to the necessary accommodation—and sometimes link this distress with their children's aggression when not accommodated [27]. Although these accommodations may contribute to the family members' well-being and daily functioning—and indeed help in the short term—they can become maladaptive over time, disrupting the children's participation in their environments and even causing more severe symptoms [28,32].

Given the association of FA with a broad array of child and family challenges attributed to ASD, it is a crucial target outcome for intervention. Intervention research examining FA outcomes with autistic children has been scarce. The related literature includes studies of autism and co-occurring anxiety disorders [31,41] and of autistic adolescents and adults and co-occurring OCD [42,43]. These studies associated FA with treatment outcomes: Russell et al. [42] found that higher FA levels predicted poorer treatment outcomes, and Storch et al. [31] found significantly reduced FA with the child's reduced anxiety. A more recent study found that parent-led cognitive behavioral therapy supported the parents' ability to manage their child's anxiety without accommodating it [44].

The literature supports the positive effects of medical cannabis treatment for autistic children. However, no research has yet examined its impact on FA. Hence, the main goals of this mixed-methods study were to (1) examine the impact of medical cannabis treatment on parent-reported FA and (2) deepen the understanding of parents' perspectives on changes in FA following cannabis treatment.

Although prior psychosocial interventions have reported changes in FA, no cannabis studies to date have included FA as an outcome. This study directly addresses that gap.

2. Materials and Methods

Primary and secondary outcomes: The pre-specified primary outcome was the frequency of family accommodation (FAS-RRB items 1–7 total score). Secondary outcomes were the child's short-term response when no accommodation was provided (FAS-RRB items 9–11) and parental distress related to accommodation (FAS-RRB item 8). Participant flow. In total, 87 families were recruited; 65 children completed the 6-month CBD-rich protocol; of these, 44 parents provided complete FAS-RRB data at baseline, 3 months, and 6 months and were included in the primary analyses.

2.1. Procedure and Participants

We used an explanatory, sequential mixed-methods design [45,46] in which the quantitative trends explicitly informed the qualitative interview guide; integration was planned a priori via connecting (building the interview topics on quantitative patterns) and weaving the two strands to produce meta-inferences. The quantitative study related to the impact on FA of medical cannabis treatment for autistic children. The follow-up qualitative phenomenological study included in-depth interviews to deepen understanding and contextualize the phenomena [47], as shown in Figure 1.

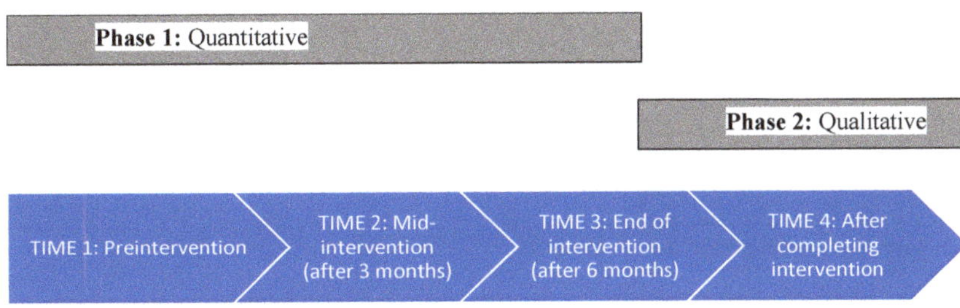

Figure 1. Sequential Mixed-Methods Research Design.

2.2. Phase 1: Quantitative Study

We conducted the quantitative research as part of an open-label study at Shamir Medical Center in Israel, recruiting participants through social media platforms and in collaboration with the Israeli Society for Autistic Children. Inclusion criteria were children aged 5 to 12 years with a medical diagnosis of ASD (based on *DSM-5* criteria) accepted by the Ministry of Health. We confirmed the ASD diagnosis using the Autism Diagnostic Observation Schedule™ [48]. Furthermore, parental reports of their children's disruptive behavioral problems (e.g., violence, restlessness, and sleep problems) during the last 6 months were an inclusion criterion. Exclusion criteria were children with known genetic syndromes causing autism symptoms or diagnosed metabolic diseases and parents with mental health problems (e.g., psychosis or drug addiction). No IQ prerequisites were set for Phase 1.

A pediatric neurologist specializing in ASD interviewed the participants' parents, and concomitant medication regimens that were in place before enrollment were expected to remain stable throughout the study. The cannabis treatment protocol was individualized for each patient using a personalized medicine approach. Participants received medical cannabis extract infused in medium chain triglyceride oil with a 20:1 CBD:THC ratio (Nitzan Spectrum®, Seach Medical Group, Jerusalem, Israel) for 6 months. This ratio was chosen based on open-label studies that found it safe and effective for autistic children [14,17,24]. Titration followed a pragmatic schedule starting at one drop/day (5.7 mg CBD, 0.3 mg THC per drop) and increased gradually as clinically indicated based on parents' reports of tolerability and target behaviors; the final dose did not exceed 10 mg/kg/day CBD (maximum 400 mg/day) and 0.5 mg/kg/day THC (maximum 20 mg/day). Dose timing was individualized according to parental feedback (e.g., higher doses at night to support sleep). Across participants, total daily doses averaged 2.87 mg/kg CBD (SD $\approx$ 1.22); observed ranges were 0.42–6.67 mg/kg CBD and 0.02–0.35 mg/kg THC.

Biweekly follow-up interviews conducted by study staff recorded comorbid symptoms, safety, and adherence; clinic visits occurred at baseline (T1), 3 months (T2), and

6 months (T3). Parent-reported adverse events were categorized (e.g., appetite change, gastrointestinal symptoms, somnolence, irritability, psychoactive effects, sleep disturbances). Parents completed the Family Accommodation Scale for Restricted and Repetitive Behaviors (FAS-RRB) [27] three times: before the medical cannabis treatment (Time 1), after 3 months of treatment (Time 2), and after 6 months of treatment (Time 3). They also completed the demographic data questionnaire at Time 1.

A total of 87 parents of autistic children (ages 5–12 years; M = 7.39, SD = 2.02; 71 boys [81.6%], 16 girls [18.4%]) were initially enrolled. Of these, 65 (74.7%) children completed the 6-month CBD-rich cannabis treatment. Twenty-two (25.3%) dropped out before completion, for reasons including adverse effects such as worsened functioning (n = 2), violence (n = 3), abdominal pain (n = 1), weight gain (n = 1), and sleep problems (n = 1); parental perception that the treatment was ineffective (n = 9); and intake difficulties or parent–child cooperation issues (n = 5) [23]. Among the completers, 44 provided complete FAS-RRB data at all three time points, forming the analytic sample. Participant flow is summarized in Figure 2.

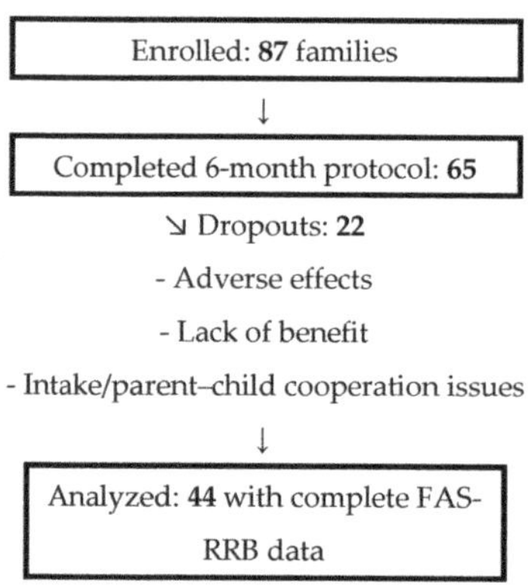

Figure 2. Participant flow.

2.3. *Phase 2: Qualitative, Time 4*

Over the 3 months following the medical cannabis treatment, an occupational therapist conducted semi-structured interviews with 15 parents selected through purposeful sampling from the full sample of the quantitative study. Inclusion criteria were (a) participation in the former study, (b) completion of the 6 months of CBD-rich cannabis treatment, and (c) language fluency. We further recommended that the parent who was most involved in the child's eating and sleeping times participate in the interview. As a result, only mothers were interviewed. We acknowledge that interviewing mothers only limits representativeness of broader family perspectives.

Parents who consented to participate in the qualitative stage were interviewed online and audio-recorded using secure university Zoom software (premium version). The interviews lasted approximately 45 min each and were transcribed after deleting all identifying details. Internal consistency for the FAS-RRB has been reported as high in autistic samples; to our knowledge, minimal important change/responsiveness have not yet been established, so we report effect sizes and exact p-values to aid interpretation.

2.4. *Measures*

2.4.1. Medical Demographic Questionnaire

This questionnaire included medical and demographic questions regarding variables such as gender, age, co-occurring diagnoses, and medications.

2.4.2. Family Accommodation Scale for Restricted and Repetitive Behaviors

The FAS-RRB [27] is an adapted version of a scale used in FA studies on OCD and anxiety disorders [30]. It assesses the frequency of accommodating behaviors that families of autistic children experience due to RRBI (e.g., "Have you changed your work habits because of your child's repetitive behaviors?"). The scale includes 11 items rated on a 5-point Likert scale from 0 (never) to 4 (daily). The first seven items relate to the frequency of accommodating behaviors and are summed to a general score from 0 to 28; higher scores indicate that more FA is needed. The eighth item addresses parental distress caused by accommodating behaviors (e.g., "Did the assistance you gave the child in these forms cause you distress?"). The last three items relate to the child's short-term response if no parental accommodation is made (e.g., "Did the child respond aggressively when you did not help him?"). Internal consistency was high for the seven FAS-RRB items ($\alpha = 0.93$) and the entire 11-item scale ($\alpha = 0.85$).

2.5. Interviews

Parents were asked open-ended questions within a semi-structured interview guide. Topics included (a) their overall experience with the treatment for themselves and their family, (b) the changes they perceived following the medical cannabis treatment, and (c) the implications for their personal and family lives and routines. They were encouraged to discuss both benefits and challenges, while the interviewer explored these issues in depth, seeking specific examples, emotions, and dilemmas the parents faced during the intervention process.

2.6. Data Analysis

The study population's demographic characteristics were described using descriptive statistics. We conducted a repeated measures analysis of variance (ANOVA) followed by a post hoc Bonferroni test to determine which periods differed significantly. The aim was to examine the cannabis treatment effects on the frequency of accommodating behaviors and the children's short-term responses. Due to the abnormal distribution of the sample, we used Friedman tests to examine the treatment's effects on parental distress and Wilcoxon signed rank tests to determine whether the differences between time-period frequencies were significant.

Three experienced occupational therapists analyzed the transcribed interviews in a three-stage systematic phenomenological approach [49]: (1) Identify meaningful text units into thematic codes, (2) group and map the codes into six categories that demonstrate commonalities and differences, and (3) merge the categories into three conceptualized major themes [50]. Each author independently coded the first three interviews into preliminary categories to map the remaining interviews and stopped interviewing upon reaching data saturation after the 15th participant [51].

Data trustworthiness was achieved by presenting rich citations from the original text (with encrypted locations), documenting detailed descriptions of the process, and journaling thoughts and feelings reflected during the interviews to identify potential bias [50]. Alongside a peer review of the data, the authors—supported by their familiarity with the phenomena and existing literature—conducted open conceptual discussions until they reached agreement.

3. Results

3.1. Quantitative

3.1.1. Descriptive Statistics

Forty-four parents of the autistic children who completed the 6-month cannabis treatment (34 boys and 10 girls; 5–12 years, M = 7.39 years, SD = 2.14) completed the FAS-RRB at all three time points. Of those parents, 40 (91%) were married and living together, and 14 (31.8%) reported that their child used prescribed medications: sleep remedies (71%), stimulants (21%), and antipsychotics (14%).

3.1.2. Family Accommodation Frequencies

We applied the repeated measures ANOVA followed by Bonferroni adjustments to avoid the possibility of alpha-error inflation. Wilk's lambda ($\Lambda = 0.649$), $F(4, 170) = 10.25$, $p < 0.001$, and $\eta p2 = 0.194$ indicated a difference in the FAS-RRB scores following treatment. The following univariate test demonstrated differences in accommodating behavior frequency and the children's short-term responses. Table 1 lists the outcome measures' means, standard deviations, *p* values, and effect sizes ($\eta p2$) from the RM univariate test.

Table 1. Means and Standard Deviations of Outcome Measures and *p* Values and Effect Sizes ($\eta 2$) of RM-Univariate Test Showing Differences in Accommodating Behavior Frequency and Child's Short-Term Response and Means and Standard Deviations of Friedman Test of Outcome Measures Showing Differences in Parental Distress.

Outcome	M (SD)			F(df = 2.86)	*p*	ηp2
	Time 1 n = 44	Time 2 n = 44	Time 3 n = 44			
Accommodating behavior frequency	16.45 (7.79)	12.34 (7.57)	12.22 (7.71)	13.58	<0.001	0.24
Child's short-term response	7.95 (3.30)	5.22 (3.70)	5.29 (3.81)	19.13	<0.001	0.31
Parental distress	2.04 (1.72) Mdn = 2	1.20 (1.40) Mdn = 1	1.613 (1.46) Mdn = 1	$\chi 2(2) = 7.56$	0.023	r = 0.45

Note. FAS-RRB scoring: FA frequency (items 1–7) summed 0–28, higher = more accommodation; child short-term response (items 9–11) summed 0–12, higher = more negative response when no accommodation is provided; parental distress (item 8) scored 0–4, higher = greater distress. Effect sizes are partial η^2 (~0.01 small, ~0.06 medium, ≥0.14 large). Pairwise post hoc tests used Bonferroni adjustment.

The post hoc Bonferroni test results revealed that the mean scores for accommodating-behavior frequency and the child's short-term response subscales were significantly higher at Time 1 (pretreatment) than at Times 2 and 3 (posttreatment). That is, FA and the children's maladaptive behavior decreased if their parents made no accommodations following the cannabis treatment. This decrease stabilized as the intervention continued: We found no significant differences between the Times 2 and 3 mean scores in either subscale.

The Friedman test indicated a significant difference between the three times in the parental distress subscale ($n = 44$, $\chi 2(2) = 7.56$, $p = 0.023$, $\Lambda = 0.085$). Specifically, the Wilcoxon signed rank tests showed a significant difference based on positive ranks between Time 1 (Mdn = 2) and Time 2 (Mdn = 1), $Z = -3.003$, $p = 0.003$, $r = 0.452$. Parental distress decreased following the cannabis treatment when no parental accommodation was made. However, we found no significant difference between the mean scores at Times 2 and 3. Thus, the apparent rebound at 6 months relative to 3 months was not statistically significant and is unlikely to be clinically meaningful as the median remained 1 at both time points.

3.2. Qualitative (Themes)

The qualitative analysis highlighted the parents' feelings of relief due to their children's behavioral improvements and reduced need for FA, as well as the subsequent effects on the parents' daily lives. The phenomenological analysis of the in-depth interviews revealed three key themes (summarized in Table 2): changes in the parents' sense of well-being, parents' ability to find and maintain meaningful employment or leisure activities, and the overall family environment.

Table 2. Summary of Manual Coding Categories.

Theme	Coding Category
1. Parental sense of well-being *"You can be more relaxed. You can enjoy your food."*	• Reduced parental stress and decreased need for constant alertness due to fewer maladaptive behaviors of the child • Consistent maintenance of daily routines, such as sleeping and eating; increased availability for other family members, including the spouse and siblings
2. Parents' ability to find and maintain meaningful occupations/jobs *"I couldn't wake up for work; I was just tired... Today, I work in the mornings, and, in the evening, I actually go to events."*	• Ability to plan the day in advance • Confidence that the child will be fine without the mother's presence
3. Parent and family environment *"[Preintervention,] we could not go to other family members that he didn't want to visit. Cannabis gave him more support; he felt more confident."*	• Child's improved ability to participate in social settings • Increased ability to leave the safe home and engage in out-of-home family activities

3.2.1. Parental Sense of Well-Being

Most (12/15) of the mothers consistently described a substantial change in the family's sense of well-being. Specifically, they described decreases in their autistic children's maladaptive behaviors, which they associated with the children's ability to be "more attentive," "calmer," and "more present" following the cannabis treatment. They described these changes as reducing the need for FA. Nevertheless, a minority (3/15) described limited or inconsistent benefits; see Theme 3 for details.

Y (mother of a 9-year-old) shared the positive change in her overall sense of well-being due to her 9-year-old son's ability to reduce his need for her constant touch to calm down. His changed needs reduced the FA, which manifested in symptom-related actions:

> *He really needed my touch. To relax, he needed my hug all the time. He used to say, "I need to calm down. Hug me now. I need to breathe, give me a hand." ... In the last year [posttreatment], I could go rest, and he would not bother me.*

N (mother of an 11-year-old) elaborated on her changed stress level and reduced need for alertness due to changes in her son's ability to participate in daily routine and family activities, such as praying with his father. She reported a reduced need for her FA, like avoiding activities that could trigger her son's stress: "You can be more relaxed. You can enjoy your food... Once these behaviors have decreased, it allows me as a human being to enjoy the situation a little bit more and not be so alert." N emphasized that the changes in her son's maladaptive behavior were significant but not a cure:

> *In the course of the intervention, I felt [the maladaptive behavior] had diminished—not perfectly at all, but in a significant way ... Something about him was positively affected. If he feels well, then we are all well.*

The interviews revealed that most of the family's day before the cannabis treatment revolved around the autistic child's needs and the required accommodations. Parents described their daily lives as unpredictable, with great difficulty maintaining routines for themselves or for their family. They mentioned frequent FA to maintain daily routines primarily for sleeping, eating, and transitioning between contexts and activities.

S (mother of an 11-year-old) elaborated on the extreme symptom-related accommodation her family used during mealtime to address her 11-year-old autistic son's needs and demands:

> *He's sitting down to eat in the living room [or] kitchen. We [the family] had to shut ourselves in a different room. Everyone needed to prepare the food and leave "his" area . . . Cannabis decreased the anxieties, so [now] he can eat next to us, which is a huge improvement for us. We don't have to run away from home anymore.*

Through her words, S demonstrated positive changes in the family's routine and sense of well-being following her child's decreased anxiety during the cannabis treatment.

Most (9/15) mothers mentioned the positive effects of this treatment on the child's ability to fall and stay asleep. The most commonly mentioned pretreatment FA was sitting with the child for long hours at night, which was incompatible with the child's age. According to the mothers, these symptom-related FAs disturbed their quality of life. L (mother of a 7-year-old) explained, "You don't sleep at night for 3 months, and you have to be constantly awake and be with him. . . And then we started cannabis, and, really, it was a huge improvement." D added that the cannabis contributed to her marriage due to her son's earlier bedtime: "The fact that he sleeps early [following the cannabis] is a lot, a lot. It gives me and my husband some time together." The child's improved ability to fall asleep and maintain sleep during the cannabis treatment positively affected the parents' well-being.

The mothers also described their FA as avoiding, delaying, or performing actions to maintain a daily routine, sometimes at the expense of the other family members. All noted that much of their pretreatment days had been occupied with their autistic child's needs; the other family members were expected to understand and support the mother. D, a mother of five, described becoming more available for her autistic son's four younger siblings due to his changed ability to understand situations and be more independent after cannabis treatment:

> *The little siblings said, "Mom, why are you always just with K? Only K! He's bigger and can do it alone. We're small, and we need your help." And today [after the cannabis], it's less, like there's a change. Today, he understands. He can play by himself; he can be alone. And then I can also spend time with my little kids and help them.*

3.2.2. Parents' Ability to Find and Maintain Meaningful Occupations/Jobs

A third (5/15) of the mothers shared how their child's decreased maladaptive behaviors and improved daily participation reduced their need for FA and enhanced their ability to engage in meaningful preferred activities, such as an occupation/job—besides merely addressing their children's needs. N elaborated on her son's improved emotional regulation, which allowed her to plan her day. She explained how her son's mood used to determine her day—whether she could go to work—and the stress around that uncertainty:

> *One day, he wakes up OK, and one day, he doesn't. I could go to sleep and think, "Tomorrow, I need to do X, Y, Z," but I could not know how the morning would look . . . I don't have this problem anymore; I don't feel this stress.*

L shared the FA her family used to do to support her son's sleep difficulties. It did not allow her to wake up in the mornings or focus on other activities because she was too exhausted: "Before [cannabis], I could plan with you and after not sleeping at night, I didn't show up. I couldn't. I could not come. I was too tired."

Both N and L reported relief that they could engage in meaningful occupations/jobs following the intervention. L added that she could even attend business meetings in the evenings—she knew the evening routine would be fine without her presence: "Today, I'm more relaxed, first of all, to bring someone to look after the kids, and I know it's going to be OK. I now work in the mornings, and in the evenings, I actually go to events!" Employment and activity changes were self-reported by mothers; no external verification (e.g., employment records) was collected.

These examples demonstrate how the mothers were less preoccupied with the autistic child's needs posttreatment. Some even asked for outsourcing support. The families' routines improved as their stress and alertness for unexpected events decreased.

3.2.3. Parent and Family Environment

Throughout the interviews, most (10/15) participants discussed their difficulty leaving the safe home and engaging in out-of-home activities. The mothers shared with pain the family's price tag for avoiding overwhelming stimulation and crowded places for the child's sake. They especially mentioned refraining from family activities such as going on vacations or to restaurants, hosting family and friends, and being hosted by others. Following the intervention, most (12/15) mothers indicated positive changes in their children's ability to self-regulate and participate in social settings. These positive changes in the child's presentation decreased the need to avoid family outings. D described: Reports distinguished between tolerance of crowded public places (e.g., restaurants) and participation in structured family outings (e.g., visiting relatives), with improvements noted in both.

> *Before [cannabis], he wouldn't stay where there were too many people. He would refuse to sit down. He would always inspect whether it suited him ... where to sit, where not to sit ... Today, there's no problem. Today, you go out, sit, it doesn't matter where. It doesn't matter if there's a lot of people.* No additional follow-up beyond the 6-month treatment period was conducted; therefore, persistence of these changes beyond this window was not assessed.

Consistent with the quantitative variability, one fifth (3/15) of the mothers reported that the cannabis had no beneficial effect on the need for FA. R, the mother of a 5-year-old autistic child, described the treatment's inconsistent effects on her child: "If I focus on the effect of the cannabis oil, the change was on and off. That is what was so hard. One day, you could be calm; one day, it feels like I haven't given anything." Indeed, an inconsistent response from the child was described as not only affecting the FA consistency but also affecting the mothers' general sense of well-being. Mothers who reported inconsistent effects did not identify specific patterns (e.g., time-of-day or dose-related triggers).

4. Discussion

As medical cannabis is increasingly used to treat autistic children, recent studies have primarily focused on examining its effects on child outcomes [13,23,52]. However, studies examining the effects of this treatment on the families of autistic children remain scarce.

The current mixed-methods study examined the effects of a 6-month medical cannabis treatment for autistic children on FA and parental well-being. Its results support the potential effectiveness of this treatment in reducing FA frequency and parental distress. Furthermore, the findings highlight mostly positive changes in the family's overall well-being, as well as the parents' ability to find and maintain meaningful occupations and engage in social interactions following the child's treatment. Given the open-label design of this study, the findings should be viewed as associations rather than causal effects, reflecting parent-reported perceptions.

These findings align with a recent study [26], which found that the benefits of cannabis treatment for autistic children extended beyond the clinical and medical scope, leading to an overall improvement in both the patient's and the family's quality of life.

Specifically, our results indicate a significant decrease in FA at 3 months (Time 2) and 6 months (Time 3) of treatment. However, the decrease between Time 2 and Time 3 was not significant. Our in-depth interviews further supported this decrease in FA posttreatment and shed light on its positive effects. The mothers appreciated being able to spend quality time with their other children and spouses. They emphasized their renewed ability to have family meals, go on family outings, and enjoy simple daily activities as a family. They also highlighted the positive impact of their enhanced ability to engage in meaningful social and professional activities.

Earlier studies demonstrated reductions in FA following other interventions for children and youth with autism. For example, Storch et al.'s [31] and Frank et al.'s [41] intervention studies with children and youth with ASD and anxiety showed that following cognitive behavioral therapy, FA decreased significantly from pre- to postintervention. These studies align with our findings, supporting the notion that interventions targeting the child's symptoms also positively affect parental factors like FA.

Of substantial importance in addition to decreased FA, our quantitative results suggest decreased parental distress after 3 months of cannabis treatment. The parents related this reduction to their children's lessened maladaptive behaviors, in turn decreasing the parents' need to accommodate constantly.

Unexpectedly, the decreased parental distress observed after 3 months of treatment (Time 2) was not sustained after 3 more months (Time 3). The opposite was true: Parental distress reemerged, although not to levels as high as at Time 1. These results may allude to a ceiling in the child's behavioral improvements following cannabis treatment, a habituation effect in the parents' response, or a placebo/expectation effect—reflected in parents' hope and excitement for a promising treatment with few or no side effects compared with previous medicines. In an open-label study, statistical regression toward the mean is also plausible and could contribute to the observed pattern.

In our study, 25.3% of participants discontinued treatment, and among those who completed the 6-month protocol, some parents reported no meaningful change in FA, as reflected in the quantitative results. Our recently published study [25] similarly found that unrealistic parental expectations and hopes pose significant adherence challenges. That work emphasized that CBD-rich cannabis treatment is not without barriers, underscoring the need for professional guidance and education for parents of autistic children regarding its potential impact. Further longitudinal research is warranted to examine whether the observed changes in child behaviors and parental accommodations can be sustained over the long term (i.e., years of treatment) and whether they persist once treatment ends.

Our findings further highlight the bidirectional effects that FA has on parents. On the one hand, the mothers elaborated on the intense necessity to satisfy their children's needs and support their participation in even basic daily activities. On the other hand, they mentioned the intense energy required to provide these accommodations. They described the hardship of the accommodating effort and the stressful effects of such accommodations on their relationships with their other children, spouses, work, leisure, and emotional well-being. These hardships suggest the crucial importance of reducing FA, as mentioned in other studies [38,40].

Previous studies have addressed this bidirectional effect and suggest that, although necessary, FA may create a vicious cycle by worsening the child's symptoms over time: The children increasingly rely on these accommodations, and their maladaptive behaviors may escalate when the FA are not provided [28,32]. Our study's quantitative results also show a significant decrease in the children's negative short-term response after 3 months of cannabis treatment when parents do not provide FA. These results might indicate the treatment's indirect role in breaking that vicious behavioral cycle by reducing the need for FA. To clarify mechanisms, future work should prospectively assess potential mediators (e.g., anxiety or sleep) that may link treatment-related reductions in FA with the child's reduced short-term negative response.

Recent research has associated higher FA levels at the beginning of intervention with poorer intervention outcomes for youth with autism and anxiety [41,53]. Based on the results of the current and previous studies, we suggest that identifying elevated FA levels at the intervention's assessment stage may be of enhanced importance and that reduced FA could be an outcome for interventions with autistic children. Including FA when evaluating intervention outcomes would provide a more comprehensive and integrated approach to assessing the interventions' impacts on children and parents/families.

4.1. Limitations

This study has several limitations that warrant consideration. First, owing to the open-label design, neither participants nor outcome assessors were blinded, and outcomes relied primarily on parent-reported measures; together these factors could inflate perceived benefits via expectancy or placebo effects. Accordingly, randomized, double-blind, placebo-controlled trials are needed to more rigorously establish efficacy.

Second, individualized dose titration and concomitant medications complicate attribution of change and obscure potential dose–response relationships.

Third, the qualitative sample comprised only mothers and was conducted within a specific cultural and health-system context, which may limit generalizability.

Fourth, COVID-19 restrictions resulted in missing follow-up questionnaires for some parents. Although 65 participants completed the treatment protocol, only 44 had complete FAS-RRB assessments at all three time points. Analyzing only complete-case data (n = 44) may introduce bias; future studies should consider multiple imputation and prespecified sensitivity analyses to address missingness.

4.2. Implications

The results of this study indicate positive—yet preliminary—implications for medical cannabis on child behavior and extend understanding of its potential effects on family/parental factors among families of autistic children. The findings also support routinely tracking family accommodation (FA) as a clinically meaningful outcome alongside parental distress and the child's short-term response when FA is withheld. Given variability across families and co-treatments, these implications should be applied cautiously and with sensitivity to context.

Author Contributions: Conceptualization, A.D., E.G. and O.S.; Methodology, A.D., E.G. and O.S.; Data curation, A.D., M.B. and E.K.; Writing—original draft, A.D.; Writing—review and editing, E.G., A.B.-S. and O.S.; Formal analysis, A.D., E.G. and O.S.; Visualization, E.G.; Supervision, E.G., A.B.-S. and O.S.; Resources, E.K., M.B. and O.S.; Software, E.K. and M.B.; Project administration, O.S. All authors have read and agreed to the published version of the manuscript.

Funding: No funding was received for conducting this study.

Institutional Review Board Statement: The study was conducted in accordance with the Declaration of Helsinki and approved by the Institutional Review Board the University of Haifa (No. 274/21 on 26 May 2021) and the Shamir Medical Center Helsinki Committee (No. ASF-0056-21 on 16 February 2021).

Informed Consent Statement: Informed consent was obtained from all subjects involved in the study.

Data Availability Statement: The data presented in this study are not publicly available due to ethical approval guidelines. The data can be requested from the corresponding author.

Acknowledgments: We thank all participants who contributed to this research, the research team at Shamir Medical Center, Israel, and Nitzan Spectrum®, Seach Medical Group, Israel, for providing the medicinal cannabis without cost.

Conflicts of Interest: The authors declare no conflicts of interest.

Abbreviations

The following abbreviations are used in this manuscript:

ANOVA	Analysis of variance
ASD	Autism spectrum disorder
CBD	Cannabidiol
DSM-5	*Diagnostic and Statistical Manual of Mental Disorders* (5th ed)
FA	family accommodations
FAS-RRB	Family Accommodation Scale for Restricted and Repetitive Behaviors
OCD	Obsessive–compulsive disorder
RRBI	Restricted and repetitive behaviors
THC	Tetrahydrocannabinol

References

1. American Psychiatric Association. *Diagnostic and Statistical Manual of Mental Disorders*, 5th ed.; American Psychiatric Association Publishing: Washington, DC, USA, 2013; ISBN 978-08-9042-575-6. [CrossRef]
2. Casanova, M.F.; Frye, R.E.; Gillberg, C.; Casanova, E.L. Comorbidity and Autism Spectrum Disorder. *Front. Psych.* **2020**, *11*, 1273. [CrossRef]
3. Lai, M.C.; Kassee, C.; Besney, R.; Bonato, S.; Hull, L.; Mandy, W.; Szatmari, P.; Ameis, S.H. Prevalence of Co-Occurring Mental Health Diagnoses in the Autism Population: A Systematic Review and Meta-Analysis. *Lancet Psychiatry* **2019**, *6*, 819–829. [CrossRef] [PubMed]
4. Adams, D.; Emerson, L.M. The Impact of Anxiety in Children on the Autism Spectrum. *J. Autism Dev. Disord.* **2021**, *51*, 1909–1920. [CrossRef] [PubMed]
5. Mannion, A.; Leader, G. Comorbidity in Autism Spectrum Disorder: A Literature Review. *Res. Autism Spectr. Disord.* **2013**, *7*, 1595–1616. [CrossRef]
6. South, M.; Rodgers, J.; Van Hecke, A. Anxiety and ASD: Current Progress and Ongoing Challenges. *J. Autism. Dev. Disord.* **2017**, *47*, 3679–3681. [CrossRef]
7. Karst, J.S.; Van Hecke, A.V. Parent and Family Impact of Autism Spectrum Disorders: A Review and Proposed Model for Intervention Evaluation. *Clin. Child Fam. Psychol. Rev.* **2012**, *15*, 247–277. [CrossRef]
8. Bridgeman, M.B.; Abazia, D.T. Medicinal Cannabis: History, Pharmacology, and Implications for the Acute Care Setting. *Pharm. Ther.* **2017**, *42*, 180–188.
9. Mechoulam, R.; Gaoni, Y. Hashish-IV: The Isolation and Structure of Cannabinolic Cannabidiolic and Cannabigerolic Acids. *Tetrahedron* **1965**, *21*, 1223–1229. [CrossRef]
10. Mechoulam, R.; Shvo, Y. Hashish-I: The Structure of Cannabidiol. *Tetrahedron* **1963**, *19*, 2073–2078. [CrossRef]
11. Iseger, T.A.; Bossong, M.G. A Systematic Review of the Antipsychotic Properties of Cannabidiol in Humans. *Schizophr. Res.* **2015**, *162*, 153–161. [CrossRef]
12. Kozela, E.; Juknat, A.; Gao, F.; Kaushansky, N.; Coppola, G.; Vogel, Z. Pathways and Gene Networks Mediating the Regulatory Effects of Cannabidiol, a Nonpsychoactive Cannabinoid, in Autoimmune T Cells. *J. Neuroinflamm.* **2016**, *13*, 136. [CrossRef]
13. Fusar-Poli, L.; Cavone, V.; Tinacci, S.; Concas, I.; Petralia, A.; Signorelli, M.S.; Diaz-Caneja, C.M.; Aguglia, E. Cannabinoids for People with ASD: A Systematic Review of Published and Ongoing Studies. *Brain Sci.* **2020**, *10*, 572. [CrossRef]
14. Aran, A.; Cayam-Rand, D. Medical Cannabis in Children. *Rambam Maimonides Med. J.* **2020**, *11*, e0003. [CrossRef] [PubMed]
15. Poleg, S.; Golubchik, P.; Offen, D.; Weizman, A. Cannabidiol as a Suggested Candidate for Treatment of Autism Spectrum Disorder. *Prog. Neuropsychopharmacol. Biol. Psychiatry* **2019**, *89*, 90–96. [CrossRef] [PubMed]

16. Aran, A.; Cassuto, H.; Lubotzky, A.; Wattad, N.; Hazan, E. Cannabidiol-Rich Cannabis in Children with Autism Spectrum Disorder and Severe Behavioral Problems: A Retrospective Feasibility Study [Brief Report]. *J. Autism Dev. Disord.* **2019**, *49*, 1284–1288. [CrossRef] [PubMed]
17. Barchel, D.; Stolar, O.; De-Haan, T.; Ziv-Baran, T.; Saban, N.; Fuchs, D.O.; Koren, G.; Berkovitch, M. Oral Cannabidiol Use in Children with Autism Spectrum Disorder to Treat Related Symptoms and Co-Morbidities. *Front. Pharmacol.* **2019**, *9*, 1521. [CrossRef]
18. Bar-Lev Schleider, L.; Mechoulam, R.; Saban, N.; Meiri, G.; Novack, V. Real Life Experience of Medical Cannabis Treatment in Autism: Analysis of Safety and Efficacy. *Sci. Rep.* **2019**, *9*, 200. [CrossRef]
19. Hacohen, M.; Stolar, O.E.; Berkovitch, M.; Elkana, O.; Kohn, E.; Hazan, A.; Hewyman, E.; Sobol, Y.; Waissengreen, D.; Gal, E.; et al. Children and Adolescents with ASD Treated with CBD-Rich Cannabis Exhibit Significant Improvements Particularly in Social Symptoms: An Open Label Study. *Transl. Psychiatry* **2022**, *12*, 375. [CrossRef]
20. Ponton, J.A.; Smyth, K.; Soumbasis, E.; Llanos, S.A.; Lewis, M.; Meerholz, W.A.; Tanguay, R.L. A Pediatric Patient with Autism Spectrum Disorder and Epilepsy Using Cannabinoid Extracts as Complementary Therapy: A Case Report. *J. Med. Case Rep.* **2020**, *14*, 162. [CrossRef]
21. Fleury-Teixeira, P.; Caixeta, F.V.; Ramires da Silva, L.C.; Brasil-Neto, J.P.; Malcher-Lopes, R. Effects of CBD-Enriched Cannabis Sativa Extract on Autism Spectrum Disorder Symptoms: An Observational Study of 18 Participants Undergoing Compassionate Use. *Front. Neurol.* **2019**, *10*, 1145. [CrossRef]
22. Kuester, G.; Vergara, K.; Ahumada, A.; Gazmuri, A.M. Oral Cannabis Extracts as a Promising Treatment for the Core Symptoms of Autism Spectrum Disorder: Preliminary Experience in Chilean Patients. *J. Neurol. Sci.* **2017**, *381*, 932–933. [CrossRef]
23. David, A.; Stolar, O.; Berkovitch, M.; Kohn, E.; Waisman-Nitzan, M.; Hartmann, I.; Gal, E. Characteristics for Medical Cannabis Treatment Adherence Among Autistic Children and Their Families: A Mixed-Methods Analysis. *Med. Cannabis Cannabinoids* **2024**, *7*, 68. [CrossRef] [PubMed]
24. Aran, A.; Harel, M.; Cassuto, H.; Polyansky, L.; Schnapp, A.; Wattad, N.; Shmueli, D.; Golan, D.; Castellanos, F.X. Cannabinoid treatment for Autism: A Proof-of-Concept Randomized Trial. *Mol. Autism* **2021**, *12*, 6. [CrossRef] [PubMed]
25. David, A.; Stolar, O.; Berkovitch, M.; Kohn, E.; Hazan, A.; Waissengreen, D.; Gal, E. Effects of Medical Cannabis Treatment for Autistic Children on Anxiety and Restricted and Repetitive Behaviors and Interests: An Open-Label Study. *Cannabis Cannabinoid Res.* **2024**, *10*, 537–548. [CrossRef]
26. Mazza, J.A.D.S.; Ferreira, L.S.; Martins-Vieira, A.D.F.; Beserra, D.D.L.; Rodrigues, V.A.; Malcher-Lopes, R.; Caixeta, F.V. Clinical and Family Implications of Cannabidiol (CBD)-Dominant Full-Spectrum Phytocannabinoid Extract in Children and Adolescents with Moderate to Severe Non-Syndromic Autism Spectrum Disorder (ASD): An Observational Study on Neurobehavioral Management. *Pharmaceuticals* **2024**, *17*, 686. [CrossRef]
27. Feldman, I.; Koller, J.; Lebowitz, E.R.; Shulman, C.; Itzchak, E.B.; Zachor, D.A. Family Accommodation in Autism Spectrum Disorder. *J. Autism Dev. Disord.* **2019**, *49*, 3602–3610. [CrossRef]
28. Shimshoni, Y.; Shrinivasa, B.; Cherian, A.V.; Lebowitz, E.R. Family Accommodation in Psychopathology: A Synthesized Review. *Indian. J. Psychiatry* **2019**, *61*, S93. [CrossRef]
29. Lebowitz, E.R.; Scharfstein, L.A.; Jones, J. Comparing Family Accommodation in Pediatric Obsessive-Compulsive Disorder, Anxiety Disorders, and Nonanxious Children. *Depress. Anxiety* **2014**, *31*, 1018–1025. [CrossRef]
30. Lebowitz, E.R.; Woolston, J.; Bar-Haim, Y.; Calvocoressi, L.; Dauser, C.; Warnick, E.; Scahill, L.; Chakir, A.R.; Shechner, T.; Hermes, H.; et al. Family Accommodation in Pediatric Anxiety Disorders. *Depress. Anxiety* **2013**, *30*, 47–54. [CrossRef]
31. Storch, E.A.; Zavrou, S.; Collier, A.B.; Ung, D.; Arnold, E.B.; Mutch, P.J.; Lewin, A.B.; Murphy, T.K. Preliminary Study of Family Accommodation in Youth with Autism Spectrum Disorders and Anxiety: Incidence, Clinical Correlates, and Behavioral Treatment Response. *J. Anxiety Disord.* **2015**, *34*, 94–99. [CrossRef]
32. Zavrou, S.; Rudy, B.; Johnco, C.; Storch, E.A.; Lewin, A.B. Preliminary Study of Family Accommodation in 4–7 Year-Olds with Anxiety: Frequency, Clinical Correlates, and Treatment Response. *J. Ment. Health* **2018**, *28*, 365–371. [CrossRef] [PubMed]
33. Ben-Sasson, A.; Podoly, T.Y.; Lebowitz, E. Family Accommodation Scale for Sensory Over-Responsivity: A Measure Development Study. *Front. Psychol.* **2022**, *13*, 2155. [CrossRef] [PubMed]
34. Ben-Sasson, A.; Podoly, T.Y.; Lebowitz, E. The Role of Pediatric Sensory Over-Responsivity and Anxiety Symptoms in the Development of Family Accommodations. *Child Psychiatry Hum. Dev.* **2023**, *56*, 131–141. [CrossRef] [PubMed]
35. Walbam, K.M. A lot to Maintain: Caregiver Accommodation of Sensory Processing Differences in Early Childhood. *J. Child Fam. Stud.* **2022**, *32*, 2199–2213. [CrossRef]
36. Adams, D.; Emerson, L.M. Family Accommodation of Anxiety in a Community Sample of Children on the Autism Spectrum. *J. Anxiety Disord.* **2020**, *70*, 102192. [CrossRef]
37. Dai, Y.G.; Carter, A.S. Characterizing Accommodations by Parents of Young Children with Autism: A Mixed Methods Analysis. *J. Autism Dev. Disord.* **2022**, *53*, 3380–3393. [CrossRef]

38. Shiloh, G.; Gal, E.; David, A.; Kohn, E.; Hazan, A.; Stolar, O. The Relations Between Repetitive Behaviors and Family Accommodation Among Children with Autism: A Mixed-Methods Study. *Children* **2023**, *10*, 742. [CrossRef]
39. Iniesta-Sepúlveda, M.; Rodriguez-Jimenez, T.; Lebowitz, E.R.; Goodman, W.K.; Storch, E.A. The Relationship of Family Accommodation with Pediatric Anxiety Severity: Meta-Analytic Findings and Child, Family and Methodological Moderators. *Child Psychiatry Hum. Dev.* **2021**, *52*, 1–14. [CrossRef]
40. Koller, J.; David, T.; Bar, N.; Lebowitz, E.R. The Role of Family Accommodation of RRBs in Disruptive Behavior Among Children with Autism. *J. Autism Dev. Disord.* **2021**, *52*, 2505–2511. [CrossRef]
41. Frank, H.E.; Kagan, E.R.; Storch, E.A.; Wood, J.J.; Kerns, C.M.; Lewin, A.B.; Small, B.J.; Kendall, P.C. Accommodation of Anxiety in Youth with Autism Spectrum Disorder: Results from the TAASD Study. *J. Clin. Child Adolesc. Psychol.* **2022**, *51*, 219–229. [CrossRef]
42. Russell, A.J.; Jassi, A.; Fullana, M.A.; Mack, H.; Johnston, K.; Heyman, I.; Murphy, D.G.; Mataix-Cols, D. Cognitive Behavior Therapy for Comorbid Obsessive-Compulsive Disorder in High-Functioning Autism Spectrum Disorders: A Randomized Controlled Trial. *Depress. Anxiety* **2013**, *30*, 697–708. [CrossRef]
43. Jassi, A.D.; Vidal-Ribas, P.; Krebs, G.; Mataix-Cols, D.; Monzani, B. Examining Clinical Correlates, Treatment Outcomes and Mediators in Young People with comorbid Obsessive–Compulsive Disorder and Autism Spectrum Disorder. *Eur. Child Adolesc. Psychiatry* **2023**, *32*, 1201–1210. [CrossRef] [PubMed]
44. Byrne, G.; Ghráda, Á.N.; O'Mahony, T. Parent-Led Cognitive Behavioural Therapy for Children with Autism Spectrum Conditions: A Pilot Study. *J. Autism Dev. Disord.* **2023**, *53*, 263–274. [CrossRef]
45. Bishop, F.L. Using Mixed Methods Research Designs in Health Psychology: An Illustrated Discussion from a Pragmatist Perspective. *Br. J. Health Psychol.* **2015**, *20*, 5–20. [CrossRef] [PubMed]
46. Grace, D. Intersectionality-Informed Mixed Methods Research: A Primer. *Health Sociol. Rev.* **2014**, *19*, 478–490.
47. Creswell, J.W.; Klassen, A.C.; Plano Clark, V.L.; Smith, K.C. *Best Practices for Mixed Methods Research in the Health Sciences*; National Institutes of Health: Bethesda, MD, USA, 2011.
48. Lord, C.; Rutter, M.; DiLavore, P.; Risi, S.; Gotham, K.; Bishop, S. *Autism Diagnostic Observation Schedule (ADOS-2)*, 2nd ed.; Western Psychological: Torrance, CA, USA, 2012.
49. Corbin, J.; Strauss, A. *Basics of Qualitative Research: Techniques and Procedures for Developing Grounded Theory*, 4th ed.; Sage: Thousand Oaks, CA, USA, 2015; ISBN 978-14-8331-568-3.
50. Howard, K.; Katsos, N.; Gibson, J. Using Interpretative Phenomenological Analysis in Autism Research. *Autism* **2019**, *23*, 1871–1876. [CrossRef]
51. Charmaz, K. *Constructing Grounded Theory*, 2nd ed.; Sage: Thousand Oaks, CA, USA, 2014; ISBN 978-14-4629-722-3.
52. Fletcher, S.; Pawliuk, C.; Ip, A.; Huh, L.; Rassekh, S.R.; Oberlander, T.F.; Siden, H. Medicinal Cannabis in Children and Adolescents with Autism Spectrum Disorder: A Scoping Review. *Child Care Health Dev.* **2022**, *48*, 33–44. [CrossRef]
53. Townsend, A.N.; Guzick, A.G.; Hertz, A.G.; Kerns, C.M.; Goodman, W.K.; Berry, L.N.; Wood, J.J.; Storch, E.A. Anger Outbursts in Youth with ASD and Anxiety: Phenomenology and Relationship with Family Accommodation. *Child Psychiatry Hum. Dev.* **2022**, *55*, 1259. [CrossRef]

children

MDPI

Systematic Review

XR Technologies in Inclusive Education for Neurodivergent Children: A Systematic Review 2020–2024

Bárbara Valverde Olivares [1], Loretto Muñoz Araya [1], José Luis Valín [1], Marcela Jarpa Azagra [2], Rocío Hidalgo Escobar [2], Isabel Cuevas Quezada [3] and Cristóbal Galleguillos Ketterer [1,*]

[1] Escuela de Ingeniería Mecánica, Pontificia Universidad Católica de Valparaíso, Valparaíso 2362807, Chile; barbara.valverde@pucv.cl (B.V.O.); loretto.munoz@pucv.cl (L.M.A.); jose.valin@pucv.cl (J.L.V.)

[2] Escuela de Pedagogía, Pontificia Universidad Católica de Valparaíso, Valparaíso 2362807, Chile; marcela.jarpa@pucv.cl (M.J.A.); rocio.hidalgo@pucv.cl (R.H.E.)

[3] Escuela de Kinesiología, Pontificia Universidad Católica de Valparaíso, Valparaíso 2362807, Chile; isabel.cuevas@pucv.cl

* Correspondence: cristobal.galleguillos@pucv.cl; Tel.: +56-32-227-3000

Highlights:

What are the main findings?

- XR technologies have been used in inclusive education primarily to support cognitive, social, and behavioral skills in neurodivergent children.
- Existing studies report improvements in engagement and task performance, although sample sizes and study designs are heterogeneous.

What are the implications of the main findings?

- XR applications may represent a valuable complement to traditional inclusive education practices.
- Further research with standardized assessment methods is necessary to validate their effectiveness and inform implementation strategies.

Abstract: Background/Objectives: Extended reality (XR) technologies have been increasingly applied in inclusive education settings to assist neurodivergent children. However, the existing evidence remains fragmented across diverse contexts and disciplines. This systematic review synthesizes current research to identify the educational purposes, implementation characteristics, and reported outcomes associated with the use of XR in inclusive educational environments. **Methods**: A comprehensive literature search was conducted in major academic databases using predefined keyword combinations related to XR, inclusive education, and neurodivergence. Peer-reviewed articles that applied XR tools in educational settings for neurodivergent children were screened against predefined inclusion and exclusion criteria. Data were extracted regarding study design, participant characteristics, XR modality, educational objectives, and outcome indicators. **Results**: The reviewed studies report heterogeneous applications of XR technologies, including virtual and augmented reality, to support cognitive, social, and behavioral skill development in neurodivergent learners. Most studies employed small sample sizes and quasi-experimental or exploratory designs. Although several studies reported improvements in engagement, communication skills, and task performance, outcome measures varied substantially and methodological rigor was limited in many cases. **Conclusions**: Current evidence suggests that XR technologies hold potential as complementary tools in inclusive education for neurodivergent children. Nonetheless, the heterogeneity of study designs and the lack of standardized assessment metrics limit the generalizability of the results. More robust empirical investigations are required to establish evidence-based guidelines for the implementation of XR in inclusive educational contexts.

Keywords: extended reality; virtual reality; augmented reality; neurodivergence; autism spectrum disorder; ADHD; child development; inclusive education; pediatric technology; educational intervention; motor development; systematic review

1. Introduction

The integration of emerging technologies in educational environments has garnered increasing attention as a means to reduce learning barriers for neurodivergent students, particularly those diagnosed with autism spectrum disorder (ASD) [1]. Neurodivergent learners often face significant challenges in traditional educational settings, including difficulties with social communication, sensory processing, executive function, and motor coordination, which can impede their academic progress and social integration [2].

Extended Reality (XR), an umbrella term encompassing virtual reality (VR), augmented reality (AR), and mixed reality (MR), has emerged as a promising educational intervention with the potential to create immersive, controlled, and adaptable learning environments [3,4]. These technologies offer unique advantages for neurodivergent learners by providing predictable, customizable environments that can be tailored to individual sensory preferences and learning needs, while allowing for systematic skill development and minimizing overwhelming sensory stimuli present in traditional classroom settings [2].

The concept of inclusive education, rooted in the principles of universal design for learning (UDL) and the United Nations Convention on the Rights of Persons with Disabilities, emphasizes the importance of creating educational environments that accommodate diverse learning needs [1]. However, implementing truly inclusive practices remains challenging, particularly given the heterogeneous nature of neurodivergent presentations and the limited resources available in many educational settings [4].

Extended Reality (XR) technologies offer unique advantages for neurodivergent learners by providing controlled, customizable, and predictable learning environments that can be systematically adjusted to match individual sensory preferences, cognitive capabilities, and motor development needs [5,6]. From a motor development perspective, XR technologies can provide safe, controlled environments for practicing complex motor skills without the physical risks associated with real-world activities [7].

The theoretical foundation for XR-based interventions in neurodivergent education draws from multiple developmental and learning theories. The motor learning theory emphasizes the importance of repetitive practice and feedback in skill acquisition, particularly relevant for children with motor coordination difficulties common in neurodivergent populations [8]. XR technologies can provide safe spaces for neurodivergent children to observe and practice motor skills and social interactions without the anxiety and unpredictability associated with real-world encounters [2].

Recent advances in XR technology have led to the development of increasingly sophisticated and accessible platforms specifically designed for neurodivergent populations, incorporating motor development principles and evidence-based assessment tools [9]. These include adaptive interfaces, real-time feedback systems, customizable sensory environments, and motor assessment protocols that can be adjusted to meet individual developmental needs [2].

Despite the growing interest and investment in XR technologies for neurodivergent education, the research literature remains fragmented and methodologically inconsistent. Previous reviews have identified several critical gaps, including limited longitudinal evaluation, insufficient diversity in participant samples, lack of standardized outcome measures for motor development assessment, and inadequate consideration of implementation factors in real-world educational settings [1,4].

Furthermore, ethical considerations specific to the use of immersive technologies with vulnerable pediatric populations require careful attention, particularly regarding motor safety and developmental appropriateness. The involvement of children, families, educators, and motor development specialists in the design and evaluation of these technologies is essential to ensure their appropriateness, acceptability, and effectiveness.

This systematic review aims to address these knowledge gaps by providing a comprehensive analysis of current research on XR technologies in neurodivergent education, with particular attention to motor development outcomes. The primary objectives are to (1) systematically identify and analyze studies investigating XR interventions for neurodivergent children in educational contexts; (2) evaluate the effectiveness of different XR modalities (VR, AR, MR) across various skill domains, with emphasis on motor development outcomes; (3) assess methodological quality and identify limitations in current research; (4) examine implementation factors including technology requirements, training needs, and motor assessment protocols; and (5) provide evidence-based recommendations for future research and practice.

2. Materials and Methods

2.1. Study Design and Registration

This systematic review was conducted according to the Preferred Reporting Items for Systematic Reviews and Meta-Analyses (PRISMA) 2020 statement [10]. The review protocol was developed a priori and included specific inclusion and exclusion criteria, search strategies, and data extraction procedures to ensure transparency and reproducibility. A completed PRISMA 2020 checklist is provided as Supplementary Materials.

2.2. Research Questions

The primary research question guiding this systematic review was as follows: how do Extended Reality (XR) technologies contribute to improving educational processes and outcomes for neurodivergent children in educational settings? Secondary questions included the following: (1) What types of XR technologies are most commonly used in neurodivergent education? (2) Which skill domains, particularly motor development, show the greatest improvement with XR interventions? (3) What are the main methodological limitations in current research? (4) What implementation factors facilitate or hinder the use of XR in educational settings?

2.3. Search Strategy

A comprehensive search strategy was developed and implemented across five major electronic databases: Scopus (Elsevier, Amsterdam, The Netherlands), IEEE Xplore (Institute of Electrical and Electronics Engineers, New York, NY, USA), PubMed/MEDLINE (National Library of Medicine, Bethesda, MD, USA), ERIC—Education Resources Information Center (National Center for Education Statistics, Washington, DC, USA), and PsycINFO (American Psychological Association, Washington, DC, USA).

Literature screening and data extraction were performed using Covidence (Covidence, Melbourne, Australia), a web-based systematic review management platform. Qualitative data analysis and thematic synthesis were conducted using NVivo 12 (QSR International, Melbourne, Australia). Statistical analysis of effect sizes was performed using SPSS Statistics version 27 (IBM Corporation, Armonk, NY, USA).

The search algorithm utilized Boolean operators (AND and OR) to combine three main concept groups with their related terms and synonyms:

Concept 1—Extended Reality Technologies: "extended reality" OR "XR" OR "virtual reality" OR "VR" OR "augmented reality" OR "AR" OR "mixed reality" OR "MR" OR "immersive technology" OR "3D environment".

Concept 2—Neurodivergent Populations: "autism" OR "autism spectrum disorder" OR "ASD" OR "ADHD" OR "attention deficit" OR "neurodivergent" OR "neurodiversity" OR "developmental disability" OR "pervasive developmental disorder".

Concept 3—Educational Context: "education" OR "learning" OR "teaching" OR "school" OR "classroom" OR "pedagogy" OR "curriculum" OR "educational intervention" OR "motor development" OR "psychomotor development".

The search was expanded to include articles published between January 2020 and December 2024 to capture the evolution of recent XR technologies while maintaining comprehensive coverage of contemporary relevant research.

2.4. Inclusion and Exclusion Criteria

Inclusion criteria:

- Peer-reviewed articles published between 2020 and 2024.
- Studies involving neurodivergent children (ages 3–18 years).
- Educational applications of XR technologies (VR, AR, or MR).
- Empirical studies including experimental designs, case studies, and observational studies.
- Articles written in English with full-text availability.
- Studies measuring educational, social, cognitive, or motor skill outcomes.

Exclusion criteria:

- Studies focused exclusively on clinical or therapeutic contexts without educational components.
- Research involving adult populations only.
- Studies without specific XR technology interventions.
- Conference abstracts, editorials, opinion pieces, and gray literature.
- Studies with insufficient methodological detail for quality assessment.
- Duplicate publications or overlapping datasets.

2.5. Study Selection Process

The study selection process followed a two-stage screening approach. Initially, three independent reviewers (B.V., L.M., and I.C.) screened the titles and abstracts against the inclusion and exclusion criteria. Subsequently, full-text articles of potentially eligible studies were independently reviewed by the same reviewers. Disagreements were resolved through discussion with a senior reviewer (C.G.K.). The selection process was documented using a PRISMA flow diagram to ensure transparency and reproducibility.

2.6. Data Extraction

A standardized data extraction form was developed and piloted on a subset of the included studies. Data extraction was performed independently by three reviewers (J.V., M.J., and I.C.) with verification by a senior reviewer (C.G.K.). Extracted data included the following:

- Study characteristics (author, year, country, study design, and duration).
- Participant demographics (sample size, age range, gender distribution, and diagnostic categories).
- Intervention details (XR technology type, hardware/software specifications, duration, frequency, and setting).
- Outcome measures (assessment tools, measurement domains, motor development assessments, and data collection methods).

- Results (quantitative and qualitative findings, and effect sizes where available).
- Implementation factors (training requirements, technical challenges, and stakeholder feedback).
- Study limitations and recommendations.

2.7. Quality Assessment

The methodological quality of the included studies was assessed using tools adapted for educational interventions. For experimental and quasi-experimental studies, the Cochrane Risk of Bias tool was adapted to include the specific criteria for educational and motor development interventions. The Cochrane Risk of Bias tool evaluates randomization processes, allocation concealment, blinding of participants and personnel, blinding of outcome assessment, incomplete outcome data, selective reporting, and other potential sources of bias. For case studies and observational research, the National Institutes of Health (NIH) Quality Assessment Tool for Case Series Studies was utilized. The NIH tool assesses study objectives, case definition, representativeness, exposure measurement, outcome assessment, follow-up length, statistical analysis, and results presentation. Quality assessment was conducted independently by three reviewers (R.H., M.J., and I.C.) with discrepancies resolved through consensus discussion.

2.8. Data Synthesis

Due to the heterogeneity of study designs, interventions, and outcome measures, a narrative synthesis approach was employed rather than meta-analysis. Data were synthesized thematically according to the following: (1) XR technology types and characteristics; (2) target skill domains and learning outcomes, with special attention to motor development; (3) participant characteristics and sample diversity; (4) intervention implementation factors; and (5) methodological quality and limitations. Quantitative data were presented using descriptive statistics where appropriate, while the qualitative findings were synthesized using thematic analysis principles. Effect sizes were calculated where sufficient data were available following Cohen's guidelines for interpretation (small: $d = 0.2$, medium: $d = 0.5$, and large: $d = 0.8$). Comprehensive characteristics of all the included studies are provided in Supplementary Table S1, and the quality assessment scores are detailed in Supplementary Table S2.

3. Results

3.1. Study Selection and Characteristics

The systematic search yielded 2156 records from Scopus (n = 856), IEEE Xplore (n = 391), PubMed (n = 542), ERIC (n = 234), and PsycINFO (n = 133). After removing duplicates (n = 287), 1869 records underwent title and abstract screening. Of these, 124 articles were selected for full-text review, resulting in 22 studies meeting all the inclusion criteria (Figure 1).

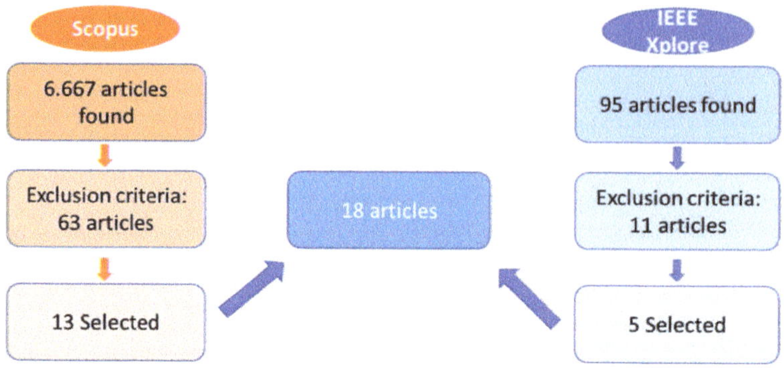

Figure 1. PRISMA flow diagram showing the study selection process for XR technologies in neurodivergent education. The systematic search yielded 2156 initial records across five databases, with 22 studies ultimately meeting the inclusion criteria for a comprehensive analysis.

3.2. Study Characteristics and Distribution

The included studies were conducted across multiple countries, with the highest representation from the United States ($n = 7$, 31.8%), followed by European countries ($n = 9$, 40.9%), Asian countries ($n = 4$, 18.2%), and other regions ($n = 2$, 9.1%). Study designs included randomized controlled trials ($n = 9$, 40.9%), pre-post intervention studies ($n = 7$, 31.8%), case studies ($n = 4$, 18.2%), and mixed-methods studies ($n = 2$, 9.1%).

3.3. XR Technology Distribution and Applications

The analysis of technology utilization revealed that virtual reality was the most frequently employed XR modality ($n = 12$, 54.5%), followed by augmented reality ($n = 7$, 31.8%) and combined VR/AR or general XR approaches ($n = 3$, 13.6%) (Table 1, Figure 2).

Table 1. Distribution of XR technologies and their primary applications in neurodivergent education.

Technology Type	Number of Studies	Primary Applications
Virtual Reality (VR)	12 (54.5%)	Social skills training, emotion recognition, motor coordination, virtual field trips, gross motor skills
Augmented Reality (AR)	7 (31.8%)	Daily living skills, object recognition, interactive learning environments, fine motor tasks
Mixed/Combined XR	3 (13.6%)	Comprehensive skill development, adaptive learning platforms, multimodal training

Virtual reality applications predominantly focused on creating immersive environments for practicing motor coordination and interpersonal interactions, while augmented reality was primarily used for enhancing real-world learning contexts with digital overlays and fine motor skill development.

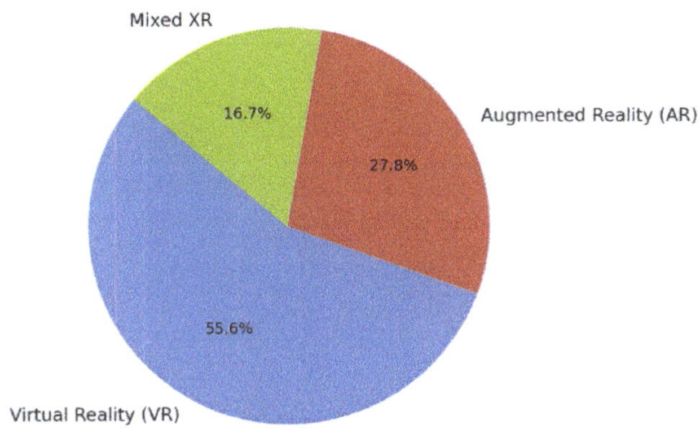

Figure 2. Distribution of XR technologies in the reviewed studies (n = 22). Virtual reality (VR) was the most commonly utilized technology (54.5%), followed by augmented reality (AR) (31.8%) and combined or mixed XR approaches (13.6%). This distribution reflects the maturity and accessibility of VR platforms for educational applications.

3.4. Participant Characteristics and Demographics

The total sample across the empirical studies comprised 412 participants, with individual study samples ranging from 18 to 95 participants (mean = 39.2, SD = 21.3). Participant ages ranged from 3 to 18 years, with a mean age of 9.8 years (SD = 3.4). The gender distribution revealed an imbalance, with male participants comprising 74.3% (n = 306) of the total sample compared to 25.7% (n = 106) female participants, reflecting the higher prevalence of neurodivergent diagnoses in males but also indicating continued underrepresentation of females in research.

Diagnostic categories were dominated by autism spectrum disorder (ASD), representing 86.9% (n = 358) of the participants. Other diagnoses included attention deficit hyperactivity disorder (ADHD) (n = 34, 8.3%) and mixed neurodevelopmental conditions (n = 20, 4.9%).

3.5. Intervention Characteristics and Implementation

Intervention durations varied considerably across the studies, with session lengths ranging from 15 to 75 min (mean = 38.6 min, SD = 16.2). Frequency of the sessions ranged from twice weekly to daily implementation, with most studies conducting sessions 2–3 times per week. Total intervention periods spanned from 2 weeks to 20 weeks (mean = 9.1 weeks, SD = 5.2).

Implementation settings were predominantly controlled environments, with 59.1% (n = 13) of the studies conducted in research laboratories or specialized technology rooms, 31.8% (n = 7) in classroom settings, and 9.1% (n = 2) in home environments with supervision.

3.6. Outcome Measures and Skill Domains

The studies targeted multiple skill domains, with motor coordination being the most frequently addressed area alongside social skills (Table 2). Outcome measurement approaches varied significantly, with some studies using standardized assessment tools while others employing custom-developed measures or observational protocols.

Table 2. Primary outcome domains and measurement approaches across included studies.

Skill Domain	Studies Reporting (%)	Common Assessment Methods
Motor coordination	14 (63.6%)	Movement Assessment Battery for Children-2, Bayley Scales of Infant Development, motion capture, and Bruininks–Oseretsky Test
Social interaction skills	13 (59.1%)	ADOS-2, Social Skills Rating System, and direct observation
Attention and engagement	9 (40.9%)	Continuous Performance Test, behavioral observation, and eye-tracking
Emotional recognition	8 (36.4%)	Facial emotion recognition tasks and physiological measures
Daily living skills	6 (27.3%)	Vineland Adaptive Behavior Scales and task completion rates
Academic skills	5 (22.7%)	Curriculum-based measures and achievement tests

3.7. *Effectiveness and Outcomes*

Overall, the included studies reported positive outcomes across multiple domains, with the effect sizes varying considerably. Motor coordination interventions showed the most consistent positive results, with 12 of 14 relevant studies (85.7%) reporting significant improvements in gross motor skills, spatial awareness, and balance. The effect sizes for motor interventions ranged from moderate to large (d = 0.6 to 1.2), with particular success in interventions targeting gross motor skills and spatial navigation.

Social skills interventions demonstrated positive outcomes in 11 of 13 studies (84.6%), with the effect sizes ranging from moderate to large (d = 0.5 to 1.1). Fine motor skill improvements were less consistently reported, with mixed results across the studies.

Attention and engagement outcomes were positive in 17 of 22 studies (77.3%), with XR environments showing particular effectiveness in maintaining sustained attention compared to traditional instructional methods.

3.8. *Implementation Factors and Stakeholder Perspectives*

The studies that included stakeholder feedback (n = 11, 50.0%) provided valuable insights into implementation facilitators and barriers. Teachers, families, and motor development specialists consistently reported high levels of student motivation and engagement when using XR technologies, with particular appreciation for the individualized and controlled nature of interventions and their potential to address motor development needs safely.

Technical challenges reported across the studies included hardware reliability issues, software compatibility problems, calibration difficulties for motor assessment tools, and the need for technical support during implementation. Cost considerations and the need for specialized training in motor development assessment were identified as significant barriers to widespread adoption.

3.9. *Methodological Quality and Limitations*

The quality assessment revealed variations in methodological rigor across the studies, with 45.5% of the studies achieving high quality ratings, 50.0% moderate quality, and 4.5% low quality. Major limitations identified included the following:

- Limited longitudinal follow-up in 77.3% of the empirical studies.
- Insufficient assessment of skill generalization to real-world contexts.
- Predominance of controlled research settings over authentic educational environments.
- Limited diversity in participant samples across neurodivergent conditions.

- Inconsistent use of standardized motor development assessment measures.
- Lack of age-stratified analysis despite broad age ranges.

The broad age range of 3–18 years encompasses vastly different developmental stages, from preschoolers to high school students, yet most studies did not stratify results by age group or developmental level.

3.10. Longitudinal Outcomes and Skill Transfer

Only five studies (22.7%) included follow-up assessments beyond immediate post-intervention measurement. Among these, four studies reported maintained improvements at 4–12 week follow-up, with particularly strong retention observed for motor skills.

Skill transfer to real-world settings was explicitly assessed in only six studies (27.3%), with mixed results. While some participants demonstrated generalization of learned motor skills to novel environments, others showed limited transfer, highlighting the need for systematic generalization programming and real-world practice opportunities.

4. Discussion

4.1. Principal Findings and Developmental Implications

This systematic review provides compelling evidence that XR technologies offer significant potential for supporting the educational and developmental needs of neurodivergent children, particularly in the domain of motor development, while simultaneously revealing critical gaps in the current research methodology and implementation practices. The predominance of positive outcomes across multiple developmental domains—including motor coordination, social communication, emotional regulation, and sustained attention—suggests that XR interventions can effectively address core challenges faced by neurodivergent learners in traditional educational settings.

The finding that 85.7% of the studies focusing on motor coordination reported significant improvements is particularly noteworthy given the prevalence of motor difficulties in neurodivergent conditions [11]. From a kinesiological perspective, XR environments provide unique opportunities for controlled motor practice, allowing for repetitive skill training with immediate feedback while minimizing the risk of injury or failure that may occur in real-world motor activities [7]. The ability to gradually adjust difficulty levels and environmental demands makes XR particularly suitable for addressing the heterogeneous motor profiles observed in neurodivergent populations.

4.2. Technology-Specific Considerations and Motor Development

The differential applications of VR versus AR technologies revealed in this review reflect their distinct capabilities for motor skill development. Virtual reality's strength in creating fully immersive, controlled environments makes it particularly suitable for gross motor skills training and spatial awareness development, where environmental variables can be systematically controlled and safety ensured [2].

Augmented reality's capacity to overlay digital information onto real-world environments appears more effective for fine motor skills and functional task training, where the goal is to enhance rather than replace real-world motor experiences [1]. This distinction has important implications for motor development specialists and educational practitioners seeking to select appropriate technologies for specific motor learning objectives.

The predominance of laboratory-based implementations rather than authentic classroom or home settings raises important questions about the ecological validity of motor skill improvements. While controlled environments are necessary for establishing motor learning efficacy, the transition to real-world educational and home settings presents additional challenges including space requirements, safety considerations, and integration with the existing motor development programs.

4.3. Motor Development Assessment and Standardization

The variability in motor assessment tools used across the studies represents a significant limitation in the current evidence base. While some studies employed gold-standard assessments such as the Movement Assessment Battery for Children-2 (MABC-2) or Bayley Scales, others relied on custom-developed measures or simple observational protocols. This methodological inconsistency limits the ability to compare outcomes across the studies and establish evidence-based guidelines for XR-based motor interventions.

Future research should prioritize the use of standardized, psychometrically sound motor assessment tools that are sensitive to the types of changes expected from XR interventions. Additionally, the development of XR-specific motor assessment protocols that can capture both quantitative movement parameters and qualitative aspects of motor performance would strengthen the evidence base considerably.

4.4. Age-Stratified Analysis and Developmental Considerations

The broad age range of 3–18 years included in most studies, without age-stratified analysis, represents a critical limitation in understanding how XR technologies may differentially benefit children at various developmental stages. Motor development follows predictable patterns throughout childhood and adolescence, with different motor skills emerging at specific developmental periods [7].

Preschool-aged children (3–5 years) develop fundamental motor skills and may benefit most from XR interventions targeting basic gross motor patterns. School-aged children (6–12 years) refine motor skills and develop more complex coordination abilities, while adolescents (13–18 years) deal with the motor challenges associated with rapid physical growth and may benefit from XR interventions targeting sport-specific or functional motor skills.

4.5. Implementation Science and Stakeholder Perspectives

The studies that included stakeholder feedback provided valuable insights into implementation facilitators and barriers from multiple perspectives. Teachers and motor development specialists reported high levels of student motivation and engagement when using XR technologies, but also expressed concerns about technical complexity, training requirements for motor assessment, and integration with the existing curricula and therapy programs.

Parent and family feedback was generally positive, with particular appreciation for the safe, controlled nature of XR motor interventions and the ability to practice motor skills without risk of injury or social embarrassment. However, concerns were raised about cost, space requirements for implementation, and the need for generalization to real-world motor activities.

4.6. Safety and Ethical Considerations in Motor Development

The use of immersive technologies for motor skill training with vulnerable pediatric populations raises important safety and ethical considerations that require systematic attention. Physical safety concerns include motion sickness, falls during VR use, inappropriate motor demands for developmental level, and the potential for overuse injuries from repetitive movements. Motor development specialists emphasize the importance of proper movement analysis and safety protocols when implementing XR-based motor interventions.

Ethical considerations include ensuring that XR motor interventions are developmentally appropriate, do not replace necessary real-world motor experiences, and are integrated appropriately with the existing motor development programs. The involvement of qualified motor development specialists in the design and implementation of XR motor interventions is essential for ensuring both safety and effectiveness.

4.7. Future Research Directions and Recommendations

Based on the findings of this review, several critical research priorities emerge for advancing the field. First, large-scale randomized controlled trials with adequate statistical power and diverse participant samples are urgently needed, with particular attention to age-stratified analyses that consider developmental motor patterns.

Second, the development and validation of standardized outcome measures specifically designed for XR-based motor interventions is essential. These measures should capture both quantitative movement parameters and functional motor outcomes relevant to daily life activities.

Third, longitudinal studies with extended follow-up periods are needed to understand the long-term developmental impacts of XR motor interventions and their retention over time. Fourth, implementation research examining factors that facilitate or hinder successful XR motor intervention adoption in real-world educational and therapeutic settings is crucial for translation to practice.

4.8. Clinical and Educational Implications

For clinicians, educators, and motor development specialists working with neurodivergent children, this review suggests that XR technologies can be valuable additions to intervention repertoires, particularly for addressing motor coordination and spatial awareness difficulties. However, XR motor interventions should be viewed as complementary to, rather than replacements for, the established evidence-based motor development practices and real-world motor experiences.

The selection of appropriate XR motor interventions should be guided by individual child characteristics, including motor development profile, sensory preferences, cognitive abilities, and specific motor learning objectives. Collaborative assessment and planning involving children, families, educators, motor development specialists, and technology specialists is essential for optimal outcomes.

4.9. Limitations of This Review

Several limitations should be acknowledged in interpreting the findings of this systematic review. Despite expanding to multiple databases, the restriction to English-language publications may have excluded relevant studies published in other languages. The focus on peer-reviewed articles may have missed important findings reported in gray literature or conference proceedings.

The heterogeneity of study designs, interventions, and outcome measures precluded meta-analytic synthesis, limiting the ability to quantify overall effect sizes with precision. The quality of evidence, while improved compared to previous reviews, remains generally moderate, reflecting the relatively early stage of research in this field but limiting confidence in the findings.

The limited number of studies that included follow-up assessments beyond immediate post-intervention represents a significant knowledge gap regarding the persistence of XR-facilitated motor and cognitive improvements.

5. Conclusions

This systematic review demonstrates that Extended Reality technologies, particularly virtual and augmented realities, represent promising tools for supporting the educational and motor development needs of neurodivergent children. The evidence indicates consistent positive outcomes across multiple domains, including motor coordination, social skills, and attention, with high levels of engagement and acceptance from students, teachers, families, and motor development specialists.

However, significant methodological limitations in the current research limit the strength of evidence and generalizability of the findings. Small sample sizes, inadequate control groups, limited follow-up periods, lack of age-stratified analyses, and inconsistent use of standardized motor assessment tools represent critical gaps that must be addressed in future research.

The successful implementation of XR technologies in neurodivergent education and motor development requires more than technological innovation alone. Comprehensive approaches that address teacher and specialist training, curriculum and therapy program integration, safety protocols, technical support, and ongoing evaluation will be essential for realizing the potential of these technologies.

Future research priorities should include large-scale randomized controlled trials with age-stratified analyses, development of standardized assessment tools for XR-based interventions, investigation of long-term outcomes and skill generalization, and examination of implementation factors in authentic educational and therapeutic settings. Additionally, greater attention to ethical considerations, demographic diversity, stakeholder involvement, and motor development expertise will be crucial for advancing the field.

While XR technologies show considerable promise for creating more inclusive and effective educational environments that support both cognitive and motor development in neurodivergent learners, realizing this potential will require sustained, systematic research efforts and collaborative partnerships between researchers, educators, technology developers, motor development specialists, and the neurodivergent community itself.

The investment in rigorous research and thoughtful implementation of XR technologies in neurodivergent education has the potential to significantly improve educational outcomes, motor development, and quality of life for this population. Systematic reviews emphasize the importance of evidence-based frameworks for technology implementation [12,13]. Furthermore, caregiver perspectives and family involvement are critical for ensuring real-world applicability and technology acceptance [14]. Advanced tools such as emotion recognition systems can enhance personalized interventions tailored to individual learner needs [15], ultimately contributing to a more inclusive and equitable educational system that addresses the comprehensive developmental needs of all learners.

Supplementary Materials: The following supporting information can be downloaded at https://www.mdpi.com/article/10.3390/children12111474/s1. File S1: PRISMA checklist and protocol registration. Table S1: Comprehensive characteristics of all 22 included studies (author, year, country, design, sample size, age range, XR technology type, intervention characteristics, and outcome measures). Table S2: Quality assessment scores for all 22 studies using Cochrane Risk of Bias and NIH Quality Assessment tools.

Author Contributions: Conceptualization, C.G.K. and B.V.O.; methodology, B.V.O., J.L.V. and I.C.Q.; validation, M.J.A., R.H.E. and I.C.Q.; formal analysis, B.V.O., C.G.K. and I.C.Q.; investigation, J.L.V., M.J.A., R.H.E. and I.C.Q.; data curation, R.H.E., B.V.O. and I.C.Q.; writing—original draft preparation, B.V.O., C.G.K. and I.C.Q.; writing—review and editing, L.M.A. and all authors; visualization, C.G.K.; supervision, C.G.K. and I.C.Q.; project administration, C.G.K. All authors have read and agreed to the published version of the manuscript.

Funding: This research received no external funding.

Institutional Review Board Statement: Not applicable. This study was a systematic review of published literature and did not involve human subjects research.

Informed Consent Statement: Not applicable.

Data Availability Statement: The data supporting this systematic review are available from the corresponding author upon reasonable request. The data are not publicly available due to access restrictions imposed by database providers (Scopus, IEEE Xplore, PubMed/MEDLINE, ERIC, and PsycINFO) and to protect the intellectual property of primary study authors.

Conflicts of Interest: The authors declare no conflicts of interest.

Abbreviations

XR	Extended Reality
VR	Virtual Reality
AR	Augmented Reality
MR	Mixed Reality
ASD	Autism Spectrum Disorder
ADHD	Attention Deficit Hyperactivity Disorder
PRISMA	Preferred Reporting Items for Systematic Reviews and Meta-Analyses
MABC-2	Movement Assessment Battery for Children-2
UDL	Universal Design for Learning
NIH	National Institutes of Health

References

1. Khowaja, K.; Banire, B.; Al-Thani, D.; Sqalli, M.T.; Aqle, A.; Shah, A. Augmented reality for learning of children and adolescents with autism spectrum disorder: A systematic review. *IEEE Access* **2020**, *8*, 78779–78807. [CrossRef]
2. Frolli, A.; Savarese, G.; Di Carmine, F.; Bosco, A.; Saviano, E.; Rega, A.; Carotenuto, M.; Ricci, M.C. Children on the autism spectrum and the use of virtual reality for supporting social skills. *Children* **2022**, *9*, 181. [CrossRef] [PubMed]
3. Cleary, F.; Power, M.; Kennedy, S.; O'Donnell, M.; Walsh, R.; Connor, S.; Murphy, K.; Sullivan, P.; O'Brien, J.; Lynch, M. XR interventions to improve motor skills development among autistic children: A systematic review. *IEEE Access* **2024**, *12*, 23456–23470.
4. Kennedy, S.; Power, M.; Cleary, F. Inclusivity gaps in XR educational systems for autistic populations. *Comput. Educ.* **2024**, *198*, 104756.
5. Savarese, G.; Frolli, A.; Bosco, A.; Saviano, E.; Ricci, M.C.; Carotenuto, M.; Rega, A.; Di Carmine, F.; Panuccio, G.; Leone, E. Neuropsychological responses to immersive social training in children with ASD. *Children* **2023**, *11*, 216.
6. Tecău, A.S.; Chitu, I.B.; Constantin, C.P.; Popescu, M.R.; Sava, A.; Leordean, D.; Bogdan, C.; Rotariu, M.; Gheorghe, S.; Micu, D. Teacher perceptions on XR technologies in inclusive classrooms. *Children* **2023**, *10*, 1336.
7. Cuevas, I.; Valencia Narbona, M.; de la Fuente, H.; González, A. Desarrollo psicomotor de niños y niñas prematuros (as) por síndromes hipertensivos del embarazo y por otras causas. *RETOS* **2023**, *64*, 123–136. [CrossRef]
8. Grynszpan, O.; Weiss, P.L.; Perez-Diaz, F.; Gal, E.; Sowa, M.; Martin, N.; Couillet, B.; Conoir, M.; Cormier, B.; Tardieu, H. Innovative technology-based interventions for autism spectrum disorder: A meta-analysis. *Autism* **2014**, *18*, 346–361. [CrossRef] [PubMed]
9. Huertas Celdrán, A.; García-Higuera, J.M.; Riofrío-Luzcando, A.; López-López, P.; Martín-González, F.; Pérez-Fernández, M.J.; Rodríguez-Contreras, R.; Fernández-Torres, M.; Sánchez-Sáez, J.; Alonso-García, V. Designing adaptive XR platforms for autism interventions. *J. Ambient. Intell. Humaniz. Comput.* **2023**, *14*, 3456–3470.
10. Page, M.J.; McKenzie, J.E.; Bossuyt, P.M.; Boutron, I.; Hoffmann, T.C.; Mulrow, C.D.; Shamseer, L.; Tetzlaff, J.M.; Akl, E.A.; Brennan, S.E.; et al. The PRISMA 2020 statement: An updated guideline for reporting systematic reviews. *BMJ* **2021**, *372*, n71. [CrossRef] [PubMed]
11. Loomes, R.; Hull, L.; Mandy, W.P.L. What is the male-to-female ratio in autism spectrum disorder? A systematic review and meta-analysis. *J. Am. Acad. Child Adolesc. Psychiatry* **2017**, *56*, 466–474. [CrossRef] [PubMed]
12. Al-Thani, D.; Khowaja, K.; Banire, B.; Sqalli, M.T.; Aqle, A.; Shah, A.; Al-Mazrouei, S.; Al-Kaabi, J.; Al-Mansouri, H.; Mohammed, Y. Augmented reality for learning of children and adolescents with autism spectrum disorder (ASD): A systematic review. *IEEE Access* **2024**, *12*, 45673–45692.
13. Banire, B.; Al-Thani, D.; Salim, S.S. A framework for designing assistive augmented reality systems for children with autism. *IEEE Access* **2017**, *5*, 9508–9517.

14. Bosco, A.; Saviano, E.; Frolli, A.; Carotenuto, M.; Ricci, M.C.; Savarese, G.; Di Carmine, F.; Rega, A.; Leone, E.; Panuccio, G. Caregiver perspectives on XR interventions for children with ASD. *J. Autism Dev. Disord.* **2023**, *53*, 1456–1468.
15. Chitu, I.B.; Tecău, A.S.; Constantin, C.P.; Popescu, M.R.; Bogdan, C.; Sava, A.; Gheorghe, S.; Rotariu, M.; Leordean, D.; Micu, D. AR-based emotional recognition tools for children with ASD. *Children* **2023**, *10*, 436. [PubMed]

children

MDPI

Review

Can Functional Cognitive Assessments for Children/Adolescents Be Transformed into Digital Platforms? A Conceptual Review

Yael Fogel [1,*], Naomi Josman [2], Ortal Cohen Elimelech [2] and Sharon Zlotnik [3]

1 Department of Occupational Therapy, Ariel University, Ariel 4070000, Israel
2 Department of Occupational Therapy, Faculty of Social Welfare and Health Sciences, University of Haifa, Haifa 3498838, Israel; njosman@univ.haifa.ac.il (N.J.); ocoheneli@staff.haifa.ac.il (O.C.E.)
3 Department of Occupational Therapy, Zefat Academic College, Jerusalem St 11, Safed 1320611, Israel; sharon.zl@zefat.ac.il (S.Z.)
* Correspondence: yaelfo@ariel.ac.il (Y.F.); Tel.: +972-52-6262455

Highlights:

What are the main findings?

- Most functional cognitive assessments (n = 13) for children and adolescents with high ecological validity remain unavailable in digital formats, highlighting a significant gap between traditional tools and technology-based solutions.
- Digitization of these assessments offers potential benefits, such as improved accessibility, precision in data collection, and scalability; however, replicating real-life contexts and capturing strategy use digitally remains challenging.

What is the implication of the main finding?

- Innovative digital tools are needed that successfully achieve high ecological validity by preserving real-world context and observation of strategies, while maximizing digital availability through advanced technologies (e.g., VR, mobile platforms).
- The proposed conceptual framework can guide clinicians, researchers, and developers in prioritizing features for future technology-enhanced assessments, promoting evidence-based, context-sensitive evaluation practices.

Abstract: Background/Objectives: Functional cognition, integrating cognitive abilities during real-life task performance, is essential for understanding daily functioning in children and adolescents. Traditional paper-based cognitive assessments in controlled environments often lack ecological validity. Although performance-based assessments more accurately represent functioning in natural contexts, most have not been transformed into digital formats. With technology increasingly embedded in education and healthcare, examining the extent/nature of adaptations, benefits, and challenges of digitizing these tools is important. This conceptual review aimed to (1) examine the extent/nature of traditional performance-based cognitive assessments adapted into digital platforms, (2) compare ecological validity/scoring metrics of traditional and digital tools, and (3) identify opportunities and propose recommendations for future development. Methods: We used an AI-based tool (Elicit Pro, Elicit Plus 2024) to conduct a literature search for publications from the past decade, focusing on transformations of traditional assessments into digital platforms for children and adolescents. This initial search yielded 240 items. After screening, 45 were retained for manual review. Studies were extracted based on their discussion of the assessments (traditional or digital) and assessment tools used. Ultimately, 13 papers that met the inclusion criteria were evaluated based on units of analysis. Results: The analysis yielded three units. The first unit focused on digital transformation trends:

four assessments (31%) were converted to digital platforms, two (15%) were developed as native digital tools, and the majority (seven, 54%) remained traditional. In the second unit, assessments were evaluated according to ecological validity and digital availability, demonstrating that assessments with high ecological validity tended not to be digitally accessible. The third unit synthesized scoring metrics, identifying eight distinct cognitive domains. Conclusions: Digitizing functional cognitive assessments offers greater accessibility, precision, and scalability, but replicating real-world contexts remains challenging. Emerging technologies may enhance ecological validity and support development of effective, technology-enhanced assessment practices.

Keywords: performance-based assessment; ecological validity; executive functions; cognitive assessment

1. Introduction

Cognitive abilities play a pivotal role in performing daily activities, from simple routines to complex tasks that require executive and metacognitive skills. For individuals with cognitive impairments, even basic activities of daily living (ADLs) may present significant challenges [1,2]. In occupational therapy and related disciplines, the concept of *functional cognition*, the integration of cognitive abilities while performing real-life tasks, has become increasingly relevant [3,4].

Although there is no universally accepted definition of *functional cognition*, it is generally conceptualized as the dynamic interplay between cognitive processes (e.g., attention, memory, executive functions [EFs]), performance skills (e.g., motor abilities), and environmental and task demands [5–7]. Functional cognition is best evaluated through direct task performance rather than isolated cognitive testing because direct tasks more accurately reflect an individual's capacity to manage everyday demands [8–10].

Assessing functional cognition is a cornerstone of understanding daily performance, particularly in children and adolescents, whose participation in ADLs and instrumental ADLs is still developing [6,7,11]. Unlike traditional cognitive tests that evaluate isolated domains, functional cognition assessments emphasize the integration of cognitive abilities, such as attention, memory, and EFs, with motor skills, environmental demands, and task complexity [5–7]. As such, they provide a more ecologically valid picture of the child's or adolescent's ability to function in real-life contexts.

Ecological validity describes how accurately an assessment predicts performance in natural environments [12]. It includes two essential components: representativeness and generalizability. *Representativeness* describes how closely the assessment reflects real-life situations, rather than artificially controlled tasks in a laboratory. *Generalizability* is the degree to which the performance in the assessment predicts functioning in everyday settings [3,4]. In this sense, performance-based assessments that simulate or observe actual daily activities offer significant advantages over traditional formats, particularly in capturing the real-world impact of cognitive challenges.

Thus, functional cognition is best evaluated in the context of actual task performance, that is, *occupational performance*, rather than through decontextualized or standardized conditions [8,9]. Performance-based approaches, including direct observation in naturalistic environments or the use of simulated tasks, provide more accurate insight into the interaction between cognitive processes, motor abilities, and environmental demands [13].

Moreover, such context-sensitive assessments align with professional standards and national expectations for demonstrating meaningful outcomes in clinical practice [14]. They also support identifying concrete intervention targets in domains such as schoolwork, play, social participation, and self-care, where cognitive demands intersect with emotional, behavioral, and contextual factors [9].

Traditional assessments of functional cognition and EFs in children and adolescents have relied predominantly on standardized tests and proxy-report questionnaires, typically using paper-and-pencil formats. These assessments are generally administered in structured, controlled environments like clinics or schools [15]. A common example is the Behavior Rating Inventory of Executive Function, widely used to assess EF-related behaviors in home and school contexts through parents' and teachers' reports [16]. Another widely applied tool is the Delis–Kaplan Executive Function System, which evaluates a range of verbal and nonverbal EFs in children and adults through standardized tasks [17]. Although these traditional assessments are established and effective for identifying cognitive deficits, they do not fully reflect how children and adolescents function in their natural, everyday environments, thus limiting the assessments' ecological validity.

In contrast, performance-based assessments focus on real-world tasks and appear to offer greater ecological validity. These tools aim to provide a more in-depth understanding of an individual's functional cognitive abilities by capturing their use of strategies, performance patterns, habits, routines, and contextual and environmental supports rather than evaluating isolated cognitive domains such as attention, memory, or EFs [14,18]. Because these assessments simulate or directly observe performance in meaningful daily activities, they are seen as more representative of actual functioning and recognized as valuable alternatives to traditional approaches [3,4]. Performance-based assessments are particularly beneficial when conducted in real-life or simulated contexts that account for the dynamic interplay between cognitive processes, motor skills, and environmental demands [13].

Bridging these two approaches, the Cognitive Functional Evaluation-Extended model [19,20] integrates traditional cognitive tests with performance-based measures to provide a comprehensive and context-sensitive evaluation of functional cognitive in children and adolescents. This model combines the assessment of cognitive abilities, daily performance, and environmental influences to reflect the dynamic and interactive nature of cognitive functioning. It enables clinicians to develop a holistic understanding of a child's cognitive capabilities and how these abilities manifest in everyday life, supporting more targeted and ecologically valid interventions.

The environments in which individuals function today—including schools, healthcare centers, workplaces, and social settings—are increasingly embedded with technology [21,22]. Considering these rapid technological developments, growing attention has been directed toward creating instruments that use digital platforms to assess functional cognition. Over the past decade, platforms such as virtual reality (VR) environments, wearable sensors, desktop-based software, and mobile applications have been shown to enhance the ecological validity of cognitive assessments by facilitating real-time evaluation in more naturalistic contexts [23].

Technology-based assessments offer a range of benefits. They provide increased accessibility, allow the simulation of diverse and complex real-life scenarios, and support data collection that is more precise and objective through automated scoring and advanced analytics [24]. In addition, the expansion of telerehabilitation and remote healthcare services has opened new avenues for evaluating cognitive functioning outside of traditional clinical settings, making assessments more flexible and scalable [25,26].

Despite their promise, technology-based assessment tools pose several important challenges that must be addressed. These include the need for rigorous methodological precautions to ensure validity, reliability, and consistency in measuring outcomes [11,25,27]. Furthermore, for these tools to justify the resources required for their development and implementation, they must not only replicate the capabilities of traditional assessments but also provide added value by improving measurement sensitivity, relevance, or efficiency [28].

Although research on the feasibility of converting existing cognitive assessment tools into technology-based platforms is ongoing, most studies have focused on general cognitive tests. These efforts have explored whether digital platforms can maintain or enhance the accuracy of assessment outcomes and the potential benefits and limitations of such conversions compared to traditional methods [29]. However, to our knowledge, there has been no specific investigation into the transformation of performance-based assessments of functional cognition into digital tools. Hence, there is a significant gap in the current literature, particularly given the recognized ecological value of performance-based approaches and the increasing integration of technology into educational and healthcare environments.

Against this backdrop, our conceptual review explores the feasibility, effectiveness, and potential advantages of transforming traditional performance-based assessments of functional cognition into digital platforms, focusing specifically on assessments for children and adolescents. Figure 1 illustrates the components of functional cognition and their interrelations. The figure leans on the established definition of functional cognition to better describe this complex term.

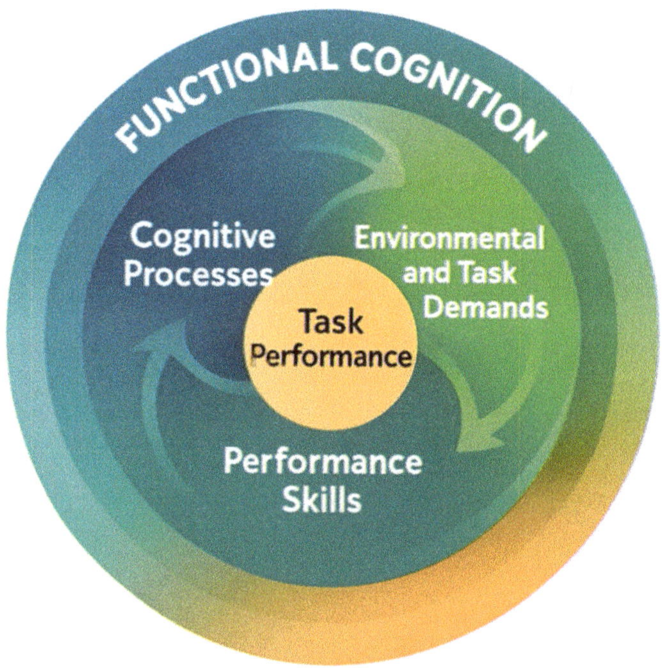

Figure 1. The components and interrelations of functional cognition.

Building on the current literature and theoretical perspectives, this review aims to contribute to the evolving discussion on how technological innovations can support more context-sensitive and developmentally appropriate cognitive assessments. By highlighting emerging directions and identifying key considerations for future development, the review aspires to advance more accurate, effective, and ecologically valid assessment tools that can be integrated into real-world clinical and educational settings. Hence, the specific objectives of this conceptual review are to

1. Examine the current extent and nature of adaptations of traditional performance-based cognitive assessments into digital platforms.
2. Compare the ecological validity and scoring metrics of traditional tools versus digital platforms.
3. Identify opportunities and propose evidence-informed recommendations for the future development of digital platforms for functional cognition assessment in children and adolescents.

2. Materials and Methods

This study follows Jaakkola's [30] template for constructing a conceptual review. In this method, the researchers classify and organize concepts into categories based on shared characteristics to facilitate clearer understanding and analysis. To gather and perform an initial search and analysis of relevant literature for this review, we utilized Elicit [https://elicit.com/] using the Pro license. Elicit is an AI-powered research assistant designed to facilitate evidence synthesis by retrieving, summarizing, and structuring information from academic sources. Elicit searches across over 126 million academic papers from a corpus of open-access and non-open-access studies across all academic disciplines [https://support.elicit.com/en/categories/146369, accessed on 29 September 2025]. The study selection process was performed by three independent researchers. An AI-assisted search, completed in September 2025, identified an initial 240 items. After a title and abstract screening, 45 were retained for manual review. Following a full-text analysis, 13 studies met the final inclusion criteria. The implementation of artificial intelligence tools adheres to the TITAN guidelines (for details, see Supplementary Materials).

The data extraction procedure involved the following steps:

1. Structured search query: The query was entered into the Elicit "Find Papers" feature, which retrieves relevant academic articles based on the prompt, "Find papers related to the following topic—transforming traditional functional cognitive assessments into digital platforms: feasibility, effectiveness, and potential advantages for children and youth."
2. Filtering and refining results: using built-in filters for publication year (e.g., last 10 years to focus on recent advancements), as well as English-language publication
3. Extracting key information in the following categories: (a) title, authors, and publication year, link to full text, and number of its citations; (b) abstract summary; (c) performance-based (yes/no); (d) transformation to digital platform (yes/no); (e) remote administration (yes/no); and (f) advantages and disadvantages.
4. Based on this selection, another thorough manual process was applied. This second analysis focused on identifying manuscripts that discussed performance-based cognitive assessments on either traditional or digital platforms. Of the initial 240 papers, the resulting data totaled 45 papers, which were exported into a spreadsheet for further in-depth manual analysis performed by all the researchers.
5. To mitigate potential biases from the AI-assisted search, such as the under- or over-retrieval of certain literature, a thorough manual review of all results was conducted. This manual screening involved excluding papers that discussed only intervention tools (e.g., computer programs, mobile applications, web and video conferencing platforms, computerized cognitive behavioral therapy interventions, cognitive training, and neuro-feedback) and not assessment tools. Non-performance-based cognitive assessments, such as interviews, were also excluded. Papers were also excluded if they involved participants other than children or adolescents or the researchers had not identified the selection as an academic manuscript. Thirteen papers covering various assessment methods, including traditional paper-and-pencil tests, tablet-based

assessments, computerized neuropsychological tests, game-based assessments, and remote teleassessments, remained.

From the 13 articles that met the inclusion criteria, one unique assessment tool was identified and analyzed from each. Therefore, this study is based on the analysis of 13 assessment tools, with each tool counted only once. This analysis process also involved multiple stages: (1) Screening: Abstracts were reviewed to ensure relevance. (2) Full-text review: Articles meeting the criteria were reviewed in detail. (3) Discussions about performance-based assessments were further analyzed for the advantages or disadvantages of transformation. (4) Data extraction: We identified key concepts to establish the units of analysis. These key concepts were structured into tables and categorized, as detailed in the Results.

3. Results

Three key units of analysis emerged in our analysis of data from all 13 assessments regarding challenges and implications of digital cognitive assessment platforms: (a) digital transformation trends, (b) ecological validity and digital platforms, and (c) scoring metrics across cognitive domains.

3.1. Trends in Adapting Traditional Performance-Based Cognitive Assessments into Digital Platforms

Table 1 presents an overview of 13 cognitive performance-based assessment tools targeting various populations of children and adolescents, assessment methodologies, and their digital-platform transformations. Among those assessments, four (31%)—the Children's Memory Test (CMT), Tower of London, Weekly Calendar Planning Activity (WCPA), and Wisconsin Card Sorting Test for children (WCST)—had been converted to digital platforms. In addition, two (15%) assessments—the Adaptive Cognitive Evaluation Explorer (ACE-X) and Cambridge Neuropsychological Test Automated Battery (CANTAB)—had been digitized natively. The other seven (54%), particularly EF and general cognitive assessment tools, remained entirely traditional.

The 13 assessments addressed diverse populations, focusing on general cognitive abilities, attention deficit hyperactivity disorder, autism spectrum disorders, EF deficits, learning disabilities, and neurodevelopmental delays. Newly added tools, such as the WCPA [31] and the Children's Cooking Task (CCT) [32], provided ecologically valid measures of functional cognition, emphasizing real-world EF challenges.

Table 1. An overview of 13 cognitive performance-based assessments.

Assessment	Purpose: To …	Description	Population: Developed for …	Scoring Metric	Age Range (Years)	Psychometric Properties: Reliability and Validity Types Assessed	Digital Platform
Weekly Calendar Planning Activity (WCPA) [33]	examine impact of EFs difficulties on the ability to perform daily activities involving multiple steps	Participants enter a list of appointments on a weekly schedule according to specified rules. There are three difficulty levels.	adults and adapted for children and adolescents	Number of accurate meetings, rules followed, number of strategies, planning time, total time, efficiency score	6–21	Interrater reliability [34], test–retest reliabilities among college student [35], discriminate validity [31,35,36]. There is normative data for adolescents 12–18 years [37].	No digital version available
Test of Everyday Attention for Children (TEA-Ch) [38]	measure multiple aspects of attention. The second edition (TEA–Ch2) [39] provides a simplified arrangement for ages 5 to 7 years and an extended arrangement for ages 8 to 15 years.	A battery of game-like assessments comprising nine distinct tasks	adults and adapted for children and adolescents	Sustained attention, selective attention, and attentional control	6–16	Test–retest reliability [40], convergent validity [40], discriminate validity [41,42], construct validity [41–43]	Computer program measures reaction times, accuracy, and scores as part of TEA-Ch2
Behavioral Assessment of the Dysexecutive Syndrome for Children (BADS-C) [44]	evaluate EF through tasks that simulate real-life scenarios and problem-solving demands.	A battery of tasks, including the Playing Cards, Water, and Key Search tests and three versions of the Zoo Map Test.	adults and adapted for children and adolescents	Total time, planning time, and number of errors	8–16	Interrater reliability [44], ecological validity, construct validity [45], construct validity (e.g., [46]), discriminate validity (e.g., [47], concurrent validity [47]. Norms are available from 7 years old [44].	No digital version available

Table 1. *Cont.*

Assessment	Purpose: To . . .	Description	Population: Developed for . . .	Scoring Metric	Age Range (Years)	Psychometric Properties: Reliability and Validity Types Assessed	Digital Platform
Children's Cooking Task [48]	examine EF, problem-solving, and sequencing skills through a cooking task simulation.	Participate in preparing a chocolate cake and juice using the recipe provided.	adults and adapted for children and adolescents	Goal accomplishment, dangerous behavior, need for adult assistance, total time, total number of errors additions, omissions, comments/ questions, estimation errors, substitution sequence errors, control errors, context neglect, environmental adherence, purposeless actions and displacements, dependency, inappropriate behavior	8–20	Internal consistency, test–retest reliability, discriminant validity, concurrent validity [32,48]	No digital version available
Do-Eat performance-based assessment [49]	evaluate areas of strength and difficulty in activities of daily living and instrumental activities of daily living among children with various disorders and help define therapeutic goals for occupational therapy intervention focusing on motor, EF, sensory, and emotional skills	Conducted in a natural setting, involving three tasks: make a sandwich, prepare chocolate milk, and complete a certificate of achievement.	children with neurodevelop-mental disorders	Total time, total score, cue scores, sensory motor skills, EF skills (attention, initiation, sequencing, shifting, spatial organization, temporal organization, inhibition, problem-solving, remembering instructions), and task performance.	5–8	internal consistency, interrater reliability, construct validity, concurrent validity [49,50]	No digital version available

Table 1. *Cont.*

Assessment	Purpose: To . . .	Description	Population: Developed for . . .	Scoring Metric	Age Range (Years)	Psychometric Properties: Reliability and Validity Types Assessed	Digital Platform
Children's Kitchen Task assessment [51]	assess EFs and process skills during cooking activities, focusing on problem-solving and error detection.	A Play-Do task accompanied by written and pictorial instructions. The child receives examiner-provided cues as needed to successfully complete the activity.	adults and adapted for children and adolescents	Total time, total score, number of cues, organization score	8–12	Interrater reliability, internal consistency [51,52]	No digital version available
Preschool Executive Task Assessment [53]	assess EFs among young children and determine the level of assistance they need to accomplish the task	The child is instructed to draw a caterpillar picture. The child receives a box containing the necessary equipment and a comprehensive illustrated instruction book.	preschool children	Total time, total cues, total score, performance measure (working memory, organization, emotional ability, distractibility)	3–6	Interrater reliability [53], concurrent validity [52,54]	No digital version available
Children's Memory Test (CMT) [55]	measure aspects of memory like immediate and delayed recall and meta-memory abilities in children (version 2, CMT-2, is available)	Memory task that involves four scenes relating to everyday living situations, each containing 20 pictures of objects.	adults and adapted for children and adolescents	Immediate recall, delayed recall, meta-memory (performance, prediction, performance estimation), and strategy used	5–16	Internal consistency, content validity, construct validity, concurrent validity [56]	Transferred to digital format

Table 1. *Cont.*

Assessment	Purpose: To ...	Description	Population: Developed for ...	Scoring Metric	Age Range (Years)	Psychometric Properties: Reliability and Validity Types Assessed	Digital Platform
Cambridge Neuropsychological Test Automated Battery (CANTAB) [57]	assess cognitive abilities, such as visual memory, visual attention, and working memory/planning	Computerized neuropsychological tests that assess various cognitive functions. In this flexible battery, the researcher can select a subtask based on the participant's interests.	adults and adapted for children and adolescents	Attention and psychomotor speed (mean reaction time, correct responses, false alarms, omission errors, sensitivity index, response variability, movement time, EF (number of problems solved, total errors, mean initial thinking time between/within errors, total stages completed, pre-extradimensional shift errors, total trials completed, strategy score, emotional/social cognition: number of correctly identified emotions, accuracy per emotion (e.g., happiness, fear),memory, total correct responses, trials to success/trials to criterion, mean correct latency,% correct, delayed recall accuracy (e.g., reaction time).	4–90.	Internal consistency, construct validity [58], discriminant validity [59]	Developed as digital
Tower of London Test [60]	measure planning and problem-solving abilities	Solve a problem using two wooden towers and diameter balls by reaching the examiner's tower abstraction within a specified time and number of moves. Different difficulty levels and versions (different numbers of balls) exist.	children with neurodevelopmental disorders	Total score, planning time, task level achieved, execution time	6–80 (digital version intended for 5–53)	Cronbach's alpha convergent validity, discriminant validity [61]	Transferred to digital format

Table 1. *Cont.*

Assessment	Purpose: To ...	Description	Population: Developed for ...	Scoring Metric	Age Range (Years)	Psychometric Properties: Reliability and Validity Types Assessed	Digital Platform
Wisconsin Card Sorting Test for children (WCST) [62]	assess abstract reasoning, cognitive flexibility, and EFs by evaluating the ability to adapt to changing sorting rules	Four stimulus cards and 128 response cards with printed objects that differ in number, color, and shape: The child matches the response cards to the stimulus cards with correct or incorrect feedback. A short form with 64 cards is available.	adults and adapted for children and adolescents	Total number of correct answers, total errors, perseverative responses, perseverative errors, non-perseverative errors, categories completed, number of trials to complete the category, % conceptual level response, failure to maintain set.	6.5–89.0	Norms are available for children 6 months–6 years [62]	Transferred to digital format
The Birthday Task Assessment [63]	assess performance in a complex, multistep task requiring EF abilities	A role-playing scenario related to a birthday party. The child must complete three tasks of varying difficulty according to specific rules: prepare two sandwiches with peanut butter and jelly, wrap two birthday presents, and prepare a card for the birthday party.	children with neurodevelop-mental disorders.	Total time, broken rules, errors (omission, object substitution, action addition, total errors)	8–16	Interrater reliability [63]	No digital version available
Adaptive Cognitive Evaluation Explorer (ACE-X) [64]	assess cognitive abilities, including working memory, attention, and cognitive flexibility. The assessment was adapted from the Adaptive Cognitive Evaluation-Classroom (ACE-C).	This mobile EF assessment tool includes 15 tasks in real-world settings. An incorporated algorithm enables repeatedly administering the same tasks without losing sensitivity to low performance levels.	anyone 7–107 years experiencing cognitive difficulties	Processing speed, working memory, inhibitory control, and cognitive flexibility	7–107	Intraclass correlation coefficients, test–retest reliability, concurrent validity [64]	Developed as digital

3.2. Ecological Validity of Traditional Tools Versus Digital Platform Assessments

The digital transformation of assessments necessitates an evaluation of their ecological validity and digital platforms. Figure 2 presents a conceptual map illustrating the positioning of functional cognitive assessments for children and adolescents along two key dimensions: ecological validity and digital platforms. The vertical axis reflects how well each tool simulates real-life tasks, ranging from low (lab-based tasks) to high (real-life or role-play scenarios mimicking daily functioning). The horizontal axis classifies tools by their digital platforms: non-digital (paper-based only), transferred to digital (originally analog, now also in digital format), or developed as native digital platforms. Assessments such as the WCPA, Do-Eat, and Birthday Task Assessment are in the top-left quadrant, indicating high ecological validity with no digital availability. Assessments like the CMT and Test of Everyday Attention for Children (TEA-Ch) are in the moderate-middle quadrant, suggesting partial contextual relevance and availability in transferred digital formats. Only the ACE-X is in the top-right quadrant, representing both high ecological validity and a native digital format. Conversely, lab-based tools, such as the Tower of London, WCST, and CANTAB, occupy the lower cells, reflecting lower contextual relevance despite varying digital availability.

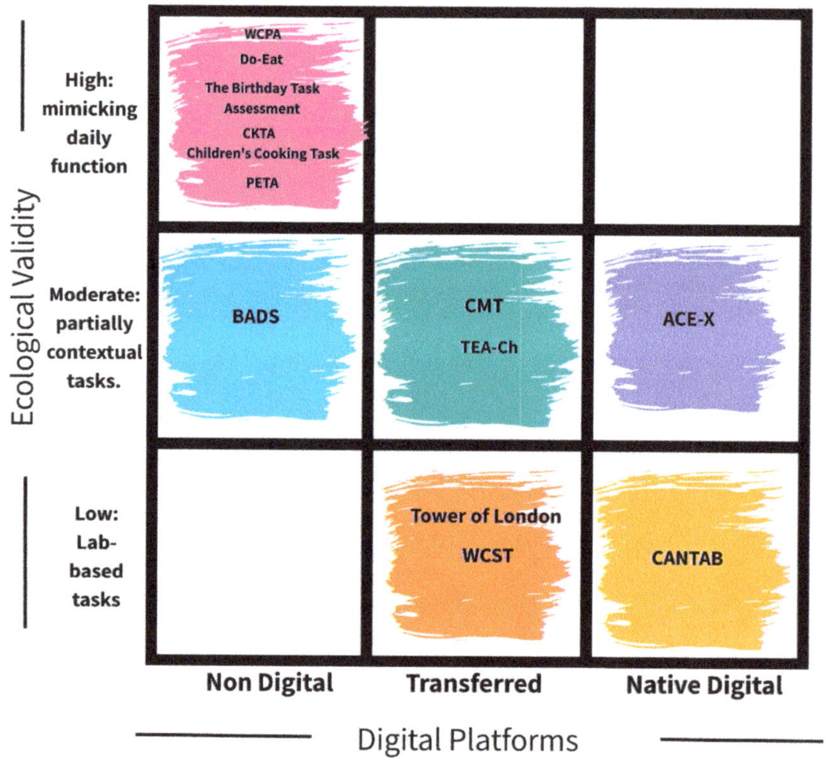

Figure 2. Conceptual map of functional cognitive assessments.

3.3. Scoring Metrics Across Cognitive Domains

We conducted a classification process based on content analysis of the assessment characteristics to better understand the distribution of scoring metrics used across assessment tools for functional cognition in children and youth. We reviewed and categorized each assessment according to the type of cognitive functions it evaluated, with specific attention to whether performance-based scoring metrics were used to quantify ability. Guided by widely accepted theoretical frameworks in neuropsychology and rehabilitation sciences, we identified eight core cognitive domains for grouping the assessments. These domains reflect the primary constructions evaluated by most tools in the reviewed table and are consistent with contemporary EF and cognitive performance models.

3.3.1. Rationale for the Eight-Domain Classification

The eight-domain classification was designed to reflect the multifaceted nature of functional cognition, recognizing that successful performance of daily activities requires coordinated use of multiple cognitive abilities. By grouping assessment tools according to their primary focus, such as EFs, attention, memory, or sequencing and organization, this framework clarifies which abilities an assessment directly measures and which measures only infers indirectly through performance patterns, strategy use, or errors.

3.3.2. The Seven Domains

- Executive functions: This broad category encompasses planning, inhibition, self-monitoring, cognitive flexibility, and strategy use. Most instruments reviewed assessed at least one executive component, justifying the domain's centrality.
- Attention: Sustained, selective, and divided attention were clustered as a distinct domain, given that several assessments exclusively targeted attentional capacity independent of broader executive processes.
- Processing speed: Assessments measuring reaction time, information processing efficiency, and cognitive fluency were grouped under this domain.
- Problem-solving and planning: This domain included assessments that required multistep reasoning, hypothesis generation, and goal-directed behavior (e.g., Tower of London, WCPA).
- Sequencing and organization: Specific to everyday tasks requiring ordered steps and spatial-temporal organization, this domain emerged from assessments such as the Do-Eat and cooking tasks.
- Memory: This domain encompasses immediate recall and the ability to hold and manipulate information during task performance. It included encoding, storage, and information retrieval processes essential for everyday functioning. Assessment tools that capture this domain include the CMT, ACE-X, and selected CANTAB subtests.
- Emotional/social cognition: Although assessed less frequently than the other domains, we retained this domain to reflect assessments that include affect recognition and social reasoning, particularly in computerized batteries like the CANTAB.

We mapped each assessment tool to one or more identified domains, depending on the tool's primary constructs and subtests. Assessments appearing in multiple domains were counted in each relevant category. To quantify the frequency of scoring metrics used across domains, we calculated the number of distinct assessments that utilized scoring metrics within each domain. A bar chart was then constructed (Figure 3) to represent this distribution visually. Each bar in the chart corresponds to a cognitive domain; the bar length indicates the number of assessments using scoring metrics in this domain. The names of the assessment tools contributing to each domain are displayed alongside the bars for clarity and transparency.

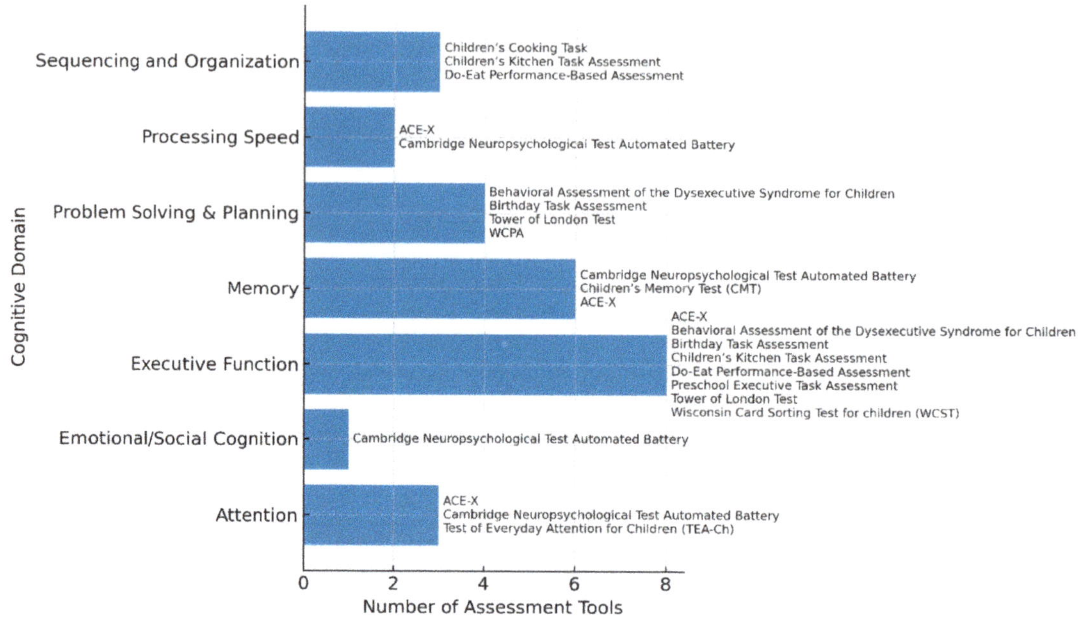

Figure 3. Frequency of assessment tools using scoring metrics across eight cognitive domains.

4. Discussion

This conceptual review aimed to evaluate the transformation of traditional functional cognitive assessments into digital platforms. The data extraction yielded three primary units of analysis: digital transformation trends, ecological validity and digital availability, and scoring metrics across cognitive domains.

4.1. Digital Transformation Trends

This study examined 13 functional cognition assessments in the context of daily life. These assessments, designed for children and adolescents with various conditions (e.g., neurodevelopmental disorders), cover a wide age range. They have been standardized and validated for reliability and validity. Interestingly, very few are digitally available, and many were not originally developed for digital formats. This lower digital availability likely reflects the difficulty of capturing daily settings digitally and its inadequacy for evaluating certain cognitive abilities. Assessments such as the CCT [32] and the Do-Eat [49] assess cognitive performance in complex daily activities using daily scenarios, a feature that is difficult to replicate on a digital platform. Likewise, the WCPA [31,37] relies on direct observation of performance and strategy use, two crucial elements that could be compromised if the assessment were digitized.

Specifically, *cognitive strategies*—mental action plans individuals use to approach challenging tasks systematically—are considered integral to typical learning and performance. These strategies can often be observed during or immediately after the execution of a task and are crucial for children and adolescents to acquire motor skills and achieve occupational performance [65,66]. Their need for a therapist's direct observation makes transforming these traditional assessments into digital platforms particularly challenging.

Conversely, technological platforms offer inherent advantages, such as enhanced data precision and efficiency. They can capture fine-grained performance metrics (e.g., reaction times, eye-tracking) by recording micro-level behavioral data [67]. Furthermore, digital platforms can reduce therapist workload and enable large-scale data collection. As Condy et al. [68] demonstrated, tablet-based assessments allow efficient testing with reduced therapist involvement.

However, according to previous studies, therapists may not be comfortable moving away from traditional methods due to concerns about accuracy and personal interaction [69,70]. Considering the potential of technological platforms, assessments that are indeed digitally available could be incorporated into clinical practice.

4.2. Ecological Validity and Digital Availability

Positioning the assessments along two axes—one examining ecological validity, and the other digital examining availability—allows analysis of their practical utility. Our analysis revealed a key challenge: Assessments that effectively represent real-world daily performance through engaging, ecological scenarios are often the most difficult to replicate in a digital environment without compromising validity.

Our findings illustrate this digital trend, showing that assessments with high ecological validity (e.g., WCPA, Do-Eat, Birthday Task) tend to lack digital availability. The ACE-X was an exception, demonstrating ecological validity and native digital format. Other assessments, including the CMT and TEA-Ch, fell in the middle; they showed partial contextual relevance and availability in transferred digital formats. The Tower of London, WCST, and CANTAB had lower contextual relevance despite their varying degrees of digital availability.

Innovative technological advancements, particularly in VR, have opened new avenues for enhancing the ecological validity of cognitive assessments [71]. Current VR environments show promise for improving ecological validity because they offer more realistic evaluations of daily cognitive abilities. The VR-based tasks have demonstrated correlations with traditional EF tests but better reflect everyday behavioral functioning [15]. Therefore, incorporating more advanced technology into such assessments may increase the ability to transform them into digital platforms.

4.3. Scoring Metrics Across Cognitive Domains

The scoring metrics classification process resulted in seven core cognitive domains: EFs, attention, processing speed, problem-solving and planning, sequencing and organization, memory, and emotional/social cognition. These classifications clarify the specific cognitive constructs each assessment addresses. They also highlight which abilities are directly observable during task performance and which are inferred indirectly from performance patterns, strategy use, or errors.

Recognizing the variability across these domains underscores the multifaceted nature of functional cognition and the diverse skill set children and adolescents need to navigate daily life successfully [5,72]. Within the context of this review, the eight-domain framework serves as a comparative tool for mapping assessments, identifying coverage gaps, and guiding the selection or development of tools—particularly in the transition from traditional to digital platforms—to ground clinical and research decisions in a comprehensive understanding of cognitive demands.

4.4. Limitations and Future Directions

There are several limitations to this study. First, the review identified only 13 studies. Although this small number likely reflects the general scarcity of digitally available ecological assessments, future research could include, for instance, gray literature, such as doctoral dissertations and conference proceedings, which may report on emerging digital tools before they appear in peer-reviewed publications. Second, the complex definition of *functional cognition* complicates the application of inclusion criteria. Because the term is relatively new [3,4,73], we included many studies based on our interpretation that they measured functional cognition—even if they did not explicitly use the term. It would be useful if future studies developed criteria for measuring functional cognition. Finally, future studies should establish the validity and reliability of these digital tools by examining their measurement invariance, usability, and social validity with children and caregivers in naturalistic settings, which could contribute to the future development of digital functional cognitive assessments.

5. Conclusions

Although research has explored the digitalization of traditional assessments, the specific transformation of performance-based functional cognition assessments into digital tools remains a gap in the literature. Transforming functional cognitive assessments into digital formats represents a significant opportunity to enhance their accessibility, accuracy, and inclusivity [74,75]. However, to justify investment in their development and implementation, technology-based tools should not only replicate but also enhance traditional assessment features [28].

The conceptual model developed in this review is grounded in three core evaluative dimensions: technological availability, ecological validity, and scoring metrics across cognitive domains. By integrating these dimensions, our model offers a structured framework for mapping and comparing functional cognitive assessments for children and adolescents. Positioning tools along the axes of ecological validity and digital availability and overlaying their distribution of scoring metrics allows clearer differentiation between assessments that may appear similar in purpose but diverge in their capacity to capture real-world cognitive performance or to leverage technological platforms.

This perspective facilitates identifying gaps, such as the absence of highly ecologically valid tools in native digital formats. It provides a basis for examining how well existing assessments align with contemporary clinical, educational, and technological demands.

Building on this framework, the model sharpens our ability to distinguish between specific assessments, highlighting their relative strengths, limitations, and potential for digital transformation. The findings derived from this framework have direct implications for practice and future development. For therapists, this model can guide the selection of the most appropriate assessments. For technology developers, it can inform the incorporation of more advanced tools capable of capturing nuanced behavioral observations in realistic daily contexts. For certain tools, such as the WCPA, it may be possible to incorporate digital features through a data-logging platform that records responses on a touchscreen or captures user actions via video, thereby supporting more efficient scoring and reducing the cognitive load of the examiner.

Finally, for researchers, the model encourages the continued exploration of traditional assessments' ecological validity while recognizing the unique research advantages of computerized tools, particularly VR-based platforms that automatically record process-oriented data. Such tools save valuable interaction time with participants while providing detailed step-by-step insights into functional cognition and its underlying cognitive components, most notably EFs, thereby enhancing the efficiency and depth of cognitive evaluation.

Supplementary Materials: The following supporting information can be downloaded at: https://www.mdpi.com/article/10.3390/children12101384/s1, TITAN Guideline Checklist. Reference [76] is cited in Supplementary Materials.

Author Contributions: Conceptualization, N.J., Y.F., O.C.E. and S.Z.; methodology, N.J., Y.F., O.C.E. and S.Z.; software, N.J., Y.F., O.C.E. and S.Z.; validation, N.J., Y.F., O.C.E. and S.Z.; formal analysis, N.J., Y.F., O.C.E. and S.Z.; investigation, N.J., Y.F., O.C.E. and S.Z.; resources, N.J., Y.F., O.C.E. and

S.Z.; data curation, N.J., Y.F., O.C.E. and S.Z.; writing—original draft preparation, N.J., Y.F., O.C.E. and S.Z.; writing—review and editing, N.J., Y.F., O.C.E. and S.Z.; visualization, N.J., Y.F., O.C.E. and S.Z.; supervision, N.J., Y.F., O.C.E. and S.Z.; project administration, N.J., Y.F., O.C.E. and S.Z.; funding acquisition, N.J., Y.F., O.C.E. and S.Z. All authors have read and agreed to the published version of the manuscript.

Funding: This research received no external funding.

Institutional Review Board Statement: Not applicable.

Informed Consent Statement: Not applicable.

Data Availability Statement: The original contributions presented in this study are included in the article/Supplementary Materials. Further inquiries can be directed to the corresponding author.

Conflicts of Interest: The authors declare no conflicts of interest.

Abbreviations

The following abbreviations are used in this manuscript:

ADL	Activity of daily living
ACE-X	Adaptive Cognitive Evaluation Explorer
BADS	Behavioral Assessment of the Dysexecutive Syndrome
CANTAB	Cambridge Neuropsychological Test Automated Battery
CCT	Children's Cooking Task
CMT	Children's Memory Test
EFs	Executive functions
TEA-Ch	Test of Everyday Attention for Children
VR	Virtual reality
WCPA	Weekly Calendar Planning Activity
WCST	Wisconsin Card Sorting Test

References

1. Wesson, J.; Clemson, L.; Brodaty, H.; Reppermund, S. Estimating functional cognition in older adults using observational assessments of task performance in complex everyday activities: A systematic review and evaluation of measurement properties. *Neurosci. Biobehav. Rev.* **2016**, *68*, 335–360. [CrossRef] [PubMed]
2. Edemekong, P.F.; Bomgaars, D.; Sukumaran, S.; Levy, S.B. *Activities of Daily Living*; StatPearls Publishing: Treasure Island, FL, USA, 2019.
3. Lee, Y.; Randolph, S.B.; Kim, M.Y.; Foster, E.R.; Kersey, J.; Baum, C.; Connor, L.T. Performance-based assessments of functional cognition in adults, part 1—Assessment characteristics: A systematic review. *Am. J. Occup. Ther.* **2025**, *79*, 7904205130. [CrossRef] [PubMed]
4. Lee, Y.; Randolph, S.B.; Kim, M.Y.; Foster, E.R.; Kersey, J.; Baum, C.; Connor, L.T. Performance-based assessments of functional cognition in adults, part 2—Psychometric properties: A systematic review. *Am. J. Occup. Ther.* **2025**, *79*, 7904205140. [CrossRef] [PubMed]
5. Giles, G.M.; Edwards, D.F.; Morrison, M.T.; Baum, C.; Wolf, T.J. Screening for functional cognition in postacute care and the Improving Medicare Post-Acute Care Transformation (IMPACT) Act of 2014. *Am. J. Occup. Ther.* **2017**, *71*, 7105090010p1–7105090010p6. [CrossRef]
6. Wolf, T.J.; Edwards, D.F.; Giles, G.M. *Functional Cognition and Occupational Therapy: A Practical Approach to Treating Individuals with Cognitive Loss*; AOTA Press: Bethesda, MD, USA, 2019.
7. Edwards, D.F.; Wolf, T.J.; Marks, T.; Alter, S.; Larkin, V.; Padesky, B.L.; Spiers, M.; Al-Heizan, M.O.; Giles, G.M. Functional cognition: Conceptual foundations for intervention in occupational therapy. *Am. J. Occup. Ther.* **2019**, *73*, 7303205010p1–7303205010p18.
8. American Occupational Therapy Association. Occupational therapy practice framework: Domain and process, 3rd ed. *Am. J. Occup. Ther.* **2014**, *68*, S1–S48. [CrossRef]
9. American Occupational Therapy Association. Occupational therapy practice framework: Domain and process, 4th ed. *Am. J. Occup. Ther.* **2020**, *74*, 7412410010p1–7412410010p87. [CrossRef]

10. Toglia, J.; Foster, E. *The Multicontext Approach: A Metacognitive Strategy-Based Intervention for Functional Cognition*; MC CogRehab Resources: Hastings on Hudson, NY, USA, 2021.
11. Cermak, S.A.; Toglia, J. Cognitive development across the life-span: Development of cognition and executive functioning in children and adolescents. In *Cognition, Occupation, and Participation Across the Lifespan: Neuroscience, Neurorehabilitation, and Models of Intervention in Occupational Therapy*, 4th ed.; Katz, N., Toglia, J., Eds.; AOTA Press: Bethesda, MD, USA, 2018; pp. 9–27.
12. Wallisch, A.; Little, L.M.; Dean, E.; Dunn, W. Executive function measures for children: A scoping review of ecological validity. *OTJR* **2017**, *38*, 6–14. [CrossRef]
13. Gomez, I.N.B.; Palomo, S.A.M.; Vicuña, A.M.U.; Bustamante, J.A.D.; Eborde, J.M.E.; Regala, K.A.; Ruiz, G.M.M.; Sanchez, A.L.G. Performance-based executive function instruments used by occupational therapists for children: A systematic review of measurement properties. *Occup. Ther. Int.* **2021**, *2021*, 6008442. [CrossRef]
14. Giles, G.M.; Edwards, D.F.; Baum, C.; Furniss, J.; Skidmore, E.; Wolf, T.; Leland, N.E. Making functional cognition a professional priority. *Am. J. Occup. Ther.* **2020**, *74*, 7401090010p1–7401090010p6. [CrossRef]
15. Lalonde, G.; Henry, M.; Drouin-Germain, A.; Nolin, P.; Beauchamp, M.H. Assessment of executive function in adolescence: A comparison of traditional and virtual reality tools. *J. Neurosci. Methods* **2013**, *219*, 76–82. [CrossRef]
16. Gioia, G.A.; Isquith, P.K.; Guy, S.C.; Kenworthy, L. *Behavior Rating Inventory of Executive Function*; Psychological Assessment Resources: Lake Magdalene, FL, USA, 2000.
17. Delis, D.C.; Kaplan, E.; Kramer, J.H. *Delis–Kaplan Executive Function System Examiner's Manual*; Psychological: New York, NY, USA, 2001.
18. Josman, N.; Rosenblum, S. A metacognitive model for children with atypical brain development. In *Cognition, Occupation, and Participation Across the Life Span: Neuroscience, Neurorehabilitation and Models for Intervention in Occupational Therapy*; Katz, N., Ed.; AOTA Press: Bethesda, MD, USA, 2018; pp. 223–248.
19. Hartman-Maeir, A.; Katz, N.; Baum, C.M. Cognitive functional evaluation (CFE) process for individuals with suspected cognitive disabilities. *Occup. Ther. Health Care* **2009**, *23*, 1–23. [CrossRef]
20. Bar-Haim Erez, A.; Katz, N. Cognitive functional evaluation. In *Cognition, Occupation and Participation Across the Lifespan: Neuroscience, Neurorehabilitation and Models of Intervention in Occupational Therapy*, 4th ed.; Katz, N., Toglia, J., Eds.; AOTA Press: Bethesda, MD, USA, 2018; pp. 69–85.
21. Paganin, G.; Simbula, S. New technologies in the workplace: Can personal and organizational variables affect the employees' intention to use a work-stress management app? *Int. J. Env. Res. Public. Health* **2021**, *18*, 9366. [CrossRef]
22. Asensio, D.; Duñabeitia, J.A. The necessary, albeit belated, transition to computerized cognitive assessment. *Front. Psychol.* **2023**, *14*, 1160554. [CrossRef]
23. Parsons, S. Learning to work together: Designing a multi-user virtual reality game for social collaboration and perspective-taking for children with autism. *Int. J. Child. Comput. Interact.* **2015**, *6*, 28–38. [CrossRef]
24. Cook, D.J.; Schmitter-Edgecombe, M.; Jönsson, L.; Morant, A.V. Technology-enabled assessment of functional health. *IEEE Rev. Biomed. Eng.* **2018**, *12*, 319–332. [CrossRef] [PubMed]
25. Ruffini, C.; Tarchi, C.; Morini, M.; Giuliano, G.; Pecini, C. Tele-assessment of cognitive functions in children: A systematic review. *Child. Neuropsychol.* **2022**, *28*, 709–745. [CrossRef] [PubMed]
26. Zeghari, R.; Guerchouche, R.; Tran Duc, M.; Bremond, F.; Lemoine, M.P.; Bultingaire, V.; Langel, K.; De Groote, Z.; Kuhn, F.; Martin, E.; et al. Pilot study to assess the feasibility of a mobile unit for remote cognitive screening of isolated elderly in rural areas. *Int. J. Environ. Res. Public. Health* **2021**, *18*, 6108. [CrossRef]
27. Dawson, D.R.; Marcotte, T.D. Special issue on ecological validity and cognitive assessment. *Neuropsychol. Rehabil.* **2017**, *27*, 599–602. [CrossRef]
28. Diamond, A.; Ling, D.S. Conclusions about interventions, programs, and approaches for improving executive functions that appear justified and those that, despite much hype, do not. *Dev. Cogn. Neurosci.* **2016**, *18*, 34–48. [CrossRef]
29. Guo, C.; Ashrafian, H.; Ghafur, S.; Fontana, G.; Gardner, C.; Prime, M. Challenges for the evaluation of digital health solutions: A call for innovative evidence generation approaches. *NPJ Digit. Med.* **2020**, *3*, 110. [CrossRef]
30. Jaakkola, E. Designing conceptual articles: Four approaches. *AMS Rev.* **2020**, *10*, 18–26. [CrossRef]
31. Toglia, J.; Berg, C. Performance-based measure of executive function: Comparison of community and at-risk youth. *Am. J. Occup. Ther.* **2013**, *67*, 515–523. [CrossRef]
32. Fogel, Y.; Rosenblum, S.; Hirsh, R.; Chevignard, M.; Josman, N. Daily performance of adolescents with executive function deficits: An empirical study using a complex-cooking task. *Occup. Ther. Int.* **2020**, *2020*, 3051809. [CrossRef]
33. Toglia, J. *Weekly Calendar Planning Activity*; AOTA Press: Bethesda, MD, USA, 2015.
34. Weiner, N.W.; Toglia, J.; Berg, C. Weekly Calendar Planning Activity (WCPA): A performance-based assessment of executive function piloted with at-risk adolescents. *Am. J. Occup. Ther.* **2012**, *66*, 699–708. [CrossRef]
35. Lahav, O.; Ben-Simon, A.; Inbar-Weiss, N.; Katz, N. Weekly Calendar Planning Activity for university students: Comparison of individuals with and without ADHD by gender. *J. Atten. Disord.* **2018**, *22*, 368–378. [CrossRef]

36. Zlotnik, S.; Schiff, A.; Ravid, S.; Shahar, E.; Toglia, J. A new approach for assessing executive functions in everyday life, among adolescents with genetic generalised epilepsies. *Neuropsychol. Rehabil.* **2020**, *30*, 333–345. [CrossRef]
37. Zlotnik, S.; Toglia, J. Measuring adolescent self-awareness and accuracy using a performance-based assessment and parental report. *Front. Public Health* **2018**, *6*, 15. [CrossRef]
38. Manly, T.; Robertson, I.H.; Anderson, V.; Nimmo-Smith, I. *The Test of Everyday Attention (TEA-CH)*; Thames Valley Test: Bury St. Edmunds, UK, 1999.
39. Manly, T.; Anderson, V.; Crawford, J.; George, M.; Underbjerg, M.; Robertson, I.H. *Test of Everyday Attention for Children–Second Edition [TEA-Ch2]*; Pearson: London, UK, 2017.
40. Manly, T.; Anderson, A.; Nimmo-Smith, I.; Turner, A.; Watson, P.; Robertson, I.H. The differential assessment of children's attention: Yhe Test of Everyday Attention for Children (TEA-Ch), normative sample, and ADHD performance. *J. Child. Psychol. Psychiatr.* **2001**, *42*, 1065–1081. [CrossRef]
41. Malegiannaki, A.-C.; Aretouli, E.; Metallidou, P.; Messinis, L.; Zafeiriou, D.; Kosmidis, M.H. Test of Everyday Attention for Children (TEA-Ch): Greek normative data and discriminative validity for children with combined type of attention-deficit/hyperactivity disorder. *Dev. Neuropsychol.* **2019**, *44*, 189–202. [CrossRef] [PubMed]
42. Fathi, N.; Mehraban, A.H.; Akbarfahimi, M.; Mirzaie, H. Validity and reliability of the test of everyday attention for children (TEACh) in Iranian 8-11 year old normal students. *Iran. J. Psychiatry Behav. Sci.* **2016**, *11*, e2854. [CrossRef]
43. Pardos, A.; Quintero, J.; Zuluaga, P.; Fernández, A. Descriptive analysis of the Test of Everyday Attention for children in a Spanish normative sample. *Actas Esp. Psiquiatr.* **2016**, *44*, 183–192. Available online: https://actaspsiquiatria.es/index.php/actas/article/view/1097 (accessed on 15 April 2025). [PubMed]
44. Emslie, H.; Wilson, F.C.; Burden, V.; Nimmo-Smith, I.; Wilson, B.A. *The Behavioural Assessment of the Dysexecutive Syndrome for Children (BADS-C)*; Thames Valley Test: Bury St. Edmunds, UK, 2003.
45. Baron, I.S. Behavioural Assessment of the Dysexecutive Syndrome for Children (BADS-C.) by Emslie, H., Wilson, FC, Burden, V., Nimmo-Smith, I., & Wilson, BA (2003). *Child. Neuropsychol.* **2007**, *13*, 539–542. [CrossRef]
46. Engel-Yeger, B.; Josman, N.; Rosenblum, S. Behavioural Assessment of the Dysexecutive Syndrome for Children (BADS-C): An examination of construct validity. *Neuropsychol. Rehabil.* **2009**, *19*, 662–676. [CrossRef]
47. Longaud-Valès, A.; Chevignard, M.; Dufour, C.; Grill, J.; Puget, S.; Sainte-Rose, C.; Valteau-Couanet, D.; Dellatolas, G. Assessment of executive functioning in children and young adults treated for frontal lobe tumours using ecologically valid tests. *Neuropsychol. Rehabili.* **2016**, *26*, 558–583. [CrossRef]
48. Chevignard, M.P.; Catroppa, C.; Galvin, J.; Anderson, V. Development and evaluation of an ecological task to assess executive functioning post childhood TBI: The Children's Cooking Task. *Brain Impair.* **2010**, *11*, 125–143. [CrossRef]
49. Josman, N.; Goffer, A.; Rosenblum, S. Development and standardization of a Do–Eat activity of daily living performance test for children. *Am. J. Occup. Ther.* **2010**, *64*, 47–58. [CrossRef]
50. Rosenblum, S.; Frisch, C.; Deutsh-Castel, T.; Josman, N. Daily functioning profile of children with attention deficit hyperactive disorder: A pilot study using an ecological assessment. *Neuropsychol. Rehabil.* **2015**, *25*, 402–418. [CrossRef]
51. Rocke, K.; Hays, P.; Edwards, D.; Berg, C. Development of a performance assessment of executive function: The Children's Kitchen Task Assessment. *Am. J. Occup. Ther.* **2008**, *62*, 528–537. [CrossRef]
52. Fogel, Y.; Cohen Elimelech, O.; Josman, N. Executive function in young children: Validation of the Preschool Executive Task Assessment. *Children* **2025**, *12*, 626. [CrossRef]
53. Downes, M.; Kirkham, F.J.; Berg, C.; Telfer, P.; de Haan, M. Executive performance on the preschool executive task assessment in children with sickle cell anemia and matched controls. *Child. Neuropsychol.* **2019**, *25*, 278–285. [CrossRef] [PubMed]
54. Downes, M.; Berg, C.; Kirkham, F.J.; Kischkel, L.; McMurray, I.; de Haan, M. Task utility and norms for the Preschool Executive Task Assessment (PETA). *Child. Neuropsychol.* **2018**, *24*, 784–798. [CrossRef] [PubMed]
55. Toglia, J.P. Contextual Memory Test. Multicontext. 2017. Available online: https://multicontext.net/contextual-memory-test (accessed on 10 April 2025).
56. Engel-Yeger, B.; Durr, D.H.; Josman, N. Comparison of memory and meta-memory abilities of children with cochlear implant and normal hearing peers. *Disabil. Rehabil.* **2011**, *33*, 770–777. [CrossRef] [PubMed]
57. Sharma, A. Cambridge neuropsychological test automated battery. In *Encyclopedia of Autism Spectrum Disorders*; Springer: New York, NY, USA, 2013; pp. 498–515.
58. Luciana, M.; Nelson, C.A. Assessment of neuropsychological function through use of the Cambridge Neuropsychological Testing Automated Battery: Performance in 4-to 12-year-old children. *Dev. Neuropsychol.* **2002**, *22*, 595–624. [CrossRef]
59. Luciana, M.; Lindeke, L.; Georgieff, M.; Mills, M.; Nelson, C.A. Neurobehavioral evidence for working-memory deficits in school-aged children with histories of prematurity. *Dev. Med. Child. Neurol.* **1999**, *41*, 521–533. [CrossRef]
60. Shallice, T. Specific impairments of planning. *Philos. Transcr. R. Soc. Lond.* **1982**, *298*, 199–209. [CrossRef]
61. Injoque-Ricle, I.; Burin, D.I. Validez y fiabilidad de la prueba de Torre de Londres para niños: Un estudio preliminar. *Rev. Argent. Neuropsicol.* **2008**, *11*, 21–31.

62. Heaton, R.K.; Staff, P.A.R. *Wisconsin Card Sorting Test: Computer Version 2*; Psychological Assessment Resources: Odessa, FL, USA, 1993.
63. Cook, L.G.; Chapman, S.B.; Levin, H.S. Self-regulation abilities in children with severe traumatic brain injury: A preliminary investigation of naturalistic action. *NeuroRehabil* **2008**, *23*, 467–475. [CrossRef]
64. Hsu, W.Y.; Rowles, W.; Anguera, J.A.; Anderson, A.; Younger, J.W.; Friedman, S.; Gazzaley, A.; Bove, R. Assessing cognitive function in multiple sclerosis with digital tools: Observational study. *J. Med. Internet Res.* **2021**, *23*, e25748. [CrossRef]
65. Toglia, J.P.; Rodger, S.A.; Polatajko, H.J. Anatomy of cognitive strategies: A therapist's primer for enabling occupational performance. *Can. J. Occup. Ther.* **2012**, *79*, 225–236. [CrossRef]
66. Toglia, J.P. *The Multicontext Approach to Cognitive Rehabilitation: A Metacognitive Strategy Intervention to Optimize Functional Cognition*; Gatekeeper Press: Citrus Park, FL, USA, 2021.
67. Germine, L.; Reinecke, K.; Chaytor, N.S. Digital neuropsychology: Challenges and opportunities at the intersection of science and software. *Clin. Neuropsychol.* **2019**, *33*, 271–286. [CrossRef]
68. Condy, E.; Kaat, A.J.; Becker, L.; Sullivan, N.; Soorya, L.; Berger, N.; Berry-Kravis, E.; Michalak, C.; Thurm, A. A novel measure of matching categories for early development: Item creation and pilot feasibility study. *Res. Dev. Disabil.* **2021**, *115*, 103993. [CrossRef]
69. Van Patten, R. Introduction to the Special Issue—Neuropsychology from a distance: Psychometric properties and clinical utility of remote neurocognitive tests. *J. Clin. Exper Neuropsychol.* **2021**, *43*, 767–773. [CrossRef]
70. Lavigne, K.M.; Sauvé, G.; Raucher-Chéné, D.; Guimond, S.; Lecomte, T.; Bowie, C.R.; Menon, M.; Lal, S.; Woodward, T.S.; Bodnar, M.D.; et al. Remote cognitive assessment in severe mental illness: A scoping review. *Schizophrenia* **2022**, *8*, 14. [CrossRef]
71. Parsons, T.D. Virtual reality for enhanced ecological validity and experimental control in the clinical, affective and social neurosciences. *Front. Hum. Neurosci.* **2015**, *9*, 660. [CrossRef] [PubMed]
72. Dumas, C.M.; Grajo, L. Functional cognition in critically ill children: Asserting the role of occupational therapy. *Open J. Occup. Ther.* **2021**, *9*, 1–9. [CrossRef]
73. Edwards, D.; Giles, G. Special issue on functional cognition. *OTJR* **2022**, *42*, 251–252. [CrossRef] [PubMed]
74. Harris, C.; Tang, Y.; Birnbaum, E.; Cherian, C.; Mendhe, D.; Chen, M.H. Digital neuropsychology beyond computerized cognitive assessment: Applications of novel digital technologies. *Arch. Clin. Neuropsychol.* **2024**, *39*, 290–304. [CrossRef]
75. Walker, E.J.; Kirkham, F.J.; Stotesbury, H.; Dimitriou, D.; Hood, A.M. Tele-neuropsychological assessment of children and young people: A systematic review. *J. Pediatr. Neuropsychol.* **2023**, *9*, 113–126. [CrossRef]
76. Agha, R.A.; Mathew, G.; Rashid, R.; Kerwan, A.; Al-Jabir, A.; Sohrabi, C.; Franchi, T.; Nicola, M.; Agha, M.; The TITAN Group. Transparency in the Reporting of Artificial Intelligence—The TITAN Guideline. *Prem. J. Sci.* **2025**, *10*, 100082. [CrossRef]

children

MDPI

Article

Independence in Activities of Daily Living Among Autistic Toddlers: A Pilot Study Using Ecological Momentary Assessment

Shani Hillel [1,2,*], Ben Aaronson [1,3] and Yafit Gilboa [1]

[1] School of Occupational Therapy, Faculty of Medicine, The Hebrew University of Jerusalem, Jerusalem 9124001, Israel; ba1@uw.edu (B.A.); yafit.gilboa@mail.huji.ac.il (Y.G.)
[2] Department of Occupational Therapy, Faculty of Social Welfare and Health Sciences, University of Haifa, Haifa 3498838, Israel
[3] Department of Pediatrics, School of Medicine, University of Washington, Seattle, WA 98105, USA
* Correspondence: shanidov9876@gmail.com

Abstract: Background: The acquisition of adaptive skills is critical for independence and participation in activities of daily living (ADL). While caregiver perceptions provide valuable insights, most studies on autistic participation have focused on older children and relied on one-time clinic-based assessments. As a result, little is known about how autistic toddlers function in their natural environments across time. Ecological momentary assessment (EMA) is a real-time, context-sensitive method in which parents can report behaviors at multiple time points in the child's natural environment. This pilot study aimed to examine ADL independence in autistic toddlers compared to their typically developing (TD) peers, to assess the feasibility of using EMA in early childhood, and to compare EMA-based assessments with a one-time standardized report. **Methods:** 23 autistic toddlers and 28 TD toddlers (aged 18–40 months) participated in the study. Parents completed a one-time report on the self-care scales of the Pediatric Evaluation of Disability Inventory (PEDI) and the Functional Independence Measure for Children (WeeFIM) and then rated their child's independence on the WeeFIM twice a day for two weeks via their smartphones. **Results:** EMA was feasible with high response rates (ASD: 91.1%, TD: 88.55%). Autistic toddlers showed different participation profiles, with less independent performance in ADL compared to TD peers. In the autism group, the average EMA scores ($M = 16.53$, $SD = 6.58$) were significantly higher than the one-time WeeFIM scores ($M = 13.74$, $SD = 5.23$), $t\,(22) = 3.23$, $p < 0.01$, suggesting underreporting in single-time assessments. In contrast, no such difference was found in the TD group. Significant positive correlations were found between the EMA mean and the one-time WeeFIM scores in both groups ($r > 0.80$), indicating convergent validity. In the autism group only, greater variability in EMA was moderately associated with higher functional independence ($r = 0.46$, $p < 0.01$). **Conclusions:** These findings indicate that autistic toddlers demonstrated higher levels of participation in their natural environment than reflected by the one-time assessment, emphasizing the limitations of single-time-point evaluations. This underscores the importance of collecting data across multiple time points to accurately assess adaptive functioning and ADL participation. The EMA technique demonstrated in this study provides exploratory evidence of feasibility as an ecologically valid approach to assessing functional independence in autistic toddlers, offering a richer and more context-sensitive alternative to traditional one-time clinical assessments.

 https://doi.org/10.3390/children12101316

Keywords: autism; toddlers; participation; independence; activities of daily living; ecological momentary assessment; parent report

1. Introduction

Autism spectrum disorder (ASD) is a lifelong neurodevelopmental condition, characterized by differences in social communication and social interaction across multiple contexts; along with repetitive patterns of behavior, interests, or activities; and distinctive sensory processing [1]. These characteristics are increasingly discussed within a neurodiversity perspective, which emphasizes variability, strengths, and support needs, rather than focusing solely on difficulties [2]. Prevalence has been increasing worldwide [3–5]; in the United States, the most recent ADDM surveillance (2022) estimated that about 3.2% (one in 31) of 8-year-old children were identified with ASD in 2022 [6]. Autism is diagnosed more frequently in males than in females, with a male-to-female ratio of 3.4 among 8-year-olds in the U.S. [6], and a median ratio of 4.2 reported in a recent global systematic review [7]. ASD characteristics typically emerge in early childhood, with the earliest observable features appearing at 12–18 months of age [8,9]. Most autistic children can be diagnosed by 18–24 months [3,10].

According to the International Classification of Functioning, Disability and Health (ICF), participation is defined as the individual's involvement in everyday activities and routines, and is considered a key component of health and functioning [11]. Participation affects children's behavioral and emotional well-being, social relationships, and overall mental and physical health [12]. Through participation, children develop essential skills, form interpersonal relationships, achieve self-satisfaction, and gain a sense of self-worth [13]. These processes are especially critical during early childhood, a period when foundations for daily occupations such as activities of daily living (ADL) are established [14].

During the toddler years, children are expected to refine adaptive skills, including self-care tasks, and develop independence in activities such as feeding, dressing, and toileting [15]. These years are pivotal for acquiring foundational skills that support future productivity and well-being [10]. ADL in early childhood includes basic self-care activities such as self-feeding, bathing, dressing, personal hygiene, and grooming [16]. Mastery of these skills is supported by concurrent development of fine motor, gross motor, cognitive, and social-emotional abilities [17]. However, due to the unique characteristics of autism, many autistic children and their caregivers factors that may constrain participation opportunities, which can influence both the number and diversity of activities in which they engage [18,19]. Previous studies have shown that nearly 50% of young autistic children are unable to perform self-care activities independently [20], and consistently demonstrate different adaptive skill profiles, characterized by less independent performance in daily living skills relative to their TD peers [21]. These early differences in adaptive skills underscore the need for targeted early intervention to promote independence.

In addition to these challenges, differences in functional activities and adaptive functioning in autistic toddlers can serve as early markers for later developmental outcomes [22]. These differences emphasize the importance of early assessment to monitor development and guide future support and intervention planning. Knowledge of the determinants of self-care participation assists with decisions about how to intervene to support optimal independence [23].

Asking for a caregiver's perceptions of their child's ADL participation and competence can provide valuable information about the child's functioning [24]. However, most previous studies have focused on older children and relied on one-time assessments conducted in clinical settings [20,21]. Thus, little is known about the participation of autistic toddlers in their natural environments over time.

EMA is an intensive longitudinal sampling approach in which parents can report behaviors and contexts at multiple time points, as they occur in their natural environment [25,26]. While EMA methods vary in design, they all share three common characteristics [27]: (1) sampling a behavior or phenomenon over multiple occurrences; (2) observing subjects in their natural environments, increasing the ecological validity of the assessment; and (3) aiming to minimize recall bias by reporting a targeted phenomenon as close to the event as possible. Traditional standardized tools such as the PEDI [28] and WeeFIM [29] are typically administered as one-time reports. However, such parent-report measures may be influenced by parental stress, as parents of children with developmental delays are at heightened risk for chronic stress that can impair memory and comprehension [30], as well as by recall bias and context-specific factors [31]. In contrast, EMA captures multiple instances of behavior across natural settings, providing richer and potentially more valid insights into functional independence, although it does not fully eliminate recall bias [31]. Given the unique aspects of EMA, it has the potential to help bridge knowledge gaps in autism research by capturing real-time experiences that might be missed in traditional assessments [32].

EMA has been employed with the autistic population to report specific areas such as negative emotions and depression [27], social experiences [33,34] and coping [35] as well as to assess leisure participation [36]. However, these studies have focused on adolescent and adult populations. While EMA has been used in these studies to explore emotional and social concerns in autistic individuals, to our knowledge, no EMA study has focused specifically on ADL participation patterns among autistic toddlers.

The main goal of this study was therefore to track the ADL independence profiles of autistic toddlers, and compare them to TD toddlers, using EMA. Our specific aims were to: (a) assess the feasibility of EMA for collecting information regarding ADL among toddlers focusing on a twice-daily measure; (b) describe and compare the independence of the two groups in a variety of ADL; (c) compare the EMA results with standardized one-time assessments to examine their convergent validity; and (d) examine the associations between the standard one-time reports and EMA, in terms of mean and variance.

We hypothesized that: (a) EMA would prove a feasible method for collecting information about ADL participation among the two groups; (b) compared to their TD peers, autistic toddlers would show different participation profiles with less independent involvement exhibit less independent participation in the variety of ADL self-care functions; (c) EMA results would demonstrate convergent validity when compared with standardized one-time measurements; and (d) As an exploratory hypothesis, we examined whether positive correlations would be found between the EMA mean and variability and the one-time report measure.

2. Materials and Methods

2.1. Participants

The study included a sample of 51 toddlers aged 18–40 months: 23 autistic toddlers and 28 TD toddlers. The sample size was calculated based on a study by Provost et al. [37]. The sample size needed was calculated using G*power version 3.1 and based on a medium-to-large effect size (d = 0.7), a power of 0.8, and α = 0.05., with an allocation ratio of 1:1. The necessary sample size was therefore 52 participants (26 for each group). Using a convenience sampling method, the autistic toddlers were recruited from rehabilitation daycare centers in central Israel, via parent networks and professional contacts, supplemented by a snowball sampling method through media resources. The TD toddlers were recruited through acquaintances and media resources, using snowball sampling. The inclusion criterion for both groups was adequate parental understanding of the Hebrew language.

For the autism group, parents reported that their child had received a clinical diagnosis of autism by either a neurodevelopmental pediatrician, a pediatric neurologist, a child-adolescent psychiatrist, or a psychologist, according to the American Psychiatric Association DSM-5 classification [1], reported by parents. Exclusion criteria were children diagnosed with a developmental disorder other than autism; and/or interfering factors such as significant visual, hearing, or motor deficits. No standardized IQ assessments were administered.

Exclusion criteria for the TD group were any parental concerns in developmental areas of cognitive speech, motor skills, or behavior, according to the child's parental report. The sample was described by age, gender, number of siblings, parental years of education, and housing density (persons per room) as an indicator of socioeconomic status. These demographic variables were collected to characterize the sample and control for potential confounders in statistical analyses.

2.2. *Measures*

2.2.1. Demographic Questionnaire

An online demographic questionnaire specifically developed for this study included 15 questions to collect personal and socioeconomic information. The questionnaire covered the child's age at assessment (in months), gender, and number of siblings. Additionally, it collected parental education level and a measure of socioeconomic status, such as housing density (persons per room). Completion time was approximately 5–10 min.

2.2.2. Pediatric Evaluation of the Disability Inventory (PEDI; [28])

PEDI is a functional assessment instrument designed for evaluating function in children with various disabilities aged 6 months to 7.5 years. It is a judgment-based parent-structured interview used by professionals [38]. When completed by a professional, the administrator should have a background in pediatrics, experience with children with disabilities, and strong training in child development [28]. PEDI measures are both functional performance and capability in three domains: (a) self-care, (b) mobility, and (c) social functioning. The functional skills scale consists of 197 items, each scored 'unable' (0) or 'capable' (1). Administration of the full PEDI (197 items across three domains) typically requires 45–60 min. The final score is the summation of the scoring on all items and can be computed in every domain. In the current study, the Researcher used the self-care domain (73 items) only, which covers eating, grooming, dressing, and personal hygiene, ranging from 0 to 73 [28]. The researcher, a trained occupational therapist, administered the tool in Hebrew, a version that has been previously used [39]. In the present study, completion of the self-care domain typically required 15–20 min. The PEDI has high internal consistency has been found for each of the scales, with Cronbach's alpha coefficients ranging from 0.95 to 0.99 [28]. PEDI has been suggested as a gold standard measure [19].

2.2.3. Functional Independence Measure for Children (WeeFIM; [29])

WeeFIM is a pediatric functional independence measure developed for children aged 6 months to 7 years with physical and/or mental disabilities. It is administered in a semi-structured interview of around 15 min. The self-care domain used in our study includes eating, grooming, bathing, dressing, and toileting, with each task rated from 1 (requiring total assistance) to 7 (complete independence). The final score sums up all 18 items, ranging from 18 to 126 points. The final score in each category can be referenced to normal scores by age group. The WeeFIM has been widely studied and was found to have strong reliability and validity: internal consistency (Cronbach's α) is 0.90, interrater-interclass correlation is 0.73–0.94, and test–retest interclass correlation is 0.97 [40].

2.2.4. Ecological Momentary Assessment (EMA)

EMA data reported by the toddlers' parents provided ecological information about the degree of the child's dependency in ADL participation. Data was collected through a Qualtrics link sent to the parents' smartphones twice daily- after the morning routine (8:00 AM) and after the evening routine (8:00 PM), over 10 consecutive weekdays (Sunday–Thursday for two weeks). The EMA form, developed for the study population, comprised all six items of the WeeFIM self-care domain (eating, grooming, bathing, dressing upper body, dressing lower body, and toileting), plus an additional item assessing sleeping/waking as an exploratory item to capture broader daily routines. The introductory instruction read: "Kindly assess the level of independent participation of your child during the current morning/evening in the specified activities" Each item was rated on an 8-point scale: 1 = total assistance; 7 = complete independence; 8 = not relevant. "Not relevant" responses were coded as missing values and excluded from analyses. The meaning of each rating point was explained to parents during the initial session to ensure consistent interpretation. Completion time was approximately 1–3 min.

Two EMA-derived variables were calculated for each participant: (1) mean EMA score, representing the child's average independence level across all days and activities; and (2) standard deviation of EMA scores, representing variability in independence across contexts and times. Variability was examined to explore whether children whose independence fluctuated more between contexts differed in their one-time assessment scores compared to those with more consistent performance. Final EMA scores were calculated as the average of all items across all responses, and standard deviations were calculated to reflect variability in participation.

2.3. Procedure

Approval for the study was obtained from the Ethics Committee for Non-Medical Human Studies in the Faculty of Medicine, The Hebrew University of Jerusalem. Participants provided online informed consent prior to participation. Data collection took approximately 6 months. All interactions with participants were conducted by an occupational therapist. Participants completed an online demographic questionnaire and thereafter, the researcher scheduled a Zoom video meeting with each participant. In this meeting, parents received an explanation of the scales and completed the self-care domains of both the PEDI and the WeeFIM in a semi-structured interview via Zoom, conducted by a licensed occupational therapist with professional training and experience in their administration. In the second stage, every Sunday through Thursday for two consecutive weeks, participants received smartphone messages twice a day, 8 AM and 8 PM, with a link to complete the EMA questionnaire (described in Measures). Thus, each participant contributed up to 20 data points (two prompts per day for 10 days). Parents were encouraged to respond in real time. Response rates and patterns of missing data were recorded to evaluate feasibility and data completeness.

2.4. Data Analysis

The variables were analyzed using IBM SPSS software (version 26 Descriptive statistics and normality tests were conducted for all variables. Independent-samples *t* tests and chi-square tests compared the autism and TD groups on demographic variables. Feasibility of the EMA was assessed through calculation of overall and group-specific response rates, as well as examination of missing data patterns across days and time points. EMA means were calculated from available responses only, with missing values (including 'not relevant') excluded from the analyses.

Analysis of covariance (ANCOVA) was used to compare groups on the one-time report (WeeFIM), controlling age and maternal education (entered as covariates). Multivariate analysis of covariance (MANCOVA) compared the groups on specific EMA activities, as well as EMA total average and total variability, also controlling for these covariates. Follow-up ANOVAs identified the sources of significant effects. Paired-samples *t* tests compared WeeFIM and EMA scores within groups. Pearson correlation coefficients examined associations between the WeeFIM score and EMA-derived variables (mean and variability). Variability analyses were conducted to explore whether greater fluctuation in daily independence levels was associated with differences in the one-time report, providing insight into contextual effects on ADL performance. Bonferroni corrections were not applied to preserve statistical power, given the pilot nature of the study and the small sample size.

3. Results

The demographic characteristics of the two groups are presented in Table 1. Independent *t* tests and chi-square analyses revealed no significant group differences in the number of siblings, father's years of education, mother's years of education, or housing density. However, significant differences emerged in both age ($t = 5.32$, $p < 0.001$), with autistic toddlers being older than their TD peers, and gender ($\chi^2 = 4.31$, $p = 0.03$), with a higher proportion of males in the autistic group (78.2%) compared to the TD group (50%). Therefore, age was included as covariate in all subsequent hypothesis-testing analyses. Since no significant gender differences were observed in the dependent variables, gender was not included as a covariate.

Table 1. Demographic characteristics of the two groups.

Demographic Information	Autistic Group (n = 23)	TD Group (n = 28)	
Age at assessment, months; *M* (*SD*), range	32.13 (4.65), 23–40	24.93 (4.86), 18–35	$t = 5.32$ ($p < 0.001$)
Gender (% males)	18 (78.2)	14 (50)	$\chi^2 = 4.31$ ($p = 0.03$)
Number of siblings; *M*	0.87	1.07	$t = -0.68$ ($p = 0.50$)
SES			
Mother years of education; *M* (*SD*), range	15.04 (2.55), 12–20	16.71 (2.17), 15–22	$t = -2.52$ ($p = 0.15$)
Father years of education; *M* (*SD*), range	14.52 (2.27), 12–18	14.71 (3.65), 8–22	$t = -0.22$ ($p = 0.83$)
Housing density, *M* (*SD*)	0.94 (0.24)	1.06 (0.34)	$t = -1.35$ ($p = 0.18$)

Note. SES = Socioeconomic Status; Housing density—persons per room. M = mean, SD = Standard deviation.

Preliminary Analyses. Tests of normality (Shapiro–Wilk) were conducted for all dependent variables within each group. Results indicated that most variables did not deviate significantly from normality (all *ps* > 0.05), except for WeeFIM scores in the autistic group ($p = 0.008$).

3.1. Aim 1: EMA Feasibilty in the Two Groups

Parents in both groups demonstrated high response rates (autistic group: $M = 18.22$, $SD = 1.98$; *TD* group: $M = 17.71$, $SD = 2.58$), corresponding to 91.1% (Figure 1) and 88.55% (Figure 2) of the maximum possible responses, respectively. An independent *t* test revealed no significant difference between the groups in the number of responses, t (49) = 0.76, $p > 0.5$.

3.2. Aim 2: Comparison Between Groups of Independence in ADL

The conducted MANCOVA included age and mother education as covariances since they were found to be significantly different between the groups. MANCOVA yielded significant differences between the autistic group and TD groups in PEDI and WeeFIM mean scores $F\ (2, 46) = 18.45$, $p < 0.001$, $\eta^2 = 0.44$. To examine the significance source, each variable's data were subjected to univariate ANOVA. Significant differences were found in PEDI $F\ (1, 47) = 37.53$, $p < 0.001$, $\eta^2 = 0.44$, and in the WeeFIM $F\ (1, 47) = 25.12$, $p = 0.000$, $\eta^2 = 0.35$. The results of this analysis showed that the TD toddlers received significantly higher scores (indicating better performance) than the children with autism in both one-time report measures. The mean and standard deviations of the measures are presented in Table 2.

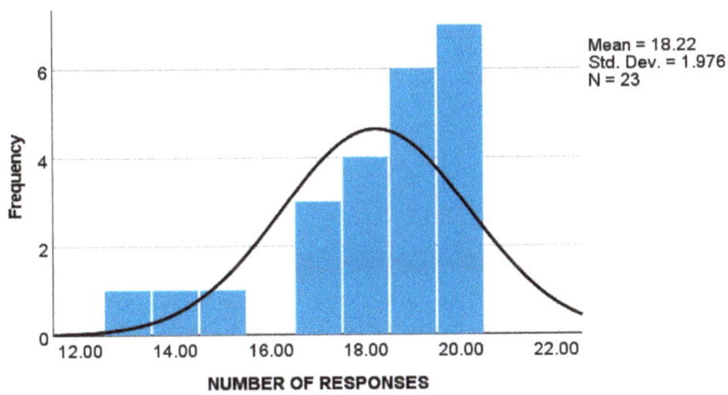

Figure 1. Histogram showing the frequencies of EMA responses in the ASD group.

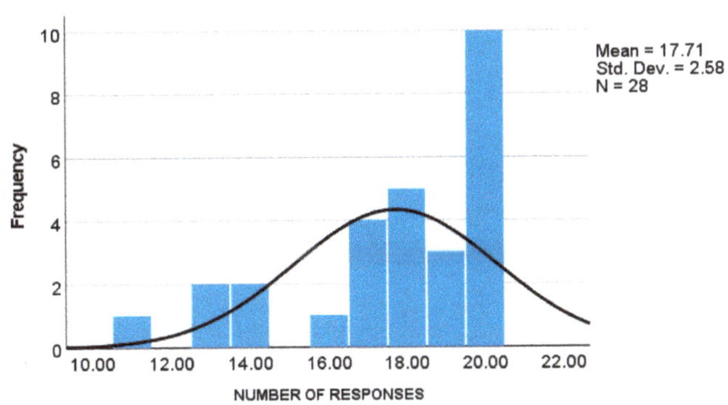

Figure 2. Histogram showing the frequencies of EMA responses in the TD group.

Table 2. Comparison of the PEDI and the WeeFIM Measures Between the Groups.

	Autistic Group (*n* = 23)		**TD Group (*n* = 28)**			
	M	*SD*	*M*	*SD*	*F*	η^2
PEDI	25.61	12.44	41.43	9.63	16.02 ***	0.44
WeeFIM	13.74	5.24	20.21	6.01	12.93 ***	0.35

Note. PEDI = Pediatric Evaluation of Disability Inventory; WeeFIM = The Functional Independence Measure for Children. *** $p < 0.001$.

To examine whether *Specific activities will differ between the groups*, The MANCOVA applied to the seven EMA variables (eating, grooming, bathing, dressing upper-body, dressing lower-body, toileting, and waking\sleeping) yielded statistically significant differences between the ASD and the TD groups $F\ (7, 41) = 3.34$, $p = 0.007$, $\eta^2 = 0.36$. Univariate ANOVAs were performed on the data for each variable. The mean and standard deviations of the measures are presented in Table 3. The results of this analysis showed that the TD children received significantly higher scores (i.e., performed better) in eating, grooming, bathing, dressing lower-body, toileting, and waking\sleeping variables. No significant group differences were found for upper-body dressing. The mean and standard deviations of the variables were also computed. The average score of the EMA was significantly higher than the TD group, and the variability of the TD group was higher, but it did not reach the significant threshold ($p = 0.073$).

Table 3. Comparison of EMA results between the two Groups.

	Autistic Group ($n = 23$)		TD Group ($n = 28$)			
	M	*SD*	*M*	*SD*	*F*	η^2
Eating	5.03	1.69	6.22	0.68	4.69 **	0.23
Grooming	2.45	1.37	3.04	1.37	5.23 **	0.25
Bathing	2.18	1.19	3.08	1.35	7.62 ***	0.33
Dressing-Upper Body	2.42	1.17	2.63	0.97	2.32	0.13
Dressing-Lower Body	2.33	1.07	3.22	1.51	7.54 ***	0.32
Toileting	2.12	1.65	2.19	1.91	6.03 ***	0.28
Waking\Sleeping	4.27	1.97	5.54	1.55	4.12 **	0.21
Total average	2.97	1.12	3.70	0.98	8.42 ***	0.35
Total variability	1.64	0.51	1.88	0.32	2.47	0.14

Note. EMA-Ecological Momentary Assessment. ** $p < 0.01$. *** $p < 0.001$.

3.3. Aim 3: Comparison of One-Time Report Measurment and EMA Results

To enable comparison between the WeeFIM one-time report and the EMA repeated measures, the waking/sleeping activity was excluded from EMA totals. A paired *t* test was conducted, and a significant difference was found only in the autistic group, with the mean score in the one-time report significantly lower than the mean score in the EMA (Table 4).

Table 4. Comparison between the WeeFIM and the EMA results within the groups.

	WeeFIM		EMA		
	M	*SD*	*M*	*SD*	*t*
Autistic group	13.74	5.23	16.53	6.58	3.23 **
TD group	20.21	6.01	20.40	6.04	0.3

Note. WeeFIM = The Functional Independence Measure for Children; EMA-Ecological Momentary Assessment. ** $p < 0.01$.

3.4. Aim 4: Relationship Between One-Time Reports and EMA Mean and Variance

Pearson correlation coefficients were calculated separately for each group (Table 5). In both groups, higher EMA mean scores were strongly and significantly associated with higher PEDI and WeeFIM scores, indicating that children who demonstrated greater independence in daily EMA also scored higher in one-time report measures.

Table 5. Correlations coefficients of one-time report measures and EMA mean and variability.

		EMA Mean	EMA Variability
Autistic group	PEDI	0.76 **	0.4
	WeeFIM	0.84 **	0.46 **
TD group	PEDI	0.79 **	−0.12
	WeeFIM	0.88 **	−0.22

Note. PEDI = Pediatric Evaluation of Disability Inventory; WeeFIM = The Functional Independence Measure for children. ** $p < 0.01$.

In the autistic group, higher EMA variability was significantly associated with higher WeeFIM scores, suggesting that children who showed more fluctuation in independence across contexts also tended to perform better in the WeeFIM. In contrast, in the TD group, correlations between independence and EMA variability were negative but not statistically significant. This difference in trends between groups is illustrated in Figure 3.

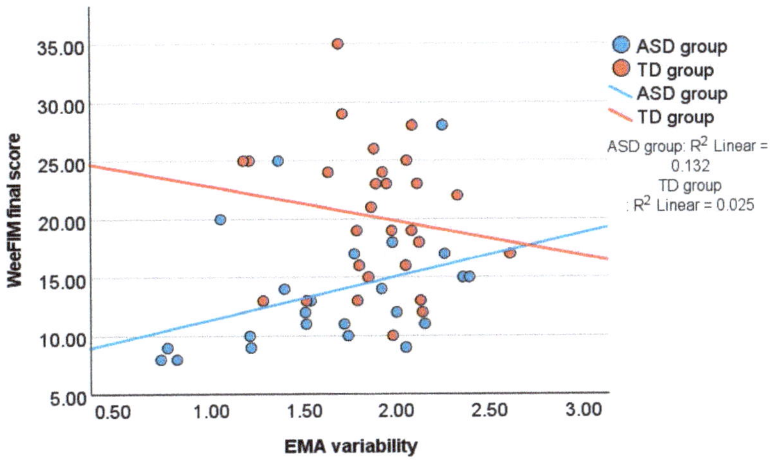

Figure 3. Correlations between the WeeFIM final score and the EMA variability.

4. Discussion

The current pilot study aimed to describe independence in ADL performance among autistic toddlers, compared to TD peers, based on parent reports via the EMA approach. EMA was found to be feasible; in fact, the participation rates in both our groups were higher than those reported in other EMA studies conducted among toddlers [26,41]. Previous literature has examined the feasibility of EMA studies using various metrics, with compliance rates being a key indicator. A meta-analysis published in 2023 [42] found that, on average, EMA studies achieved a compliance rate of 79%, though these studies typically included six prompts per day, whereas the present study used only two. In this context, the compliance rates of over 88% in both groups of the study demonstrate strong feasibility. The higher response rate may be attributed to the reminders sent to the participants with the link to the EMA questionnaire twice a day, in line with recommendations for EMA studies [43].

As expected, significant group differences were found in both the one-time reports and the EMA reports, indicating that the autistic group participated less independently in ADL than did TD toddlers. These findings can also be described as reflecting different participation profiles between the groups, rather than solely lower levels of independence. These findings are consistent with previous studies demonstrating that young autistic children show relatively lower performance in self-care tasks, compared to their age norms [21]; and that as a result, autistic children receive more adult support in performing daily self-care activities [44]. Significant differences were found in all activities except upper-body dressing. The absence of group differences in this activity may reflect contextual influences rather than true equivalence in independence. Because data collection occurred during the winter months, even TD toddlers often required parental assistance with layered clothing (e.g., coats, sweaters) [45]. Consequently, upper-body dressing may be less sensitive to developmental differences at this age due to seasonal demands, and findings should therefore be interpreted with caution.

An interesting result of our study was that only parents of autistic toddlers rated their child's participation significantly lower in their one-time report, compared to the child's average EMA score. In other words, the everyday ADL functioning of these autistic toddlers was seen to be higher than would be expected from their one-time assessments. One possible explanation for this discrepancy may be parental bias in retrospective reporting. Caregiver ratings are informant-based and not entirely free of bias and may be influenced by caregiver burden. Such biases may lead caregivers to either over- or underestimate the child's actual functioning [46]. Another possibility is that engagement in the EMA protocol may have gradually raised parents' awareness of their child's actual capabilities. Indeed, several parents from the autistic group reported that during the study, they allowed their children to be more independent in a variety of activities. This finding is in line with a previous study that asked caregivers of children with autism to answer daily questions about the child's irritability, anxiety, and mood, delivered via smartphones across 8 weeks; placebo-like effects were observed, with caregivers reporting symptoms improving over time without explicit treatment [43]. Although promising, this interpretation remains speculative and requires systematic investigation in future work.

In addition, we found that the greater variability in the EMA was associated with higher independence. As suggested by previous studies, the development of self-care functioning among autistic children is characterized by fluctuation and inconsistent performance [47,48]. These fluctuations cannot be measured using one-time reports, whereas it can be documented by EMA. Nevertheless, causality cannot be inferred, and alternative explanations such as inconsistent support, environmental variability, or measurement error should be considered. This association may also reflect methodological differences between retrospective and momentary assessments. Retrospective, one-time measures such as the WeeFIM are susceptible to recall-related biases, as they rely on parents' memory of past events rather than real-time observations [31]. In contrast, EMA enables the capture of daily fluctuations in naturalistic contexts, as highlighted in studies of youth psychopathology [49], which may help explain the observed correlation between EMA variability and WeeFIM scores in the autistic group. Given the small sample size, the observed association should be considered exploratory until replicated in larger samples.

This study has several limitations. First, the sample size was relatively small, and participants were recruited via convenience and snowball sampling, which may bias toward more motivated or well-connected families, thereby limiting the external validity of the results. Future studies should aim to recruit more representative and diverse samples. Second, autism diagnoses were parent-reported based on professional evaluations but were not independently verified, which reduces diagnostic certainty. Future research should incorporate standardized diagnostic verification procedures to enhance the robustness of findings. Third, the average age of autism diagnosis is typically higher than the average age of the current sample [3], suggesting that the children included may have had higher support needs, as they were identified and diagnosed earlier. Early diagnosis may also be associated with co-occurring lower IQ [50], which could contribute to potential bias. Fourth, no data were collected on participants' cognitive abilities (IQ) or autism symptom severity, which could have provided further insight into the observed group differences. Further research should consider controlling these factors to improve the generalizability of the findings.

Furthermore, there were significant differences between the groups in some demographic measures. Gender distribution was skewed toward males in the autistic group, consistent with the higher prevalence of autism among boys [6,7]. This imbalance may represent a potential confounder but was not included as a covariate due to the small sample size, which limited statistical power and precluded reliable adjustment for additional variables. Future studies should aim for a more balanced ratio to improve generalizability. Socioeconomic status (SES) was measured only via housing density, a narrow indicator that does not capture other SES dimensions such as income or parental occupation. Future studies should therefore incorporate multiple SES indicators (income, education, occupation) for a more comprehensive assessment. Moreover, weekend routines were not examined despite their potential influence on participation. Finally, multiple analyses were conducted without correction for multiple comparisons to preserve statistical power, given the small sample size and pilot design. This raises the possibility of Type I error, and results should therefore be interpreted with caution. Given the small sample size and absence of correction for multiple comparisons, the significant findings should be regarded as exploratory, providing valuable preliminary evidence that requires confirmation in larger samples. Despite these limitations, this pilot study indicates that EMA may be a feasible approach for assessing daily participation among autistic toddlers and points to avenues for future research.

Beyond the identified limitations, an additional noteworthy finding was that parents reported that their engagement in the study increased their child's participation, raising the possibility that EMA could serve not only as an assessment tool but also, potentially, as a supportive component within interventions aimed at enhancing daily participation. This observation aligns with the concept of reactivity, defined as the potential for behavior or experience to be affected by the act of assessing it [30]. Although this interpretation should be considered cautiously and examined systematically, it nonetheless suggests an intriguing direction for future research.

5. Conclusions

This study used EMA to evaluate independence in ADL among autistic toddlers. Autistic toddlers exhibited different participation profiles, with less independent performance in ADL compared to typically developing peers, particularly in adaptive activities. In the autistic group only, EMA scores indicated higher independence than one-time parent reports, suggesting that EMA may capture a more ecologically valid and dynamic representation of daily functioning. EMA provides exploratory evidence of feasibility as a method for ongoing, ecologically valid assessment in this population. Future studies should build on these findings by recruiting larger and more demographically balanced samples, including weekend routines, integrating parental reports with direct observations, and explicitly monitoring parental reactivity. In addition, future work should adopt neurodiversity-informed perspectives, interpreting differences in participation as reflecting diverse developmental trajectories and support needs.

Author Contributions: S.H. collected the data, analyzed the data, and drafted the manuscript. Y.G. conceptualized and designed the study, supervised the research, and guided the first author throughout the master's thesis process. B.A. contributed to content editing and language revision. All authors have read and agreed to the published version of the manuscript.

Funding: This research received no external funding.

Institutional Review Board Statement: The study was approved by the Ethics Committee for Non-Medical Human Studies at the Faculty of Medicine, The Hebrew University of Jerusalem. The code is 29082021 and the approval date is 29 August 2021. Written informed consent was obtained from the parents of all participants prior to participation.

Informed Consent Statement: All authors consent to the publication of this manuscript. Participants' parents provided consent for the anonymized data to be used in publication.

Data Availability Statement: The datasets generated and analyzed during the current study are not publicly available due to ethical and privacy restrictions but are available from the corresponding author upon reasonable request.

Acknowledgments: The authors would like to thank all the participants for their time and effort in contributing to this study.

Conflicts of Interest: The authors declare no conflicts of interest.

Abbreviations

The following abbreviations are used in this manuscript:

Abbreviation	Definition
ASD	Autism Spectrum Disorder
DSM	Diagnostic and Statistical Manual of Mental Disorders
ADL	Activities of Daily Living
PEDI	Pediatric Evaluation of Disability Inventory
WeeFIM	Functional Independence Measure for Children
EMA	Ecological Momentary Assessment
TD	Typically Developing
SES	Socioeconomic Status
G*Power	G*Power (Statistical Power Analysis Software)

References

1. American Psychiatric Association. *Diagnostic and Statistical Manual of Mental Disorders*, 5th ed.; American Psychiatric Association: Washington, DC, USA, 2013.
2. Botha, M.; Gillespie-Lynch, K. Come as you are: Examining autistic identity development and the neurodiversity movement through an intersectional lens. *Hum. Dev.* **2022**, *66*, 93–112. [CrossRef]
3. Baio, J. Prevalence of autism spectrum disorder among children aged 8 years—Autism and developmental disabilities monitoring network, 11 sites, United States, 2014. *MMWR. Surveill. Summ.* **2018**, *67*, 1–23. [CrossRef]
4. Kerub, O.; Haas, E.J.; Meiri, G.; Bilenko, N.; Flusser, H.; Michaelovski, A.; Dinstein, I.; Davidovitch, N.; Menashe, I. Ethnic disparities in the diagnosis of autism in Southern Israel. *Autism Res.* **2021**, *14*, 193–201. [CrossRef] [PubMed]
5. Malaga, I.; Blanco-Lago, R.; Hedrera-Fernandez, A.; Alvarez-Alvarez, N.; Oreña-Ansonera, V.A.; Baeza-Velasco, M. Prevalence of autism spectrum disorders in USA, Europe and Spain: Coincidences and discrepancies. *Medicina* **2019**, *79*, 4–9. [PubMed]
6. Shaw, K.A. Prevalence and early identification of autism spectrum disorder among children aged 4 and 8 years—Autism and Developmental Disabilities Monitoring Network, 16 Sites, United States, 2022. *MMWR. Surveill. Summ.* **2025**, *74*, 1–22. [CrossRef]
7. Zeidan, J.; Fombonne, E.; Scorah, J.; Ibrahim, A.; Durkin, M.S.; Saxena, S.; Yusuf, A.; Shih, A.; Elsabbagh, M. Global prevalence of autism: A systematic review update. *Autism Res.* **2022**, *15*, 778–790. [CrossRef]
8. Hyman, S.L.; Levy, S.E.; Myers, S.M. Identification, Evaluation, and Management of Children With Autism Spectrum Disorder. *Pediatrics* **2020**, *145*, e20193447. [CrossRef] [PubMed]
9. Piven, J.; Elison, J.T.; Zylka, M.J. Toward a conceptual framework for early brain and behavior development in autism. *Mol. Psychiatry* **2017**, *22*, 1385–1394. [CrossRef]
10. Zwaigenbaum, L.; Bauman, M.L.; Choueiri, R.; Kasari, C.; Carter, A.; Granpeesheh, D.; Mailloux, Z.; Smith Roley, S.; Wagner, S.; Fein, D. Early intervention for children with autism spectrum disorder under 3 years of age: Recommendations for practice and research. *Pediatrics* **2015**, *136*, S60–S81. [CrossRef]
11. World Health Organization. International Classification of Functioning, Disability, and Health: Children & Youth Version; ICF-CY. Available online: https://iris.who.int/server/api/core/bitstreams/81e04699-2930-4da2-ac97-76725c7dcc07/content (accessed on 1 June 2021).
12. Powrie, B.; Kolehmainen, N.; Turpin, M.; Ziviani, J.; Copley, J. The meaning of leisure for children and young people with physical disabilities: A systematic evidence synthesis. *Dev. Med. Child Neurol.* **2015**, *57*, 993–1010. [CrossRef]
13. Lim, C.Y.; Law, M.; Khetani, M.; Pollock, N.; Rosenbaum, P. Participation in out-of-home environments for young children with and without developmental disabilities. *OTJR: Occup. Particip. Health* **2016**, *36*, 112–125. [CrossRef] [PubMed]
14. Clark, G.F.; Kingsley, K.L. Occupational therapy practice guidelines for early childhood: Birth–5 years. *Am. J. Occup. Ther.* **2020**, *74*, 7403397010p1–7403397010p42. [CrossRef]
15. O'Brien, J.C.; Kuhaneck, H.M. *Case-Smith's Occupational Therapy for Children and Adolescents*; Elsevise: Amsterdam, The Netherlands, 2020.

16. James, S.; Ziviani, J.; Boyd, R. A systematic review of activities of daily living measures for children and adolescents with cerebral palsy. *Dev. Med. Child Neurol.* **2014**, *56*, 233–244. [CrossRef]
17. Dosman, C.F.; Andrews, D.; Goulden, K.J. Evidence-based milestone ages as a framework for developmental surveillance. *Paediatr. Child Health* **2012**, *17*, 561–568. [CrossRef]
18. Bedell, G.; Coster, W.; Law, M.; Liljenquist, K.; Kao, Y.-C.; Teplicky, R.; Anaby, D.; Khetani, M.A. Community participation, supports, and barriers of school-age children with and without disabilities. *Arch. Phys. Med. Rehabil.* **2013**, *94*, 315–323. [CrossRef]
19. Law, M.; Anaby, D.; Teplicky, R.; Khetani, M.A.; Coster, W.; Bedell, G. Participation in the home environment among children and youth with and without disabilities. *Br. J. Occup. Ther.* **2013**, *76*, 58–66. [CrossRef]
20. Jasmin, E.; Couture, M.; McKinley, P.; Reid, G.; Fombonne, E.; Gisel, E. Sensori-motor and daily living skills of preschool children with autism spectrum disorders. *J. Autism Dev. Disord.* **2009**, *39*, 231–241. [CrossRef]
21. Franchini, M.; Zöller, D.; Gentaz, E.; Glaser, B.; Wood de Wilde, H.; Kojovic, N.; Eliez, S.; Schaer, M. Early adaptive functioning trajectories in preschoolers with autism spectrum disorders. *J. Pediatr. Psychol.* **2018**, *43*, 800–813. [CrossRef]
22. Dawson, G.; Rieder, A.D.; Johnson, M.H. Prediction of autism in infants: Progress and challenges. *Lancet Neurol.* **2023**, *22*, 244–254. [CrossRef] [PubMed]
23. Schaaf, R.C.; Cohn, E.S.; Burke, J.; Dumont, R.; Miller, A.; Mailloux, Z. Linking sensory factors to participation: Establishing intervention goals with parents for children with autism spectrum disorder. *Am. J. Occup. Ther.* **2015**, *69*, 6905185005p1–6905185005p8. [CrossRef]
24. Rydz, D.; Srour, M.; Oskoui, M.; Marget, N.; Shiller, M.; Birnbaum, R.; Majnemer, A.; Shevell, M.I. Screening for developmental delay in the setting of a community pediatric clinic: A prospective assessment of parent-report questionnaires. *Pediatrics* **2006**, *118*, e1178–e1186. [CrossRef] [PubMed]
25. Stone, A.A.; Shiffman, S. Ecological momentary assessment (EMA) in behavorial medicine. *Ann. Behav. Med.* **1994**, *16*, 199–202. [CrossRef]
26. Hager, E.R.; Tilton, N.A.; Wang, Y.; Kapur, N.C.; Arbaiza, R.; Merry, B.C.; Black, M.M. The home environment and toddler physical activity: An ecological momentary assessment study. *Pediatr. Obes.* **2017**, *12*, 1–9. [CrossRef]
27. Dallman, A.R.; Bailliard, A.; Harrop, C. Identifying Predictors of Momentary Negative Affect and Depression Severity in Adolescents with Autism: An Exploratory Ecological Momentary Assessment Study. *J. Autism Dev. Disord.* **2022**, *52*, 291–303. [CrossRef]
28. Haley, S.M.; Coster, W.J.; Ludlow, L.H.; Haltiwanger, J.T.; Andrellos, P.J. *Pediatric Evaluation of Disability Inventory (PEDI): Development, Standardization and Administration Manual*; New England Medical Center Hospitals, Inc.: Boston, MA, USA, 1992.
29. Msall, M.E.; DiGaudio, K.; Rogers, B.T.; LaForest, S.; Catanzaro, N.L.; Campbell, J.; Wilczenski, F.; Duffy, L.C. The Functional Independence Measure for Children (WeeFIM) conceptual basis and pilot use in children with developmental disabilities. *Clin. Pediatr.* **1994**, *33*, 421–430. [CrossRef]
30. Woodman, A.C.; Mawdsley, H.P.; Hauser-Cram, P. Parenting stress and child behavior problems within families of children with developmental disabilities: Transactional relations across 15 years. *Res. Dev. Disabil.* **2015**, *36*, 264–276. [CrossRef]
31. Shiffman, S.; Stone, A.A.; Hufford, M.R. Ecological momentary assessment. *Annu. Rev. Clin. Psychol.* **2008**, *4*, 1–32. [CrossRef]
32. Chen, Y.; Xi, Z.; Greene, T.; Mandy, W. A systematic review of ecological momentary assessment in autism research. *Autism* **2024**, *29*, 1374–1389. [CrossRef]
33. Chen, Y.W.; Bundy, A.; Cordier, R.; Einfeld, S. Feasibility and usability of experience sampling methodology for capturing everyday experiences of individuals with autism spectrum disorders. *Disabil. Health J.* **2014**, *7*, 361–366. [CrossRef] [PubMed]
34. Chen, Y.W.; Bundy, A.C.; Cordier, R.; Chien, Y.L.; Einfeld, S.L. A cross-cultural exploration of the everyday social participation of individuals with autism spectrum disorders in Australia and Taiwan: An experience sampling study. *Autism* **2017**, *21*, 231–241. [CrossRef]
35. Khor, A.S.; Gray, K.M.; Reid, S.C.; Melvin, G.A. Feasibility and validity of ecological momentary assessment in adolescents with high-functioning autism and Asperger's disorder. *J. Adolesc.* **2014**, *37*, 37–46. [CrossRef] [PubMed]
36. Song, W.; Zheng, L.; Tichá, R.; Abery, B.; Nguyen-Feng, V.N. Leisure participation of autistic adults: An ecological momentary assessment feasibility study. *Am. J. Intellect. Dev. Disabil.* **2023**, *128*, 319–333. [CrossRef] [PubMed]
37. Provost, B.; Crowe, T.K.; Osbourn, P.L.; McClain, C.; Skipper, B.J. Mealtime behaviors of preschool children: Comparison of children with autism spectrum disorder and children with typical development. *Phys. Occup. Ther. Pediatr.* **2010**, *30*, 220–233. [CrossRef]
38. Custers, J.; Wassenberg-Severijnen, J.; Net, J.V.D.; Vermeer, A.; Hart, H.T.; Helders, P. Dutch adaptation and content validity of the 'Pediatric Evaluation Of Disability Inventory (PEDI)'. *Disabil. Rehabil.* **2002**, *24*, 250–258. [CrossRef]
39. Elad, D.; Barak, S.; Eisenstein, E.; Bar, O.; Herzberg, O.; Brezner, A. Reliability and validity of Hebrew Pediatric Evaluation of Disability Inventory (PEDI) in children with cerebral palsy~--health care professionals vs. mothers. *J. Pediatr. Rehabil. Med.* **2012**, *5*, 107–115. [CrossRef]

40. Williams, K.S.; Young, D.K.; Burke, G.A.; Fountain, D.M. Comparing the WeeFIM and PEDI in neurorehabilitation for children with acquired brain injury: A systematic review. *Dev. Neurorehabilit.* **2017**, *20*, 443–451. [CrossRef]
41. Campbell, K.L.; Wang, Y.; Kuhn, A.P.; Black, M.M.; Hager, E.R. An ecological momentary assessment study of physical activity behaviors among mothers of toddlers from low-income households. *BMC Womens Health* **2021**, *21*, 120. [CrossRef]
42. Wrzus, C.; Neubauer, A.B. Ecological momentary assessment: A meta-analysis on designs, samples, and compliance across research fields. *Assessment* **2023**, *30*, 825–846. [CrossRef]
43. Jones, R.M.; Tarpey, T.; Hamo, A.; Carberry, C.; Lord, C. Smartphone measures of day-to-day behavior changes in children with autism. *NPJ Digit. Med.* **2018**, *1*, 34. [CrossRef] [PubMed]
44. Mays, N.M.; Heflin, L.J. Increasing independence in self-care tasks for children with autism using self-operated auditory prompts. *Res. Autism Spectr. Disord.* **2011**, *5*, 1351–1357. [CrossRef]
45. Summers, J.; Larkin, D.; Dewey, D. Activities of daily living in children with developmental coordination disorder: Dressing, personal hygiene, and eating skills. *Hum. Mov. Sci.* **2008**, *27*, 215–229. [CrossRef]
46. Mlinac, M.E.; Feng, M.C. Assessment of activities of daily living, self-care, and independence. *Arch. Clin. Neuropsychol.* **2016**, *31*, 506–516. [CrossRef]
47. Wolery, M. Commentary: The environment as a source of variability: Implications for research with individuals who have autism. *J. Autism Dev. Disord.* **2000**, *30*, 379. [CrossRef]
48. Kern, P.; Wakeford, L.; Aldridge, D. Improving the performance of a young child with autism during self-care tasks using embedded song interventions: A case study. *Music Ther. Perspect.* **2007**, *25*, 43–51. [CrossRef]
49. Thunnissen, M.R.; aan het Rot, M.; van den Hoofdakker, B.J.; Nauta, M.H. Youth psychopathology in daily life: Systematically reviewed characteristics and potentials of ecological momentary assessment applications. *Child Psychiatry Hum. Dev.* **2022**, *53*, 1129–1147. [CrossRef] [PubMed]
50. Denisova, K.; Lin, Z. The importance of low IQ to early diagnosis of autism. *Autism Res.* **2023**, *16*, 122–142. [CrossRef] [PubMed]

children

MDPI

Article

ADHD Reporting in Developmental Age: The Role of the Informants

Dario Esposito *, Federica Gigliotti, Beatrice Colotti, Carlo Di Brina, Francesco Pisani and Maria Romani

Department of Human Neuroscience, Sapienza University of Rome, 00185 Roma, Italy; federica.gig@uniroma1.it (F.G.); carlo.dibrina@uniroma1.it (C.D.B.); francesco.pisani@uniroma1.it (F.P.); maria.romani@uniroma1.it (M.R.)

* Correspondence: dario.esposito@uniroma1.it

Abstract: Background: Attention-Deficit/Hyperactivity Disorder (ADHD) is a complex neurodevelopmental condition typically requiring information from multiple informants for accurate diagnosis. However, the consistency and diagnostic value of reports from teachers, parents, primary care providers (PCPs), and other professionals remain debated. This study aimed to examine the role and diagnostic accuracy of different informants in the referral and diagnostic process for ADHD in children aged 3–11. **Methods**: This retrospective study analyzed data from 120 children referred for suspected ADHD. Initial reports were obtained from teachers, parents, PCPs, and other professionals, and final diagnoses were determined through comprehensive neuropsychiatric evaluations. Diagnostic concordance and informant-specific contributions were assessed. **Results**: Of the 120 children, 64 (53.3%) received an ADHD diagnosis. Teachers were the most frequent informants, followed by parents, with fewer referrals from PCPs and other professionals. No significant differences in diagnostic accuracy were found among informants, aligning with previous studies suggesting that no single informant is superior in identifying ADHD. Notably, over 93% of referred children were diagnosed with a neuropsychiatric disorder, though not necessarily ADHD. **Conclusions**: The findings underscore the importance of combining reports from parents and teachers to capture symptom expression across different environments, which is essential for accurate ADHD diagnosis. Enhanced training for informants and a multidisciplinary approach is recommended to improve diagnostic accuracy and support early identification and intervention efforts. These results support nuanced evaluation strategies that account for informant variability and help mitigate potential misinterpretations of ADHD symptoms.

Keywords: ADHD; informants; school reporting; developmental age

1. Introduction

Attention-Deficit/Hyperactivity Disorder (ADHD) is a persistent and pervasive neurodevelopmental disorder. It is characterized by levels of hyperactivity, impulsivity, and/or inattention that are inappropriate for an individual's developmental stage. These symptoms can lead to impairments in daily functioning, particularly in areas such as academic performance, health, and social interactions. ADHD is typically diagnosed in childhood, with reported prevalence rates varying widely from 1.5% to 19.9%, though the average is approximately 5% [1,2].

The diagnosis of ADHD is complex, requiring information from multiple sources and clinical observation. Specifically, the presence of symptoms must be confirmed in at least two different settings. Parents and teachers are the most common informants, as they often have a deeper understanding of a child's daily functioning. However, pediatricians, general practitioners, and other professionals are also frequently involved in the referral process [1].

While the involvement of multiple informants is necessary for a thorough assessment, it can also result in discrepancies in the evaluation of a child's behavior. A frequently debated question in the literature is whether some informants are more reliable than others in the referral process for ADHD [3,4].

Discrepancies between informants are common in the assessment of child and adolescent psychopathology. Theoretical models such as the multi-informant model [5,6] suggest that differences in symptom reporting are not merely due to measurement error, but may reflect meaningful contextual variability—that is, variation in behavior across home, school, or clinical environments—as well as source-specific biases linked to the informant's perspective, expectations, or relationship with the child [7,8]. For instance, teachers may be more sensitive to attentional difficulties in structured settings, while parents might be better at detecting emotional or internalizing symptoms. These differences underscore the importance of integrating multiple perspectives during clinical evaluation, especially in conditions like ADHD, where symptom expression is highly context-dependent. Despite widespread recommendations for a multi-informant approach, few studies have assessed the comparative clinical validity of different informant types within real-world referral settings [5–7]. To our knowledge, this is the first study to compare, in a real clinical setting, the referrals for inattention and/or hyperactivity/impulsivity made by various informants with the final diagnoses established after a comprehensive diagnostic evaluation. This approach aims to highlight differences in assessments among various informants, as well as to identify the strengths and weaknesses of each informant type.

2. Materials and Methods

This study employed a retrospective, non-interventional design, analyzing data from patients aged three to eleven years who were referred to our child neuropsychiatry secondary care center in Central Italy. We included all children who were present for their first clinical examination at our center between January 2021 and June 2022. Following the initial visit, only those children who were registered with a primary complaint of symptoms related to hyperactivity/impulsivity and/or inattention were included for further analysis. For these patients, data were then collected regarding the individual or entity that initiated the referral for evaluation, whether it was an independent decision made by the parents or a referral suggested by another person familiar with the child (e.g., a teacher, pediatrician, or other professional). Patients seeking a second opinion, as well as those with pre-existing diagnoses of intellectual disability, autism spectrum disorder, or other complex neurodevelopmental disabilities, were excluded from the study.

Our analysis focused on several key aspects: the identification of the informants who initiated the clinical evaluation (e.g., teachers, pediatricians, or parents); the reasons for referral (i.e., hyperactivity/impulsivity, inattention, or a combination of these symptoms); and a comparison of the initial reports with the final diagnoses obtained after a standard comprehensive diagnostic evaluation.

All children underwent a comprehensive neuropsychiatric assessment conducted by a multidisciplinary team including child neuropsychiatrists and psychologists. The final diagnosis was based on DSM-5 criteria. Standardized instruments were employed, including parent- and teacher-rated ADHD symptom questionnaires, checklists for internalizing and externalizing symptoms, cognitive evaluations, and assessments of executive functioning, language development, academic skills, and graphomotor abilities.

Continuous variables are presented using the mean ± standard deviation (SD) and range, while categorical variables are presented as counts and percentages. For group comparisons, we used an unpaired Welch's *t*-test for continuous variables, selected due to the unequal variances among comparison groups. For categorical variables, either the chi-square test or Fisher's exact test (when expected frequencies were less than 5) was used. Variables with low expected counts were dichotomized into 2 × 2 contingency tables to appropriately apply the Fisher's exact test (e.g., smaller informant groups were combined with larger related categories to ensure statistical validity). A *p*-value of less than 0.05 was considered statistically significant for all comparisons. Descriptive and inferential analyses were conducted using IBM SPSS Statistics software (v. 30.0.0)

3. Results

Out of 1140 children between three and eleven years of age referred to our outpatient center for the first time between 2021 and 2022, 120 children (10.52%) met our inclusion criteria (mean age 6.83, SD: 1.82 years; 73.3% males). Table 1 summarizes the main demographic characteristics of our sample.

Table 1. Demographic data of reported children by age group, gender, and ADHD symptom presentation. [1]: percentage within the respective age group or gender; [2]: percentage of the total sample.

Reported Children	Predominant Inattentive Symptoms *n* (%)	Predominant Hyperactive/Impulsive Symptoms *n* (%)	Combined Symptoms *n* (%)	Total *n* (%)
Age Groups				
3–5 years old	8 (36.4) [1]	4 (18.2) [1]	10 (45.4) [1]	22 (18.3) [2]
6–7 years old	26 (45.6) [1]	11 (19.3) [1]	20 (35.1) [1]	57 (47.5) [2]
8–11 years old	20 (48.8) [1]	3 (7.3) [1]	18 (43.9) [1]	41 (34.2) [2]
Gender				
Male	37 (42.0) [1]	14 (16.0) [1]	37 (42.0) [1]	88 (73.3) [2]
Female	17 (53.1) [1]	4 (12.5) [1]	11 (34.4) [1]	32 (26.7) [2]
Total	54 (45.0) [2]	18 (15.0) [2]	48 (40.0) [2]	120 (100) [2]
	3–5 years old *n* (%)	**6–7 years old** *n* (%)	**8–11 years old** *n* (%)	**Total** *n* (%)
Male	18 (81.8) [1]	42 (73.7) [1]	28 (68.3) [1]	88 (73.3) [2]
Female	4 (18.2) [1]	15 (26.3) [1]	13 (31.7) [1]	32 (26.7) [2]
Total	22 (18.3) [2]	57 (47.5) [2]	41 (34.2) [2]	120 (100) [2]

The children were reported by various sources: 65 by teachers (54.17%), 30 by parents (25%), 10 by both teachers and parents (8.3%), 9 by doctors (7.5%) and 6 by other professionals (5%). In Table 2 more details are reported.

Table 2. Epidemiological and clinical data of subjects categorized by informants. Percentages refer to the respective age group, gender, reason for referral, or diagnosis. PCPs: Primary Care Practitioners. Note: The total number of children in these categories may exceed 100% (n = 120) because 8.3% of the children (n = 10) were referred by both teachers and parents and are therefore included in multiple categories.

Informants	Teachers *n* (%)	Parents *n* (%)	PCPs *n* (%)	Other Professionals *n* (%)
Age Groups				
3–5 years old (n = 22)	11 (50)	7 (31.8)	3 (13.6)	2 (9.1)
6–7 years old (n = 57)	40 (70.2)	16 (28.1)	4 (7.0)	4 (7.0)
8–11 years old (n = 41)	24 (58.5)	17 (41.5)	2 (4.9)	0
Gender				
Male (n = 88)	57 (64.8)	31 (35.2)	4 (4.5)	4 (4.5)
Female (n = 32)	18 (56.2)	9 (28.1)	5 (15.6)	2 (6.2)
Reasons for Reporting				
Inattentive Symptoms (n = 54)	33 (61.1)	15 (27.8)	6 (11.1)	3 (5.5)
Hyperactive–Impulsive (n = 18)	9 (50.0)	7 (38.9)	3 (16.7)	1 (5.5)
Combined (n = 48)	33 (68.8)	18 (37.5)	0	2 (4.2)
Diagnosis				
ADHD (n = 64)	42 (65.6)	21 (32.8)	6 (9.4)	2 (3.1)
Other Diagnosis (n 48)	28 (58.3)	16 (33.4)	2 (41.7)	4 (8.4)
No Diagnosis (n 8)	5 (6.2)	3 (3.7)	1 (1.2)	0
Total sample	75 (57.7)	40 (30.8)	9 (6.9)	6 (4.6)
ADHD Diagnosis/Reported	42/75 (56.0)	21/40 (52.5)	6/9 (66.0)	2/6 (33.3)

The diagnostic outcomes of the patients were categorized into four groups: 14 patients with ADHD only, 50 with ADHD plus at least one comorbidity, 48 with alternative diagnoses, and 8 without any clinically relevant pathology.

Overall, 64 of the 120 referred children (53.3%) were ultimately diagnosed with ADHD. This corresponds to 5.6% of all patients seen at the outpatient clinic during the study period (n = 1140). Among the 64 children confirmed with ADHD, 16 were female (which is 50% of the 32 referred girls) and 48 were male (54% of the 88 referred boys). Thus, about half of the referred children of each gender received an ADHD diagnosis. An odds ratio (OR) analysis showed that the odds of a referred boy being diagnosed with ADHD were only slightly higher than that of a referred girl (OR ≈ 1.2, 95% confidence interval [0.54–2.70]), and this difference was not statistically significant ($\chi^2(1) = 0.04$, $p = 0.85$). In other words, the diagnostic yield was comparable for boys and girls, despite the higher number of boys referred (male-to-female ratio ≈ 2.75:1, $p < 0.001$ by binomial test).

Within the ADHD-positive group (n = 64), 14 children (22%) had an exclusive ADHD diagnosis (no comorbid conditions), whereas 50 children (78%) had ADHD with comorbidities. On average, children with ADHD had 1.6 comorbid diagnoses (SD = 0.6, median = 2). The mean age at ADHD diagnosis was 6.9 years. Because the age distribution approximated normal in both the "ADHD-only" and "ADHD plus" groups (Shapiro–Wilk $p > 0.10$), we used an independent samples t-test to compare their ages. This revealed no significant age difference between children with pure ADHD and those with ADHD plus comorbidities, with a negligible effect size (Cohen's d 0.1). Thus, the age at diagnosis was similar regardless of the presence of comorbid conditions.

We explored whether the likelihood of an ADHD diagnosis varied by the child's age at referral. We grouped the referred children into three age ranges (preschool: 3–5 years; early school age: 6–7 years; and later childhood: 8–11 years). There was no statistically significant difference in ADHD diagnostic rates across these age groups ($\chi^2(2) = 5.23$, $p = 0.07$), although there was a trend suggesting a higher yield in the early school-age group.

Most of the girls reported with a hyperactive or combined presentation were diagnosed with ADHD (respectively, 74 and 72%), while most of those reported with inattentive symptoms had other comorbidities (29% with ADHD). In boys, the results were more homogenous, with about 50% of those reported with inattentive or hyperactive symptoms being diagnosed with ADHD, and 59% of those reported with combined symptoms receiving a diagnosis.

ADHD comorbidities were further divided into two groups: emotional–behavioral disorders (22 children, with a 3:1 ratio between internalizing [e.g., depression] and externalizing disorders [e.g., oppositional defiant disorder]) and other neurodevelopmental disorders (42 children, including specific learning disorder [SLD]—which was the most frequent—low intellectual functioning, and autism spectrum disorders). Fifteen children had co-occurring conditions and belonged in both groups.

Probands without ADHD can be further classified into two subsets: 48 had other diagnoses (with a mean number of disorders of 1.7; SD 0.94), and in 8 there was no clinically relevant condition (see Table 2). Among these children, 38 were diagnosed with emotional–behavioral disorders (with a ratio of approximately 2:1 between internalizing and externalizing disorders), while 27 had other neurodevelopmental disorders (with SLD being the most frequent in this group as well); 17 children had both diagnoses.

There were no statistically significant differences in ADHD diagnoses across age groups, although a trend was observed ($p = 0.07$), with most children with confirmed ADHD being referred in the age range between 6 and 7 years.

There was a significantly higher number of referrals for males compared to females ($p < 0.01$); however, no significant differences were found in the proportions of ADHD diagnoses between males and females ($p = 0.85$). Notably, symptom presentation was associated with the likelihood of an ADHD diagnosis ($p < 0.01$ for group differences). Children referred for combined-type symptoms had the highest confirmation rate of ADHD (62.5% were diagnosed), followed by those with predominantly hyperactive–impulsive symptoms (55.6% diagnosed), while those with predominantly inattentive symptoms had the lowest ADHD confirmation rate (44.4% diagnosed). The overall association between reported symptom type and diagnostic outcome corresponded to a small-to-moderate effect size (Cramér's V $\approx$ 0.17; equivalent to Cohen's $h \approx 0.36$ for the proportion difference between the highest and lowest groups), indicating that the differences, although statistically significant, were modest in magnitude. A post hoc power analysis for this comparison yielded an approximate power of 52%, suggesting a moderate ability to detect these differences given our sample size.

In our sample, the most frequently involved informants were teachers (57.7% of referrals) ($p < 0.01$), followed by parents (30.8%), while only a small percentage of children were referred by other professionals: primary care practitioners (PCPs), speech therapists, and psychologists. Table 2 provides detailed information about informants. It should be considered that 10 children were reported jointly by both parents and teachers.

In our sample, about half of patients reported for suspected ADHD by teachers (56%) or parents (52.5%) received a confirmed diagnosis of ADHD after a complete diagnostic evaluation. There was no correlation between the type of signaler and the likelihood of a correct ADHD diagnosis ($p = 0.62$). In particular, a chi-square test comparing diagnostic outcomes across the referral groups yielded $\chi^2(4) = 3.27$, $p = 0.514$. The corresponding effect size was small (Cramér's V = 0.165), with an estimated statistical power of 26%, indicating a limited ability to detect subtle differences across informants.

4. Discussion

This study explored the relationship between reports of ADHD symptoms by schools, families, and other professionals, and the final diagnoses of ADHD.

The initial sample of children suspected of inattention/hyperactivity presented with epidemiological characteristics that are consistent with the previous literature. A large majority of the children reported were indeed male (73.3%) [9,10]; most of the girls in our sample were reported for inattention, which is in line with the finding that girls are less likely to be reported for overt symptoms (hyperactivity/impulsivity) [11]. Moreover, most of the reported children were between 6 and 7 years old, probably because this is the age at which Italian children usually enter primary school, and, therefore, ADHD symptoms may become incompatible with the tasks required in a school context. In older age groups, the number of reports decreases (47% of reports at 6–7 years vs. 34% in the older age group), which is also probably associated with the gradual reduction in the more overt symptoms [12]. In accordance with this, inattention was a slightly more common reason for reporting, especially in the female group (53% of reports) and in the older age groups (49% of reports).

Children were primarily referred by teachers, with a considerably smaller proportion referred by parents (approximately 58% versus 31%). Only 8.3% of cases involved joint reporting by both parents and teachers, highlighting a low level of collaboration and shared concern between these two groups.

Teachers are widely regarded as a crucial source of information in assessing ADHD symptoms in children [13]. According to the literature, approximately 85% of clinicians rely on teacher-administered questionnaires to evaluate ADHD symptoms within the school context [13]. Several authors emphasize the value of teachers' evaluations, noting that their experience with age-appropriate behavior often aligns more closely with a clinician's perspective [7,13].

Parental reporting is equally important, as it captures the child's behavior in everyday life and provides a detailed account of their developmental history. However, parental reporting is not without limitations and biases, including a tendency to underestimate ADHD symptoms, particularly in preschool-aged children and girls [14].

A small minority of referrals in our study came from primary care providers (PCPs), such as pediatricians (6.9%), and other professionals, including psychologists, developmental therapists, and speech therapists (4.6%). PCPs play a pivotal role in ensuring appropriate referrals, acting as an essential clinical "filter" between the child, other informants, and specialized psychiatric services.

Nevertheless, PCPs face several challenges in the referral process, often stemming from a lack of specific knowledge about ADHD, misjudgments or biases regarding the disorder, and limited resources to support patients effectively [15]. International studies indicate that the percentage of PCPs who have received formal education on ADHD during their undergraduate and postgraduate training ranges from only 1% to 28% of physicians [15]. This underscores the importance of targeted educational programs, which are proven to be effective in increasing awareness and fostering a greater confidence in diagnosing and managing ADHD [16].

Another significant obstacle reported by PCPs is the scarcity of resources needed for ADHD assessments, particularly in time-constrained settings. The accurate evaluation of this multifaceted condition requires a multidisciplinary, thorough, and time-intensive diagnostic approach [16].

Among the 1140 children referred to our center, 5.6% were ultimately diagnosed with ADHD. Although influenced by referral bias, this rate is higher than the reported national average for Italy (1.1–3.1%) [17], yet consistent with the global prevalence estimates of approximately 5% [1].

Following diagnostic evaluations, the male predominance observed in initial referrals was confirmed, with boys comprising 75% of the ADHD cases. Children in the youngest age group (3–5 years) were more frequently referred by teachers ($p < 0.01$). Additionally, ADHD diagnoses accompanied by comorbidities showed a strong association with neurodevelopmental disorders, primarily learning disabilities. This finding aligns with the existing literature, which identifies ADHD as the most common comorbidity in patients with specific learning disorders (SLD); both conditions involve deficits in executive functioning [18].

Children who were "erroneously" referred for ADHD were most commonly diagnosed with emotional–behavioral disorders, with no significant gender differences. Only 30% of these children received a diagnosis of a neurodevelopmental condition, such as a specific learning disorder (SLD), without co-occurring emotional–behavioral disorders. While conditions like oppositional defiant disorder (ODD) and other externalizing disorders frequently co-occur with ADHD, they can also mimic hyperactive behaviors [19]. Additionally, anxiety and depressive symptoms in childhood can resemble both inattentive and hyperactive traits associated with ADHD [20,21].

The ratio of confirmed ADHD diagnoses to initial suspicions might suggest that parents and teachers have statistically similar "reporting abilities." Chi-square analysis revealed no significant differences in diagnostic confirmation rates among cases referred by teachers, parents, or other professionals. This aligns with the existing literature suggesting that no single group of informants is definitively superior in accurately identifying children with suspected ADHD [6,21]. Research indicates that both parents and teachers exhibit a moderate to good diagnostic accuracy for ADHD, with no significant differences in their predictive ability for a gold-standard ADHD diagnosis [22,23]. However, it should be noted that the small observed effect size and limited statistical power imply that these conclusions must be interpreted with caution. The current sample may not have been large enough to detect subtle but clinically meaningful differences between informant groups. Therefore, further research with larger and more statistically powered samples will be necessary to draw more definitive conclusions about the relative value of each informant type in the diagnostic process.

No single group of informants in our sample proved to be entirely reliable, and inconsistencies were observed across all sources. Despite teachers generating a greater number of referrals, the actual ADHD diagnosis rate remained around 50%, even when stratified by gender or age. This finding challenges the notion that specific reporters are markedly more accurate and is consistent with the recent literature on this topic [24]. However, earlier studies suggest that teacher ratings may surpass parent ratings in terms of sensitivity, specificity, and overall classification accuracy [6]. This could be attributed to the teachers' greater experience in distinguishing age-appropriate behaviors within a school context.

Importantly, due to the retrospective nature of the sample, socio-economic status, ethnicity, and parental education level were not consistently recorded and could not be included in the analysis. We acknowledge this as a significant limitation, as such variables may influence both the behavior of the informants and the clinical presentation of the child. Moreover, the retrospective design inherently introduces a potential referral bias, as the sample was composed exclusively of children who had already been referred for concerns related to attention, behavior, or development. This may limit the representativeness of the findings compared to community-based or screening populations. Additionally, the study was conducted in a single Italian tertiary center, which may affect the generalizability of results to other geographic, cultural, or clinical settings. Future research should aim to replicate these findings in multi-center and prospective samples, ideally incorporating systematic socio-demographic data collection.

Discrepancies between informants are often shaped by two interacting mechanisms: source bias—that is, systematic distortions in the informants' reports based on their expectations, roles, or relationships with the child—and contextual variability, referring to genuine differences in behavior across settings such as the home and school [4,5,8]. These concepts are well established in the multi-informant literature and suggest that the disagreement between sources does not necessarily imply error or noise but may convey clinically meaningful information.

Recent models [8] propose subtyping ADHD presentations based on the context in which symptoms manifest—such as school-only, home-only, or pervasive—arguing that context-specific patterns may have different prognostic and functional implications. Similarly, the "satellite model" described by De Los Reyes et al. [25] emphasizes the value of integrating information from multiple informants not by averaging responses but by recognizing the unique perspective each source provides within its environment. This framework challenges the notion of a single "true" report and instead supports an ecologically grounded interpretation of symptom expression.

In this light, discrepancies between parents and teachers—as observed in our study—may not undermine diagnostic validity but reflect the situational nature of ADHD symptomatology. Clinical practice should therefore move beyond a simplistic reconciliation of differences and toward an informed integration of diverse, context-sensitive data sources.

This dual-informant (parent–teacher) approach enhances the diagnostic process by capturing symptoms across different environments, a critical factor in accurately diagnosing ADHD [23].

However, it should be noted that more than 93% of patients referred for suspected ADHD were ultimately diagnosed with a neuropsychiatric disorder, even if it was not ADHD. This suggests that informants may not necessarily be misreporting in an absolute sense but may instead misinterpret symptoms and categorize them incorrectly. This underscores the value of the reporters' perspectives and emphasizes the need for a more nuanced approach to diagnosis.

These findings highlight relevant practical and policy implications. Firstly, the comparable diagnostic accuracy observed across informants reinforces the importance of systematically integrating both teacher and parent reports during the assessment process. Clinical procedures should include structured multi-informant screening tools to capture symptom consistency across different contexts. Secondly, given the teachers' prominent role in referrals, targeted training programs to enhance teachers' ability to identify ADHD symptoms, especially in under-reported groups such as girls with inattentive presentations, are recommended. Lastly, strengthening collaboration between schools, primary care providers, and specialized services can help streamline referrals, reduce diagnostic delays, and promote timely interventions through clear, multidisciplinary referral pathways.

Author Contributions: Conceptualization, B.C., C.D.B. and M.R.; methodology, D.E.; formal analysis, D.E. and B.C.; investigation, D.E., F.G. and B.C.; data curation, D.E. and F.G.; writing—original draft preparation, D.E. and B.C.; writing—review and editing, D.E., F.G., B.C., C.D.B., F.P. and M.R.; supervision, M.R.; project administration, F.P. All authors have read and agreed to the published version of the manuscript.

Funding: This research received no external funding.

Institutional Review Board Statement: The study was conducted in accordance with the Declaration of Helsinki and approved by the Institutional Review Board (or Ethics Committee) of Sapienza University of Rome (*n* 5365, 27 March 2019).

Informed Consent Statement: Informed consent was obtained from all subjects involved in the study.

Data Availability Statement: The data presented in this study are available on request from the corresponding author. The data are not publicly available due to privacy restrictions.

Conflicts of Interest: The authors declare no conflicts of interest.

References

1. Sayal, K.; Prasad, V.; Daley, D.; Ford, T.; Coghill, D. ADHD in children and young people: Prevalence, care pathways, and service provision. *Lancet Psychiatry* **2018**, *5*, 175–186. [CrossRef]
2. Danielson, M.L.; Claussen, A.H.; Bitsko, R.H.; Katz, S.M.; Newsome, K.; Blumberg, S.J.; Kogan, M.D.; Ghandour, R. ADHD Prevalence Among U.S. Children and Adolescents in 2022: Diagnosis, Severity, Co-Occurring Disorders, and Treatment. *J. Clin. Child Adolesc. Psychol.* **2024**, *53*, 343–360. [CrossRef]
3. De Los Reyes, A.; Kazdin, A.E. Informant Discrepancies in the Assessment of Childhood Psychopathology: A Critical Review, Theoretical Framework, and Recommendations for Further Study. *Psychol. Bull.* **2005**, *131*, 483–509. [CrossRef]
4. Kennerley, S.; Jaquiery, B.; Hatch, B.; Healey, M.; Wheeler, B.J.; Healey, D. Informant discrepancies in the assessment of attention-deficit/hyperactivity disorder. *J. Psychoeduc. Assess.* **2018**, *36*, 136–147. [CrossRef]
5. Narad, M.E.; Garner, A.A.; Peugh, J.L.; Tamm, L.; Antonini, T.N.; Kingery, K.M.; Epstein, J.N. Parent-teacher agreement on ADHD symptoms across development. *Psychol. Assess.* **2015**, *27*, 239–248. [CrossRef]
6. Tripp, G.; Schaughency, E.; Clarke, B. Parent and teacher rating scales in the evaluation of attention-deficit hyperactivity disorder: Contribution to diagnosis and differential diagnosis in clinically referred children. *J. Dev. Behav. Pediatr.* **2006**, *27*, 209–218. [CrossRef]
7. Murray, A.L.; Speyer, L.G.; Hall, H.A.; Valdebenito, S.; Hughes, C. Teacher versus parent informant measurement invariance of the Strengths and Difficulties Questionnaire. *J. Pediatr. Psychol.* **2021**, *46*, 1249–1257. [CrossRef]
8. Murray, A.L.; Ribeaud, D.; Eisner, M.; Murray, G.; McKenzie, K. Should We Subtype ADHD According to the Context in Which Symptoms Occur? Criterion Validity of Recognising Context-Based ADHD Presentations. *Child Psychiatry Hum. Dev.* **2019**, *50*, 308–320. [CrossRef]
9. Ayano, G.; Yohannes, K.; Abraha, M. Epidemiology of attention-deficit/hyperactivity disorder (ADHD) in children and adolescents in Africa: A systematic review and meta-analysis. *Ann. Gen. Psychiatry* **2020**, *19*, 21. [CrossRef]
10. Gaub, M.; Carlson, C.L. Gender differences in ADHD: A meta-analysis and critical review. *J. Am. Acad. Child Adolesc. Psychiatry* **1997**, *36*, 1036–1045. [CrossRef]
11. Rucklidge, J. Gender differences in attention-deficit/hyperactivity disorder. *Psychiatr. Clin. N. Am.* **2010**, *33*, 357–373. [CrossRef]
12. Döpfner, M.; Hautmann, C.; Görtz-Dorten, A.; Klasen, F.; Ravens-Sieberer, U.; The BELLA Study Group. Long-term course of ADHD symptoms from childhood to early adulthood in a community sample. *Eur. Child Adolesc. Psychiatry* **2015**, *24*, 665–673. [CrossRef]
13. Staff, A.I.; Oosterlaan, J.; van der Oord, S.; Hoekstra, P.J.; Vertessen, K.; de Vries, R.; van den Hoofdakker, B.J.; Luman, M. The validity of teacher rating scales for the assessment of ADHD symptoms in the classroom: A systematic review and meta-analysis. *J. Atten. Disord.* **2021**, *25*, 1578–1593. [CrossRef]
14. Meyer, B.J.; Stevenson, J.; Sonuga-Barke, E.J.S. Sex differences in the meaning of parent and teacher ratings of ADHD behaviors: An observational study. *J. Atten. Disord.* **2017**, *24*, 1847–1856. [CrossRef]
15. French, B.; Kelly, A.; Stallard, P. Primary care physicians' knowledge and practices regarding ADHD. *J. Atten. Disord.* **2019**, *23*, 456–464. [CrossRef]
16. Tatlow-Golden, M.; Prihodova, L.; Gavin, B.; Cullen, W.; McNicholas, F. What do general practitioners know about ADHD? Attitudes and knowledge among first-contact gatekeepers: Systematic narrative review. *BMC Fam. Pract.* **2016**, *17*, 129. [CrossRef]

17. Reale, L.; Bonati, M. ADHD prevalence estimates in Italian children and adolescents: A methodological issue. *Ital. J. Pediatr.* **2018**, *44*, 108. [CrossRef]
18. Margari, L.; Buttiglione, M.; Craig, F.; Cristella, A.; de Giambattista, C.; Matera, E.; Operto, F.F.; Simone, M.; Tesei, A. Neuropsychopathological comorbidities in learning disorders. *BMC Neurol.* **2013**, *13*, 198. [CrossRef]
19. Kadesjö, C.; Hägglöf, B.; Kadesjö, B.; Gillberg, C. Attention-deficit-hyperactivity disorder with and without oppositional defiant disorder in 3- to 7-year-old children. *Dev. Med. Child Neurol.* **2003**, *45*, 693–699. [CrossRef] [PubMed]
20. Charles, J.; Fazeli, M. Depression in children. *Aust. Fam. Physician* **2017**, *46*, 901–907. [PubMed]
21. Ramsawh, H.J.; Chavira, D.A.; Stein, M.B. Burden of anxiety disorders in pediatric medical settings: Prevalence, phenomenology, and a research agenda. *Arch. Pediatr. Adolesc. Med.* **2010**, *164*, 965–972. [CrossRef] [PubMed]
22. Bied, A.; Biederman, J.; Faraone, S. Parent-based diagnosis of ADHD is as accurate as a teacher-based diagnosis of ADHD. *Postgrad. Med.* **2017**, *129*, 375–381. [CrossRef] [PubMed]
23. Martel, M.; Schimmack, U.; Nikolas, M.; Nigg, J. Integration of symptom ratings from multiple informants in ADHD diagnosis: A psychometric model with clinical utility. *Psychol. Assess.* **2015**, *27*, 1060–1071. [CrossRef]
24. Tahıllıoğlu, A.; Bilaç, Ö.; Uysal, T.; Ercan, E.S. Who predict ADHD with better diagnostic accuracy?: Parents or teachers? *Nord. J. Psychiatry* **2021**, *75*, 214–223. [CrossRef]
25. Charamut, N.R.; Racz, S.J.; Wang, M.; De Los Reyes, A. Integrating multi-informant reports of youth mental health: A construct validation test of Kraemer and colleagues' (2003) Satellite Model. *Front. Psychol.* **2022**, *13*, 911629. [CrossRef]

children

MDPI

Review

Sleep Disorders in Children with Rett Syndrome

Christopher Harner [1], Thomas A. Gaffey [2], Shannon S. Sullivan [3], Manisha Witmans [4], Lourdes M. DelRosso [5] and Mary Anne Tablizo [3,5,*]

1 College of Science, California State University, Turlock, CA 95382, USA
2 Department of Psychology, University of Notre Dame, Notre Dame, IN 46556, USA; tgaffey@nd.edu
3 Division of Pediatric Pulmonology and Sleep Medicine, Department of Pediatrics, School of Medicine Stanford, Stanford University, Lucile Packard Children's Hospital, Stanford, CA 94305, USA
4 Division of Pulmonology, Department of Pediatrics, University of Alberta, Edmonton, AB T6G 2R3, Canada
5 Division of Sleep Medicine, Department of Internal Medicine, UCSF, Fresno, CA 93701, USA
* Correspondence: mtablizo@stanford.edu

Abstract: Rett syndrome (RTT) is an X-linked neurodevelopmental disorder marked by neurological regression, autonomic dysfunction, seizures, and significant sleep and breathing abnormalities. About 80% of affected individuals, especially young children, experience sleep disturbances such as insomnia, sleep-disordered breathing, nocturnal vocalizations, bruxism, and seizures. Breathing irregularities during sleep—like apnea, alternating hyperventilation, and hypoventilation—are common, with both obstructive and central sleep apnea identified through polysomnography. This review focuses on the prevalent sleep disorders in children with Rett syndrome and highlights current recommendations for the management of sleep disorders.

Keywords: Rett syndrome; neurodevelopmental disorder; sleep disorder

1. Introduction

Rett syndrome (RTT) is a rare, progressive X-linked genetic neurodevelopmental disorder marked by behavioral and neurological regression, dysautonomia, seizures, and motor deficits. The disorder was first described by Dr. Andreas Rett in 1966 [1] and reported in the international community by Hagberg et al. in 1983 [2]. Classic Rett syndrome (RTT) is characterized by four primary neurological criteria: loss of purposeful hand movements, loss of acquired spoken language, an abnormal gait, and stereotypic or repetitive hand movements [3]. Classic RTT is additionally marked by a brief period of normal development, followed by loss of acquired skills such as hand use and speech, deceleration of head growth, and breathing irregularities [3]. Individuals with variant or atypical RTT meet at least 2 of these main neurological criteria, along with 5 out of 11 supportive criteria. Supportive criteria may include symptoms such as bruxism, breathing irregularities while awake, sleep disturbances, abnormal muscle tone, peripheral vasomotor instability, episodes of screaming or inappropriate laughter, scoliosis or kyphosis, cold and small hands and feet, reduced pain sensitivity, intense eye contact, and growth retardation [3]. Among atypical RTT, three subsets may be identified, including a preserved speech variant, a congenital variant, and an early seizure variant [3]. Although RTT predominantly affects females, there are rare cases in males with an additional X chromosome or somatic mosaicism [4].

RTT occurs in approximately 1 in 10,000 live female births [5] and accounts for up to 10% of cases of severe intellectual disability due to genetic causes in females [6].

Sleep disturbance is a critical aspect of the disorder, and understanding sleep in RTT contributes to a comprehensive understanding of this syndrome, given the negative physical and mental health impacts on affected individuals as well as their caregivers. Studies revealed that an estimated 80% of those with RTT experience sleep-related difficulties [7], underscoring the need for effective interventions. These sleep disturbances have negative effects on daytime behavior, cognition, and overall development of the child and contribute significantly to caregiver burden [8].

Despite sleep's significant impact on child development and quality of life, evidence-based treatment options for sleep disorders in pediatric patients with RTT remain limited, with few achieving substantial improvements. This review synthesizes selected peer-reviewed research to examine prevalent sleep disturbances in children with Rett syndrome, objective findings in polysomnography (PSG), current management strategies, and provide evidence-based insights on its management for healthcare providers. Several studies suggested that there are variations in sleep problems associated with mutation type. Hence, we will start by describing the genetic mutations linked with RTT [7].

Articles were chosen based on clinical relevance, recency, and quality of methodology. This work is not intended as a systematic review, but it aims to comprehensively summarize key evidence and practical recommendations. Because of the paucity of evidence and research on RTT, case reports were also included in the treatment of sleep disturbances. This review further highlights the need for more registry-based comprehensive research to develop treatment options for this vulnerable population.

2. Genetics of Rett Syndrome

Pathogenic variants in the MECP2 gene located in the Xq28 chromosomal region were first associated with RTT in 1999. Over 900 mutations (pathogenic and benign) in MECP2 have now been identified, with substantial phenotypic variation [9,10]. The MECP2 gene is a key player in regulating DNA methylation and gene transcription, and thus mutations may have broad downstream consequences [11]. In particular, MECP2 plays important roles in neuronal development, dendritic branching, and brain morphology [12]. Functional impacts of mutations in MECP2 include alterations in synaptic function, neuronal connectivity, and gene expression patterns in brain regions implicated in RTT [13].

Most cases arise sporadically through de novo mutations. MECP2 mutations are associated with a spectrum of clinical presentations, ranging from asymptomatic female carriers with complete skewing of X chromosome inactivation [14] to males who develop severe neonatal-onset encephalopathy [3].

Research studies established that approximately 95% of classical RTT cases and 58–75% of atypical RTT cases have mutations in MECP2 [15]. Recent discoveries have unveiled mutations in loci other than MECP2, which have been linked to atypical RTT [3]. Mutations in genes such as cyclin-dependent kinase-like 5 (CDKL5) and forkhead box G1 (FOXG1) have been implicated in clinical presentations resembling RTT, underscoring the genetic heterogeneity of conditions that share similar clinical features [15,16]. Additionally, MECP2 mutations have also been identified without the clinical features of RTT, and it is important to note that MECP2 mutations are neither necessary nor sufficient for diagnosis, which remains clinical [3].

There is evidence that particular genetic mutations may be associated with heightened sleep dysfunction [17–19], though sleep complaints of one type or another are nearly universal in those with RTT. The associations between particular genetic mutations and specific sleep problems are addressed in the relevant sections of this paper. Understanding the underlying genetics and neurobiology of the disorder may help pave the way for the development of targeted therapies [20] to address specific mechanisms of dysfunction.

3. Sleep Disturbances in Rett Syndrome

Impaired sleep patterns are part of the supportive diagnostic criteria for RTT, and disturbed sleep has been noted from the earliest descriptions of the syndrome [21,22]. In some cases, sleep disturbances may be one of the earliest presenting symptoms. Approximately 80% of children with RTT experience sleep disturbances, with variable occurrence throughout life but generally a higher prevalence [7] in early childhood [17], consistent with the observation that heightened behavioral symptoms occur around the regression period [23]. Sleep disturbance is most prevalent in children up to 7 years of age, with a greater than 90% probability of any sleep disturbance. Thereafter, studies indicate some reduction in sleep disturbance in later childhood and adolescence [24,25]. Sleep disturbances in children with RTT include insomnia (both initiating and maintaining sleep), abnormal breathing in sleep, sleep vocalizations such as laughing and screaming, bruxism, sleep-related seizures, and excessive daytime sleepiness.

3.1. Disturbances in Sleep Initiation and Maintenance

Insomnia, defined as difficulty initiating or maintaining sleep, is a leading sleep disturbance for RTT patients [26–28]. In a study involving caregivers of 364 patients with RTT with confirmed MECP2 mutations, registered in the International Rett Syndrome Phenotype Database (InterRett), who completed the validated Sleep Disturbance Scale for Children (SDSC), findings indicated that over 80% of RTT patients experienced night wakings, and nearly half of this group experienced night wakings often. The median age of this sample was 14.5 years (range: 2.1–57.2 years), all but two were female, and 93.4% lived at home [19]. In this group, over 60% of the patients also experienced difficulty falling asleep. Younger children and those with the p.Arg294 mutation exhibited the most significant difficulties in sleep initiation and maintenance. Recent evidence showed that longer sleep onset latency is associated with impaired daytime interactivity among individuals with RTT which has underscored the important impacts of sleep disturbances on next-day function [29]. In a recent actigraphic study of 29 individuals with RTT and their caregivers, shorter total sleep times (TST), as well as low sleep efficiency, long sleep-onset latency, elevated wake after sleep onset (WASO), and fragmented sleep were demonstrated in both older and younger subjects [30]. A limitation of much of the current literature on sleep in RTT is that although sleep disruptions are commonly reported, associated or co-occurring findings are not well elucidated. At least one expert review reflects that, for example, disrupted sleep patterns may be related to hunger, gastroesophageal reflux, or constipation [31], but such associations have not been systematically measured in most cases.

Difficulty initiating sleep, night waking, and excessive daytime sleepiness in individuals with Rett syndrome (RTT) may be related to abnormalities in circadian rhythm regulation. Clinically, dysregulation of the sleep-wake cycle with delayed sleep onset and daytime sleeping is observed in RTT individuals. A study conducted by Piazza et al. [32] on 20 girls with RTT aged 1–32 years (mean age: 9 years; median age: 8 years) showed increased total sleep, significantly less nighttime sleep, delayed sleep onset, and significantly more daytime sleep. Nighttime sleep duration was negatively correlated with age, while daytime sleep duration was positively correlated with age. These findings suggest that there is almost an inverted pattern of sleep.

Excessive daytime sleepiness with daytime naps has been reported, particularly in older girls and women, likely from disrupted nighttime sleep and delayed sleep phase disorder. The sleep disturbances occurred across age and mutation groups in the Australian population-based sample. The prevalence of daytime napping increased with age [7]. Daytime napping was commonly reported in cases with p.R270X, p.R255X, and p.T158M mutations [7]. In the Boban et al. study described earlier, napping was reported in 42.8% of individuals, with over a third of individuals napping sometimes or often [19].

Evidence indicates that MECP2, CDKL5, and FOXG1 may play a role in regulating specific brain areas and neurotransmitters that affect the sleep-wake cycle [26]. Animal models of RTT have shown highly fragmented sleep and abnormal circadian rhythms with blunting of the circadian cycle [33]. The MECP2 gene is expressed in the suprachiasmatic nucleus, and photic stimulation causes phosphorylation [34]. There may be other genes involved that also affect the circadian rhythm, resulting in disorganization of the entire circadian rhythm both centrally at the suprachiasmatic nucleus as well as peripherally to the organs.

3.2. Abnormal Nocturnal Breathing

The classical respiratory alterations of RTT include breath-holding and irregular breathing, with over 80% of affected individuals experiencing respiratory abnormalities during their lifespans [35]. MECP2 is expressed throughout the brainstem, including regions in the pons and medulla, which is important for control of breathing. It is thought that aberrant MECP2-associated transcriptional control leads to alterations in normal breathing patterns and classical breath-holding, hyperventilation, and overactive expiration in individuals with RTT [35,36]. Additionally, altered chemosensory responsiveness to hypoxia and hypercapnia has been identified in RTT, further complicating abnormal respiratory patterns. It is estimated that 75% of children with RTT develop breath-holding during wakefulness before 6 years of age, with hyperventilation following 2–3 years later [35]. It has been demonstrated that the uncoupling between breathing and heart rate control indicative of autonomic dysregulation is more pronounced in waking than in sleep in girls with RTT with alteration in the MECP2 gene. This dysregulation has been demonstrated in sleep as well and may represent a risk for sudden death in patients with RTT [37]. Abnormal breathing, including apnea, gasping, alternating hyperventilation, and hypoventilation, is common during sleep [38,39] in RTT, although there is variability between individuals and over time within individuals [40]. Polysomnography studies in RTT have shown both obstructive and central sleep apnea along with associated hypoxia (Figure 1A and B) [11].

In addition to respiratory control abnormalities, characteristics such as low tone may influence craniofacial development and scoliosis, which can complicate abnormal breathing in sleep. Abnormal breathing may lead to sleep fragmentation and awakenings, which exacerbate symptoms of insomnia and daytime symptoms, including mood and behavioral dysfunction. In one study, parents noted a greater impact of breathing abnormalities for individuals with the p.Arg294* variant [41], though the genetic variant did not seem to modify the Rett Syndrome Behaviour Questionnaire (RSBQ) score in another study [22].

3.3. Other Sleep Abnormalities (Vocalizations, Abnormal Movements, Bruxism, and Nocturnal Seizures)

Sleep-related vocalizations, movements, and bruxism are routinely observed in RTT. Among children with RTT in the 0–7-year age group, night laughing and night screaming have been reported to be extremely common, occurring at rates of 77% and 49%, respectively [24], with the prevalence and frequency of night laughter and screaming more likely in genotypes involving a large deletion of the MECP2 gene. After adjusting for age, the likelihood of experiencing any sleep disturbance was highest in individuals with large deletions (94%) and p.R270X (92%) and p.R294X (91%) mutations. Night laughing was especially prevalent in individuals with large deletions (90%) and the p.R168X mutation (78%), while persistent night laughing was moderately common among those with p.R106W (49%) and p.R168X (42%) mutations. Night screaming was most frequently reported in individuals with the p.R270X (57%), p.R306C (51%), and large deletion (51%) mutations [24].

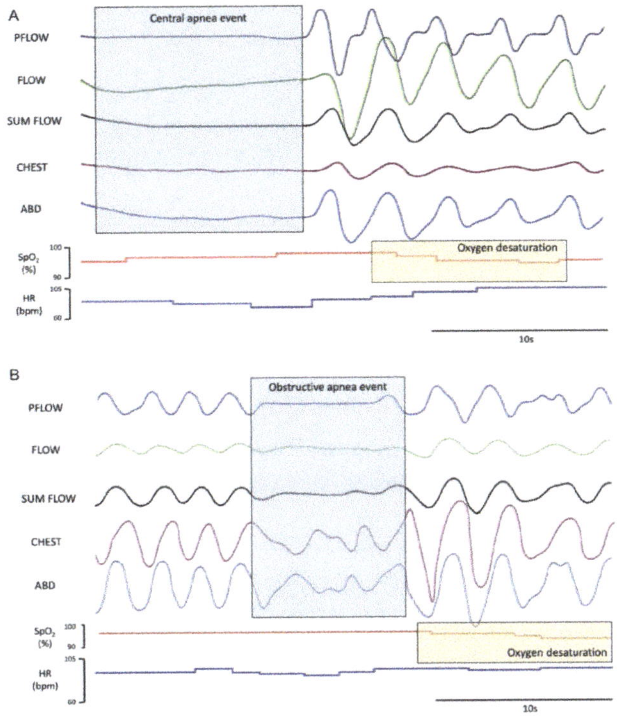

Figure 1. Sleep-disordered breathing in RTT [35]. Polysomnography studies on RTT have shown both obstructive (**B**) and central sleep apnea (**A**) with associated hypoxia [35].

Similarly, in the Boban et al. study described above, of 364 caregivers of individuals with RTT with a median age of 14.5 years, night laughing was reported for 58% of them, while night screaming, at 47.5% was slightly less commonly reported [19], and nocturnal bruxism (teeth grinding) was experienced by more than two thirds of individuals. Longitudinal evidence indicates some reduction in these symptoms over time, though persistence is common, especially among those with more severe and frequent symptoms at baseline [24].

Seizures are another common occurrence in RTT, with epilepsy occurring in 48–90% of affected individuals [42,43]. Nocturnal seizures may become more evident in later childhood or early adolescence [44], and seizure activity may be refractory and can become severe, including nocturnal electrical status epilepticus [45]. Boban et al. reported a rate of 52.8% of RTT individuals indicating the occurrence of nocturnal seizures, with 10.7% experiencing nocturnal seizures often. Patients with severe seizure activity were noted to be more likely to have poor sleep quality, suggesting that management of comorbidities is needed [19,26].

4. Sleep Impacts on Mental and Behavioral Health and Quality of Life

Addressing sleep disturbances is crucial, as they significantly impact mental and behavioral health in individuals with RTT. Insomnia and excessive daytime sleepiness showed the strongest associations with overall RSBQ scores and subscales related to mood, breathing, nighttime behaviors, and anxiety, reflecting the critical role of sleep in behavioral and mental health in RTT. Poor sleep negatively affects both mental health and quality of life [17]. Furthermore, both insomnia and daytime sleepiness have strong relationships with the RSBQ general mood subscale, as well as nighttime behaviors, breathing problems, and fear and anxiety subscales [17]. This link between sleep dysfunction and behavioral and emotional status in RTT is consistent with other studies, including evidence from the International Rett Syndrome Database demonstrating a relationship between poor sleep (insomnia and excessive daytime sleepiness) and heightened anxiety among 210 individuals with RTT aged 6–51 years [18]. Sleep disturbances in RTT also have a profound impact on overall quality of life. Longitudinal evidence indicates that quality of life in RTT has also been shown to be linked to sleep, with increased sleep disturbances associated with quality of life reduction [46]. Frequent sleep disturbances in individuals with RTT have been linked to later lower caregiver well-being scores [47], highlighting the long-term burden that disrupted sleep can place on families. In a recent study evaluating the frequency of sleep symptoms and burden on RTT individuals and their caregivers, sleep disturbances were again reported to be common (with 71.8% reporting sleep disturbances), but notably, the burden of illness was measured to be high for caregivers, being almost twice the rate for individuals with RTT, even though the overall symptoms were rated to be of mild-to-moderate severity. The authors concluded that the burden of sleep disturbances for caregivers was disproportionate to clinical severity [47]. Another explanation could be that clinical severity may be misrepresented based on the aspects that were evaluated.

5. Sleep Measurement and Objective Findings in Rett Syndrome

Common measures of sleep in children with RTT include sleep diaries (filled out by caregivers or family members), actigraphy, and in-lab polysomnography. Both sleep diaries and actigraphy offer the advantage of measuring sleep-wake cycles across many nights, commonly 2–3 weeks or longer. Although both sleep diaries and actigraphy [48] have been used to assess sleep in individuals with RTT, recently, the discordance between sleep diaries and actigraphy has been investigated, indicating 14.8% bedtime discordance and 22.6% wake time discordance of 45 min or greater between the two methods [49]. In the sample of 38 individuals (aged 2–26 years, mean of 13.1 years), missing data (instances where either diary entries or actigraphy data were incomplete or unavailable) were also common. Greater levels of missing data and discrepancies between diary-reported and actigraphy-recorded sleep patterns were correlated with higher clinical severity of Rett syndrome symptoms and a lower reported quality of life. The direction of difference between diaries and actigraphy was variable, and the study highlights limitations for both types of longitudinal sleep measures.

In contrast, polysomnography allows objective measurement of sleep features in a laboratory setting and is important for the detection of co-occurring parasomnia, sleep fragmentation, seizure activity and sleep-related breathing dysfunction and for identifying sleep or wake status and sleep architecture. Because studies are performed in a laboratory setting, some sleep features such as sleep onset latency and nighttime wakings may not reflect routine experience in the home setting. In addition, one night of monitoring may also not provide sufficient information for this complex sleep-wake dysregulation.

Polysomnography studies in RTT have shown both obstructive and central sleep apnea along with associated hypoxia (Figure 1). In a small polysomnography study of 13 pediatric patients (mean age: 10 years) with RTT, all individuals exhibited episodes of hyperpnea followed by pauses while awake, and 9 of the subjects had obstructive sleep apnea (OSA) with a mean AHI of 8.77 ± 8.82. Among these, 4 of these patients had severe OSA, and 1 had severe OSA combined with central apnea. The most common presenting symptoms were snoring (77%) and witnessed apnea (53.8%) [50]. In a larger study aggregating PSG data from 11 studies meeting eligibility criteria and reporting on 69 individuals with RTT and a mean age of $8.9 +/- 5.2$ years, the mean AHI was found to be 12.25 ± 23.89, roughly split between central and obstructive apneas, with an oxygen desaturation index of 18.62 ± 31.9 [51]. Epilepsy and scoliosis appeared to be common in this study group, though data on these co-occurring conditions were missing for nearly half the aggregated sample.

Polysomnographic recordings in RTT also indicate reduced sleep efficiency and differences in sleep architecture, in addition to the breathing abnormalities discussed above. In the aggregated sample of 69 individuals with RTT and published PSG data, sleep efficiency (SE), which represents the percentage of time asleep from lights off to lights on in a laboratory setting, was reduced compared with same-age typically developing individuals, and impaired sleep continuity was also reported [51]. PSG evidence of disrupted sleep in children with RTT has also been reported by Carotenuto et al., who used a case-control approach for 13 individuals with RTT (mean age: 8.1; SD: +/− 1.4 years) and found significantly increased stage shifts per hour, awakenings per hour (averaging 6.3 versus 1.9 awakenings per hour in unaffected individuals), and elevated Wake After Sleep Onset (WASO) rates [52]. Similarly, SE was reported to be reduced in a study of 17 girls (mean age: 9.5 ± 2.8 years) [40] at 66 ± 19%, with only 3 girls presenting SE values above 80%, and WASO was also elevated.

Sleep architecture in RTT has also been reported to be altered, characterized by a decrease in rapid eye movement (REM) and a commensurate increase in non-REM (NREM) sleep, particularly N3 (slow wave), though concomitant sleep breathing disorders were seen in this study group, with a mean apnea-hypopnea index of 19 ± 37 events per hour [38]. Zhang and Spruyt, in their aggregated report on 74 PSGs of RTT individuals across 11 studies, also found increased N3 sleep and reductions in REM sleep, hypothesizing that aberrant sleep cycling, possibly associated with a poor REM "on switch" and preponderance in slow and high-voltage sleep, characterizes sleep in RTT. However, in this study, concomitant sleep-disordered breathing was also quite common, and the authors reported a mean AHI of 11.92 ± 23.67/h in these aggregated cases [51]. The increase in the percentage of slow-wave sleep in these reports contrasts with an earlier report on reduced slow-wave sleep in RTT (though increased delta power was observed within N3 sleep cycles) involving a retrospective case-control study of 10 girls with RTT (age range: 2–9 years) [53]. SE was again reduced in RTT compared with the unaffected girls.

Elevated periodic limb movements (PLMs) have also been noted in PSG, with Carentuto reporting an elevated mean periodic limb movement index (PLMI) in 13 girls with RTT compared with matched controls, with the girls with RTT having a PLMI of 9.5 events per hour, compared with 2.8 events per hour for the controls [38,52].

Recent work by Davis et al. (2023) [54] identified altered phase-amplitude coupling (PAC) during slow-wave sleep (SWS) as a potential circuit-level biomarker of sleep-wake dysregulation. In a cohort of children with RTT, PAC between slow-wave and theta (SW:T) and slow-wave and spindle (SW:S) activity showed disrupted topography, with ectopic coupling outside the typical vertex region. This abnormal coupling pattern was not only distinct from typically developing controls but also correlated positively with overall clinical severity, as measured by the Clinical Global Impression-Severity scale, which assesses communication, motor function, seizures, and autonomic features. These findings suggest that altered SWS dynamics may reflect broader neurodevelopmental impairment in RTT and could serve as a noninvasive biomarker for disease severity and progression [54].

Heart rate variability in Rett syndrome, as observed via PSG, is characterized by reduced overall variability and a shift toward sympathetic dominance and vagal withdrawal. This was demonstrated in a 2024 study where individuals with RTT exhibited a consistent shift in sympatho-vagal balance toward sympathetic dominance and vagal withdrawal during both wakefulness and all sleep stages. This alteration in autonomic regulation in RTT has potential implications for cardiovascular health. These findings underscore the need for further research to explore the broader physiological and clinical consequences of this dysautonomia [55].

Taken together, objective findings based on PSG in individuals with RTT demonstrated significant sleep abnormalities and poor sleep quality. Common findings include reduced SE, increased arousals and WASO, elevated PLMs, increased N3 and disrupted sleep architecture, with diminished REM sleep. Abnormal breathing patterns—characterized by episodes of hyperpnea and apnea and both obstructive and central apneas with associated hypoxemia—are also frequently observed. These findings underscore the pervasive and multifaceted nature of sleep-disordered breathing in RTT.

6. Sleep-Directed Therapies

Overall management approaches in RTT involve addressing symptoms and, when possible, preventing progression. Therapies for RTT involve multiple systems and targets and are reviewed in detail elsewhere [31], though it is worth noting that some therapies targeting other disease manifestations may themselves have influences on sleep (for example, antiepileptic or mood-targeted medications). In March 2023, trofinetide, a synthetic analog of a naturally occurring brain peptide and insulin-like growth factor 1 (IGF-1)-related compound thought to act on NMDA receptors, was approved by the United States Food and Drug Administration (FDA) [56] for treating children aged 2 years or older, and there are several other agents currently in clinical trials [57,58]. Trials of trofinetide have demonstrated good efficacy in improving scores on the Clinical Global Impression-Improvement scale and RSBQ, with a specific effect only on the General Mood subscale and Repetitive Face Movement subscale, but no effects were documented on other subscales [59]. While sleep-specific outcomes were not primary endpoints in trofinetide's clinical trials, improvements in Rett Syndrome Behavior Questionnaire (RSBQ) subscales—particularly general mood and nighttime behaviors—suggest potential indirect benefits for sleep. A 2023 review by Bricker and Vaughn also described a case report in which a patient with RTT experienced sleep improvement after initiating trofinetide, though the authors noted that further studies are needed to evaluate trofinetide's direct effects on sleep in this population [60].

Managing sleep complaints and disorders in RTT requires both a pragmatic and multimodal approach, including behavioral therapies, appropriate medications, and addressing co-morbid conditions that impact sleep. These strategies should be age-based and focused on enhancing sleep consistency and stability, as well as quality and daytime status. Despite growing interest in effective interventions for sleep disorders in RTT, an outcome-driven evidence base for specific sleep-targeted therapies in RTT is sparse, hindering definitive treatment algorithms. At least one observational study using data from 320 families in the Australian Rett Syndrome Database examined the long-term management of sleep disturbances in Rett syndrome over a 12-year period. Despite limitations—such as missing data on specific sleep disorders (e.g., napping, seizures, apnea, and bruxism), potential overestimation of prevalence, and limited assessment of treatment effectiveness the study highlights the persistent and burdensome nature of sleep disturbances in RTT. It also reveals that clinical management remains inconsistent and largely based on clinician experience, emphasizing the need for individualized care strategies [24].

More recently, expert-led consensus guidelines for primary providers on managing RTT was published in 2020 [61], and comprehensive care guidelines, which include recommendations for sleep, can also be found on the International Rett Syndrome Foundation (IRSF) website [62]. The 2020 guidelines indicate that at a baseline visit and every six months, care providers for patients with RTT should review sleep onset and maintenance, respiratory symptoms, and the frequency of nocturnal interventions by caregivers, as well as review bed and bedroom safety [61]. Similarly, IRSF guidelines recommend screening for disrupted sleep by asking specific questions about bedtime, the time required to fall asleep, wake time, nocturnal awakenings, sleep disturbances, and the sleep environment [62] The IRSF guidelines also recommend screening for snoring, respiratory pauses, gasping, restless sleep, and abnormal behaviors and recommend referring to a specialist as appropriate [62]. Additional details on treatments for specific sleep conditions are summarized below.

6.1. Disturbances in Sleep Initiation and Maintenance

Behavioral strategies remain the cornerstone of managing sleep disturbances and insomnia and are considered first-line treatments. Given the high prevalence of sleep disturbances in individuals with RTT, foundational interventions such as establishing consistent bedtime routines with regular bedtimes and wake times and optimizing the sleep environment—minimizing noise, reducing light exposure, and maintaining a cooler and comfortable room temperature—are essential. While these interventions have not been rigorously studied specifically in the RTT population, they are widely used and serve as a key starting point for addressing sleep disturbances, especially in pediatric neurodevelopmental disorders [63,64]. In addition, consistent exposure to morning light, reducing maladaptive sleep associations, reinforcing limit-setting behaviors, and promoting structured daytime routines that incorporate physical activity and regular meals help promote normal sleep [26,44].

If daytime naps are employed, which may be age-appropriate or a useful tool for excessive daytime sleepiness, then they should be scheduled as part of a routine and undertaken while considering nocturnal sleep patterns [32]. Detailed sleep hygiene and behavioral sleep strategies are available [65,66], and it is important to note that in children with RTT, some trial and error of what works best and individualized care for each child may be necessary to find optimal strategies. In a report by Boban et al. which analyzed caregiver responses for 364 RTT individuals, including 274 taking no medications for sleep, sleep behavioral and hygiene strategies were employed by approximately two thirds of their families, and better use of sleep hygiene practices was associated with significantly lower odds of moderate or major impacts on the family (odds ratio: 0.60; 95% confidence interval: 0.37–0.98) and lower scores for disordered initiation and maintenance of sleep [28]. Similarly, in an older small study on three individuals with RTT, the behavioral strategy of bedtime fading was effective in advancing bedtime and promoting more regular sleep patterns by increasing the appropriate nighttime sleep duration, reducing inappropriate daytime sleep, and reducing problematic nighttime behaviors (e.g., nocturnal awakenings) [32]. This experience is reinforced by retrospective analysis indicating that among children with rare genetic neurodevelopmental disorders, implementing behavioral strategies improved sleep disturbances in the substantial majority of the patients studied, and improvements were maintained at long-term follow-up [67,68]. In RTT in particular, qualitative studies involving caregivers have indicated that a stable sleep routine improves sleep disturbance in individuals with RTT and establishes daily routines with reduced daytime stress [67].

While sleep hygiene is foundational, and behavioral therapy is accepted as first-line therapy for sleep disturbances, not all individuals with RTT will achieve adequate sleep without additional intervention, and pharmacological intervention may be considered. Given that individuals with RTT may also have respiratory abnormalities, abnormal cardiorespiratory autonomic function, and prolonged QTc intervals, caution is advised regarding safety when selecting pharmacologic agents for sleep disturbances [63].

The use of melatonin in RTT for sleep dysfunction was first reported several decades ago in a study on 4 weeks of oral melatonin administration at a dose of 2.5–7.5 mg (depending on body weight) among nine subjects with RTT in a placebo-controlled randomized crossover trial [69]. In this study, sleep onset latency (SOL) was reduced by 19.1 +/− 5.3 min, and the total sleep time (TST) and SE improved in those with worse baseline values. It should also be noted that the majority of the girls in this study were concomitantly taking anti-epileptic medications. More recently, the use of melatonin was reported to be associated with significantly improved sleep quality in RTT children in a survey study including 287 parent respondents [27]. It is worth noting that in the United States, melatonin supplements are available over the counter, and recent studies indicate large discrepancies between the labeled and actual melatonin content of many commercially available products. For example, one study found a range of actual content of melatonin that was 74–347% of the labeled content for 25 melatonin gummy products [70].

A variety of prescription medications (see Table 1) have also been reported for sleep disturbances in RTT, though little evidence exists to support specific pharmacologic therapies, and no evidence-based guidelines exist. Despite the lack of evidence, prescribing medications to help manage sleep symptoms on an individual basis is relatively common [71]. Medications used off-label and reported in RTT patients to manage sleep symptoms include (not in order of preference) clonidine, an α2-adrenoreceptor agonist; GABA-agonists such as clonazepam or zolpidem; and gabapentin [4]. Notably, clonidine and some other sedating agents may pose cardiac risks in individuals with Rett syndrome, particularly those with MECP2 mutations. These risks include QT interval prolongation, which can increase the likelihood of life-threatening arrhythmias and has been implicated in cases of sudden unexpected death in RTT. Trazodone, an atypical antidepressant that inhibits the uptake of serotonin and also has antihistamine activity and α1-adrenergic antagonism, may have the risk of QTc-interval prolongation [63], a consideration in RTT. Consensus guidelines for the care of RTT have suggested the consideration of melatonin to assist with the initiation of sleep and trazodone or clonidine to help maintain sleep [61]. Boban et al.'s survey conducted among 364 caregivers of children with RTT found that overall, 90 were on sleep medications, with the most common being 42 individuals on melatonin (either alone or as polytherapy), while 14 (3.9%) were on clonidine monotherapy, 12 (3.3%) were on trazodone monotherapy, with 15 (4.1%) reporting other medications for sleep (clonazepam, as well as other benzodiazepines and GABA-agonist hypnotics, chloral hydrate, diazepam, oxazepam, antihistamines such as diphenhydramine, cyproheptadine, hydroxyzine, antiepileptics, antipsychotics, antidepressants, and others including dextromethorphan, baclofen, magnesium, and medicinal cannabis), and 21 (5.8%) were on polytherapy [28]. The specifics on approaches for considering the more commonly encountered of these therapies are available [63,72], and consideration of off-target impacts and side effects in light of individual co-existing conditions is key. Other sedating medications such as atypical antipsychotics, antidepressants, antihistamines, and chloral hydrate are used less frequently but have been reported in children with neurodevelopmental disorders, particularly in cases of refractory insomnia [63]. An older study of the supplement L-carnitine reported an impact on sleep in RTT in an open-label trial with 21 girls and women with RTT (age range: 7–41 years; mean age of 14.4 years and median age of 10 years) compared with a control group of 62 individuals with Rett of a similar age for a 6 month period. Compared with the controls, treatment with L-carnitine led to significant improvements in sleep efficiency ($p = 0.027$), especially in the subjects with a baseline sleep efficiency of less than 90% [73]. In this investigation, daytime energy levels also improved. However, a follow-up investigation involving L-carnitine for sleep is lacking.

Pharmacology and considerations for the use of these agents have been published, though overall, there is little evidence for outcomes, and the likelihood of adverse events [63,71] must be evaluated [4]. Specialist involvement is recommended in approaching prescription medication management.

Managing co-existing conditions is an important aspect of improving sleep quality and insomnia symptoms. Evaluation and treatment of co-existing GERD and gastrointestinal dysmotility and constipation, which are incredibly common in RTT [74], as well as anxiety and mood disturbance, nocturnal breathing abnormalities, and restless legs syndrome, may contribute significantly to improved sleep quality. Alongside this awareness is the possibility that certain medications used to manage comorbid conditions may further impact sleep, sometimes negatively. Effective management of these medical issues, coupled with physician awareness of the potential sleep-related side effects of prescribed therapies, is essential for improving overall sleep outcomes.

Managing mood disturbances can significantly improve sleep. One case report [75] suggests the utility of selective serotonin reuptake inhibitors (SSRIs) in combination with a serotonin 1A agonist to manage mood issues and self-aggressiveness. One case report involved an 11-year-old girl with RTT who presented with a year-long history of sleep disturbances and self-harming behaviors. She had severe sleep disturbances, often sleeping only 4 h/night, which did not improve while on anti-migraine, anti-epileptic medications, risperidone, olanzapine, or clonidine. A trial of escitalopram yielded immediate improvements, with reduced self-harm and improved sleep (11 h nightly) lasting 3 months. However, SSRI-induced bruxism emerged, necessitating a dose reduction, which worsened behavioral issues and sleep disturbances [75].

6.2. Sleep-Related Movement Disorders

Sleep-related movement disorders, particularly restless legs syndrome (RLS), warrant consideration in the sleep evaluation of individuals with RTT, especially given the high prevalence of iron deficiency in this population. Expert consensus guidelines and those from the International Rett Syndrome Foundation recommend laboratory assessment for iron status, including fasting ferritin, serum iron, total iron-binding capacity, and transferrin saturation, when symptoms suggestive of RLS are present [61,62]. RLS is characterized by an urge to move the legs at rest, often accompanied by unpleasant sensations, with symptoms worsening in the evening and improving with movement, yet in young children, non-verbal children, or children with RTT, diagnosing RLS presents unique challenges, in which case supportive factors such as behaviors observed by the parent or caregiver, family history of RLS, personal history of anemia, and periodic limb movements of sleep (PLMS) on polysomnography may provide support for the diagnosis of pediatric RLS [76]. Importantly, iron deficiency is a known risk factor for RLS, and studies on RTT have reported iron deficiency anemia or depleted ferritin levels in up to 20% of individuals with RETT, further supporting routine screening [77]. The current guidelines for the treatment of RLS in children recommend iron supplementation as a first-line treatment [78].

6.3. Sleep-Related Breathing Disorders

Fu et al. recommended conducting an overnight sleep study for RTT individuals with snoring or pauses in breathing [61]. More recently, Italian expert consensus guidance on managing respiratory complications of RTT likewise states that nocturnal polygraphy and transcutaneous carbon dioxide monitoring are indicated in patients with congenital RTT and all RTT individuals presenting one or more of the following symptoms: snoring, obstructive apnea, hypotonia, or scoliosis [79]. If disordered breathing is identified, Cherchi et al. recommend noninvasive ventilation as tolerated, with consideration of noninvasive ventilation for all RTT patients with sleep respiratory disorders and those with hypotonia with associated hypercapnia. Beyond noninvasive ventilation, other therapeutic options have been contemplated [79]. For example, in light of the high degree of variability in breathing abnormalities even in the same individuals over time, it has been suggested that adenotonsillectomy be considered for sleep-related breathing disorders even when obstructive apneas do not predominate if they are present, and this therapy appeared to be reasonably common among children with RTT referred to a sleep specialist in a single-center retrospective chart review study [39,50]. That said, adenotonsillectomy is not fully curative, and persistent abnormal breathing has been reported [38].

Other reported therapies include medications such as acetazolamide and nasal steroids [50]. A retrospective study examined the use of acetazolamide, a carbonic anhydrase inhibitor, for treating SRBD in two patients. Both started at 5 mg/kg/dose, with serum bicarbonate levels monitored weekly, targeting ~15 mEq/L. The first patient, with an AHI of 21.2 events/h (mostly obstructive but suspected to have a central component), showed complete resolution of respiratory events (AHI: 0.3) after 17 months and no longer required daytime naps. The second patient, treated for breath-holding spells and nighttime apnea, initially required a dose increase to 8 mg/kg/dose (250 mg) to stabilize bicarbonate levels at 19 mEq/L. The breathing abnormalities resolved, and acetazolamide was stopped after 3 years of clinical improvement [50]. In the same retrospective study, a patient with mild OSA (OAHI: 2.8) was treated with nasal mometasone spray for one year, leading to improved snoring and reduced daytime naps. Despite no change in AHI on a repeat PSG three years later, the patient remained symptom-free [50].

SSRIs have also shown potential in improving respiratory abnormalities during sleep and wakefulness in individuals with RTT. Rodent models suggest that SSRIs can induce MECP2 gene expression and restore CO_2 chemosensitivity, which is impaired in RTT patients [80]. In Mecp2-null male mice, citalopram (an SSRI) restored CO_2 sensitivity, highlighting a therapeutic approach for RTT-related respiratory issues. While research studies on the use of SSRIs in RTT are lacking, case reports indicate promising results. In one case, an 11-year-old girl with hyperventilation and apneic attacks was successfully treated with 10 mg fluoxetine (an SSRI) twice daily, which significantly reduced hyperventilation and breath-holding episodes, and further improvement occurred after adding buspirone [81]. Another case reported on an 11-year-old female RTT patient with severe respiratory symptoms, including frequent apneic events during sleep, who was treated with tandospirone (a 5-HT1A agonist) and fluvoxamine (an SSRI) and experienced reduced apneic events, improved hand stereotypy, and reduced dysphagia [82]. These findings suggest that serotonergic agents may help address respiratory issues and associated behaviors in RTT linked to impaired serotonergic brain transmission. However, formal research studies are needed to confirm their efficacy.

This finding highlights a potential therapeutic approach for addressing respiratory abnormalities in RTT. As breathing disorders are common in RTT, increased interest in these agents has arisen [4].

Finally, research into neuromodulation suggests that substances that enhance GABAergic mechanisms may reduce breath-holding events and breathing irregularities in RTT and may restore chemosensitivity [35,80,83], suggesting promising avenues for the future.

6.4. Additional Recommendations

Given that individuals with Rett syndrome (RTT) may live into the fifth decade of life [84], often with a wide range of complex medical comorbidities—including autonomic dysregulation, motor impairments, epilepsy, swallowing difficulties, sleep disturbances, respiratory abnormalities, and gastrointestinal and orthopedic complications—there is a critical need to improve care strategies aimed at enhancing the quality of life for affected individuals.

Non-pharmacological strategies to manage problematic sleep in children with developmental disabilities, including RTT, are increasingly recognized as essential components of care. A comprehensive review by Spruyt and Curfs [85] evaluated 90 studies involving over 1400 children, with nearly half of the studies focusing on syndromes such as RTT. The most common interventions included bedtime routines, sleep scheduling, behavioral reinforcement techniques, and environmental adjustments such as sleep hygiene and sleep ecology. The review also highlighted the benefit of modifying the sleep environment (e.g., weighted materials, sensory-friendly bedding, and dim lighting) to promote continuous and effective sleep. Sleep ecology—including use of textured blankets, swaddling, and protective railings—was addressed in 21 studies, with success reported in two-thirds of them. Importantly, individualized interventions in the home setting were the most commonly reported and successful ones [85].

A recent preclinical study by Hung et al. demonstrated that music-based interventions improved social behavior and modulated neurobiological pathways in *mecp2* null/y mice, a model of RTT [86]. It also improved breathing patterns, and decreased the frequency of epileptic seizures. Specifically, mice exposed to daily music sessions showed enhanced social novelty behaviors and increased expression of brain-derived neurotrophic factor (BDNF) mRNA in the prefrontal cortex, along with elevated BDNF protein levels in the hippocampus. The intervention also upregulated FNDC5 gene expression, a known upstream modulator of BDNF, independent of TrkB signaling. These findings suggest that music may ameliorate RTT-associated social deficits through neuroplastic mechanisms involving BDNF/FNDC5 pathways. Although further studies in humans are needed, this study supports incorporating music-based therapies as a complementary approach to enhance social functioning, improve breathing pattern and emotional regulation in individuals with RTT and potentially alleviate sleep disturbances in individuals with Rett Syndrome.

Although a definitive cure for Rett syndrome (RTT) remains elusive, recent advancements in gene therapy have opened promising avenues for treatment. Approaches aimed at restoring normal *MECP2* gene function—the primary gene implicated in RTT—are showing particular promise, including the potential to improve associated sleep disturbances. In addition, ongoing research into pharmacological therapies targeting downstream pathways affected by *MECP2* mutations offers hope for symptom relief and meaningful improvements in quality of life for individuals with RTT [16].

Table 1. Medications used on RTT patients based on small studies, parent surveys, and case reports.

Drug Name	Class or Mechanism	Common Indication	Evidence in RTT Studies	Considerations in RTT
Melatonin	Synthetic exogenous hormone; regulates circadian rhythm	Insomnia, delayed sleep phase onset	Most commonly used in RTT based on parent survey [27,28]. One randomized crossover trial showed decreased SE and increased TST [69].	OTC, variable dosing practices
Clonidine	α2-adrenergic agonist	FDA approved for ADHD, >6 years old; off label for insomnia, RLS: indicated for antihypertensive in adults	Often used off-label as sedative in neurodevelopmental disorders [4,28].	Can lower blood pressure

Table 1. *Cont.*

Drug Name	Class or Mechanism	Common Indication	Evidence in RTT Studies	Considerations in RTT
Trazodone	Serotonin antagonist and reuptake inhibitor	Antidepressant for adults, off-label for insomnia	Mild sedative effects; discussed in behavioral comorbidity context [28,61].	QTc prolongation risk; priapism, limited pediatric data [63,68]; no FDA indication for pediatric patients
Gabapentin	GABA analog	Anticonvulsant, RLS, neuropathic pain, off -label for insomnia	Occasionally used as sedative for comorbid conditions in RTT with RLS and seizures; few data specific to pediatric RTT [4].	Sedation and mood effects should be monitored [4]
Clonazepam, diazepam, oxazepam	Benzodiazepine; GABA-A receptor agonist	Anticonvulsant, insomnia, anxiety, muscle relaxant	Based on parent survey, for dual use as sedative and for epilepsy management [4,28].	Dependence risk; respiratory depression in high doses [4]
Diphenhydramine	First-generation antihistamine	Allergies, off label OTC sleep aid	Based on parent survey, used as sedating option in refractory insomnia in 1 study [28].	Can cause paradoxical agitation; not for chronic use [28]
Hydroxyzine	First-generation antihistamine	Sedation premedication for procedure, anxiety, pruritus (approved for pediatric use)	Based on parent survey, used for insomnia [28].	Hypersedation, stupor, nausea, and vomiting
Cyproheptadine	Antihistamine	Allergies, appetite stimulant	Based on parent survey, used for insomnia [28].	Daytime sleepiness, weight gain
Escitalopram	SSRI	Antidepressant for >12 years old, general anxiety disorder for adults	One case report shows dramatic sleep and mood improvement in RTT [75].	Bruxism reported; dosing must be carefully titrated
Carnitine	Amino acid and nutritional supplement	Nutritional supplement	Open-label trial with 21 subjects showing improved SE and TST [73].	Older study and no follow up, 2001
Trofinetide	Synthetic analog of a naturally occurring brain peptide; insulin-like growth factor 1 [63,64]	Indicated for RTT for >2 years old; proposed mechanism of action is to promote synaptic maturation	Improved scores on RSBQ and clinical Global Impression Improvement scale. One case report with sleep improvement [59].	No direct evidence of improved sleep

These medications were used off-label and with no evidence to support their pharmacologic use in RTT. Their use should be carefully tailored to individual patient needs and comorbidities and monitored by clinicians familiar with RTT.

7. Conclusions

Children with RTT face a significantly increased risk of sleep disturbances, which impact not only the affected children but also their caregivers. These sleep issues underscore the need for further research to develop patient-specific treatments, particularly in the era of precision medicine. Sleep-related disturbances in RTT are diverse, necessitating interventions that address multiple aspects of sleep dysfunction [32]. By unraveling these complexities, researchers, clinicians, and families can work collaboratively to advance our understanding of the disorder and pave the way for more effective diagnostic, therapeutic, and supportive interventions. As we continue to learn more about RTT, we inch closer to improving the lives of those affected by this condition by improving their sleep.

Author Contributions: Conceptualization: C.H., T.A.G., S.S.S., M.W. and M.A.T.; methodology C.H., T.A.G., S.S.S. and M.A.T.; formal analysis C.H., T.A.G., S.S.S., M.W., L.M.D. and M.A.T.; investigation C.H., T.A.G., S.S.S., M.W., L.M.D. and M.A.T.; data curation C.H., T.A.G., S.S.S., M.W., L.M.D. and M.A.T.; writing—original draft preparation C.H., T.A.G., S.S.S., M.W. and M.A.T.; writing—review and editing C.H., T.A.G., S.S.S., M.W., L.M.D. and M.A.T.; visualization C.H., T.A.G., S.S.S., M.W., L.M.D. and M.A.T.; supervision S.S.S. and M.A.T.; project administration S.S.S., M.W. and M.A.T.; funding acquisitio no funding needed. All authors have read and agreed to the published version of the manuscript.

Funding: This research received no external funding.

Conflicts of Interest: The authors declare no conflict of interest.

References

1. Rett, A. On a unusual brain atrophy syndrome in hyperammonemia in childhood. *Wien. Med. Wochenschr.* **1966**, *116*, 723–726. [PubMed]
2. Dunn, H.G. Importance of Rett syndrome in child neurology. *Brain Dev.* **2001**, *23*, S38–S43. [CrossRef] [PubMed]
3. Neul, J.L.; Kaufmann, W.E.; Glaze, D.G.; Christodoulou, J.; Clarke, A.J.; Bahi-Buisson, N.; Leonard, H.; Bailey, M.E.S.; Schanen, N.C.; Zappella, M.; et al. Rett syndrome: Revised diagnostic criteria and nomenclature. *Ann. Neurol.* **2010**, *68*, 944–950. [CrossRef] [PubMed]
4. Persico, A.M.; Ricciardello, A.; Cucinotta, F. The psychopharmacology of autism spectrum disorder and Rett syndrome. *Handb. Clin. Neurol.* **2019**, *165*, 391–414. [CrossRef]
5. Laurvick, C.L.; de Klerk, N.; Bower, C.; Christodoulou, J.; Ravine, D.; Ellaway, C.; Williamson, S.; Leonard, H. Rett syndrome in Australia: A review of the epidemiology. *J. Pediatr.* **2006**, *148*, 347–352. [CrossRef]
6. Armstrong, D.D. Review of Rett syndrome. *J. Neuropathol. Exp. Neurol.* **1997**, *56*, 843–849. [CrossRef]
7. Young, D.; Nagarajan, L.; de Klerk, N.; Jacoby, P.; Ellaway, C.; Leonard, H. Sleep problems in Rett syndrome. *Brain Dev.* **2007**, *29*, 609–616. [CrossRef]
8. Corchón, S.; Carrillo-López, I.; Cauli, O. Quality of life related to clinical features in patients with Rett syndrome and their parents: A systematic review. *Metab. Brain Dis.* **2018**, *33*, 1801–1810. [CrossRef]
9. Amir, R.E.; Van den Veyver, I.B.; Wan, M.; Tran, C.Q.; Francke, U.; Zoghbi, H.Y. Rett syndrome is caused by mutations in X-linked MECP2, encoding methyl-CpG-binding protein 2. *Nat. Genet.* **1999**, *23*, 185–188. [CrossRef]
10. Townend, G.S.; Ehrhart, F.; van Kranen, H.J.; Wilkinson, M.; Jacobsen, A.; Roos, M.; Willighagen, E.L.; van Enckevort, D.; Evelo, C.T.; Curfs, L.M.G. MECP2 variation in Rett syndrome-An overview of current coverage of genetic and phenotype data within existing databases. *Hum. Mutat.* **2018**, *39*, 914–924. [CrossRef]
11. Zhang, X.; Smits, M.; Curfs, L.; Spruyt, K. Sleep Respiratory Disturbances in Girls with Rett Syndrome. *Int. J. Environ. Res. Public Heal.* **2022**, *19*, 13082. [CrossRef] [PubMed]
12. Lombardi, L.M.; Baker, S.A.; Zoghbi, H.Y. MECP2 disorders: From the clinic to mice and back. *J. Clin. Investig.* **2015**, *125*, 2914–2923. [CrossRef] [PubMed]
13. Alexandrou, A.; Papaevripidou, I.; Alexandrou, I.M.; Theodosiou, A.; Evangelidou, P.; Kousoulidou, L.; Tanteles, G.; Christophidou-Anastasiadou, V.; Sismani, C. De novo mosaic MECP2 mutation in a female with Rett syndrome. *Clin. Case Rep.* **2019**, *7*, 366–370. [CrossRef] [PubMed]
14. Wan, M.; Lee, S.S.J.; Zhang, X.; Houwink-Manville, I.; Song, H.-R.; Amir, R.E.; Budden, S.; Naidu, S.; Pereira, J.L.P.; Lo, I.F.; et al. Rett Syndrome and beyond: Recurrent spontaneous and familial MECP2 mutations at CpG hotspots. *Am. J. Hum. Genet.* **1999**, *65*, 1520–1529. [CrossRef]
15. Gold, W.A.; Krishnarajy, R.; Ellaway, C.; Christodoulou, J. Rett Syndrome: A Genetic Update and Clinical Review Focusing on Comorbidities. *ACS Chem. Neurosci.* **2018**, *9*, 167–176. [CrossRef]
16. Palmieri, M.; Pozzer, D.; Landsberger, N. Advanced genetic therapies for the treatment of Rett syndrome: State of the art and future perspectives. *Front. Neurosci.* **2023**, *17*, 1172805. [CrossRef]
17. Downs, J.; Wong, K.; Leonard, H. Associations between genotype, phenotype and behaviours measured by the Rett syndrome behaviour questionnaire in Rett syndrome. *J. Neurodev. Disord.* **2024**, *16*, 59. [CrossRef]
18. Kay, C.; Leonard, H.; Smith, J.; Wong, K.; Downs, J. Genotype and sleep independently predict mental health in Rett syndrome: An observational study. *J. Med. Genet.* **2023**, *60*, 951–959. [CrossRef]

19. Boban, S.; Wong, K.; Epstein, A.; Anderson, B.; Murphy, N.; Downs, J.; Leonard, H. Determinants of sleep disturbances in Rett syndrome: Novel findings in relation to genotype. *Am. J. Med. Genet. Part A* **2016**, *170*, 2292–2300. [CrossRef]
20. Zito, A.; Lee, J.T. Variable expression of MECP2, CDKL5, and FMR1 in the human brain: Implications for gene restorative therapies. *Proc. Natl. Acad. Sci. USA* **2024**, *121*, e2312757121. [CrossRef]
21. Hagberg, B. Clinical manifestations and stages of rett syndrome. *Ment. Retard. Dev. Disabil. Res. Rev.* **2002**, *8*, 61–65. [CrossRef] [PubMed]
22. Naidu, S.; Murphy, M.; Moser, H.W.; Rett, A.; Opitz, J.M.; Reynolds, J.F. Rett syndrome—natural history in 70 cases. *Am. J. Med. Genet.* **1986**, *25*, 61–72. [CrossRef] [PubMed]
23. Lee, J.; Leonard, H.; Piek, J.; Downs, J. Early development and regression in Rett syndrome. *Clin. Genet.* **2013**, *84*, 572–576. [CrossRef] [PubMed]
24. Wong, K.; Leonard, H.; Jacoby, P.; Ellaway, C.; Downs, J. The trajectories of sleep disturbances in Rett syndrome. *J. Sleep Res.* **2015**, *24*, 223–233. [CrossRef]
25. Halbach, N.; Smeets, E.; Steinbusch, C.; Maaskant, M.; van Waardenburg, D.; Curfs, L. Aging in Rett syndrome: A longitudinal study. *Clin. Genet.* **2013**, *84*, 223–229. [CrossRef]
26. Tascini, G.; Dell'ISola, G.B.; Mencaroni, E.; Di Cara, G.; Striano, P.; Verrotti, A. Sleep Disorders in Rett Syndrome and Rett-Related Disorders: A Narrative Review. *Front. Neurol.* **2022**, *13*, 817195. [CrossRef]
27. Leven, Y.; Wiegand, F.; Wilken, B. Sleep Quality in Children and Adults with Rett Syndrome. *Neuropediatrics* **2020**, *51*, 198–205. [CrossRef]
28. Boban, S.; Leonard, H.; Wong, K.; Wilson, A.; Downs, J. Sleep disturbances in Rett syndrome: Impact and management including use of sleep hygiene practices. *Am. J. Med. Genet. Part A* **2018**, *176*, 1569–1577. [CrossRef]
29. Zhang, X.; Smits, M.; Curfs, L.; Spruyt, K. Sleep and the Social Profiles of Individuals With Rett Syndrome. *Pediatr. Neurol.* **2024**, *152*, 153–161. [CrossRef]
30. Huang, C.-H.; Wong, L.-C.; Chu, Y.-J.; Hsu, C.-J.; Wang, H.-P.; Tsai, W.-C.; Lee, W.-T. The sleep problems in individuals with Rett syndrome and their caregivers. *Autism* **2024**, *28*, 3118–3130. [CrossRef]
31. Gold, W.A.; Percy, A.K.; Neul, J.L.; Cobb, S.R.; Pozzo-Miller, L.; Issar, J.K.; Ben-Zeev, B.; Vignoli, A.; Kaufmann, W.E. Rett syndrome. *Nat. Rev. Dis. Prim.* **2024**, *10*, 84. [CrossRef] [PubMed]
32. Piazza, C.C.; Fisher, W.; Moser, H. Behavioral treatment of sleep dysfunction in patients with the rett syndrome. *Brain Dev.* **1991**, *13*, 232–237. [CrossRef] [PubMed]
33. Dragich, J.M.; Kim, Y.; Arnold, A.P.; Schanen, N.C. Differential distribution of the MeCP2 splice variants in the postnatal mouse brain. *J. Comp. Neurol.* **2007**, *501*, 526–542. [CrossRef] [PubMed]
34. Zhou, Z.; Hong, E.J.; Cohen, S.; Zhao, W.-N.; Ho, H.-Y.H.; Schmidt, L.; Chen, W.G.; Lin, Y.; Savner, E.; Griffith, E.C.; et al. Brain-Specific Phosphorylation of MeCP2 Regulates Activity-Dependent Bdnf Transcription, Dendritic Growth, and Spine Maturation. *Neuron* **2006**, *52*, 255–269. [CrossRef]
35. Ramirez, J.-M.; Karlen-Amarante, M.; Wang, J.-D.J.; Huff, A.; Burgraff, N. Breathing disturbances in Rett syndrome. In *Handbook of Clinical Neurology*; Elsevier: Amsterdam, The Netherlands, 2022; Volume 189, pp. 139–151. [CrossRef]
36. Lugaresi, E.; Cirignotta, F.; Montagna, P. Abnormal breathing in the Rett syndrome. *Brain Dev.* **1985**, *7*, 329–333. [CrossRef]
37. Weese-Mayer, D.E.; Lieske, S.P.; Boothby, C.M.; Kenny, A.S.; Bennett, H.L.; Ramirez, J. Autonomic dysregulation in young girls with Rett Syndrome during nighttime in-home recordings. *Pediatr. Pulmonol.* **2008**, *43*, 1045–1060. [CrossRef]
38. Amaddeo, A.; De Sanctis, L.; Arroyo, J.O.; Khirani, S.; Bahi-Buisson, N.; Fauroux, B. Polysomnographic findings in Rett syndrome. *Eur. J. Paediatr. Neurol.* **2019**, *23*, 214–221. [CrossRef]
39. Bassett, E.; Heinle, R.; Johnston, D. Sleep Apnea in Patients With Rett Syndrome: Roles for Polysomnography and Adenotonsillectomy. *J. Child. Neurol.* **2016**, *31*, 1633–1634. [CrossRef]
40. Patel, A.A.; Glaze, D.G. Sleep and sleep disorders in Rett syndrome. In *Neurological Modulation of Sleep*; Elsevier: Amsterdam, The Netherlands, 2020; pp. 339–345. [CrossRef]
41. Mackay, J.; Downs, J.; Wong, K.; Heyworth, J.; Epstein, A.; Leonard, H. Autonomic breathing abnormalities in Rett syndrome: Caregiver perspectives in an international database study. *J. Neurodev. Disord.* **2017**, *9*, 15. [CrossRef]
42. Glaze, D.G.; Percy, A.K.; Skinner, S.; Motil, K.J.; Neul, J.L.; Barrish, J.O.; Lane, J.B.; Geerts, S.P.; Annese, F.; Graham, J.; et al. Epilepsy and the natural history of Rett syndrome. *Neurology* **2010**, *74*, 909–912. [CrossRef]
43. Dolce, A.; Ben-Zeev, B.; Naidu, S.; Kossoff, E.H. Rett syndrome and epilepsy: An update for child neurologists. *Pediatr. Neurol.* **2013**, *48*, 337–345. [CrossRef] [PubMed]
44. Bricker, K.; Vaughn, B.V. Rett syndrome: A review of clinical manifestations and therapeutic approaches. *Front. Sleep* **2024**, *3*, 1373489. [CrossRef]
45. Nissenkorn, A.; Gak, E.; Vecsler, M.; Reznik, H.; Menascu, S.; Ben Zeev, B. Epilepsy in Rett syndrome—The experience of a National Rett Center. *Epilepsia* **2010**, *51*, 1252–1258. [CrossRef]

46. Mendoza, J.; Downs, J.; Wong, K.; Leonard, H. Determinants of quality of life in Rett syndrome: New findings on associations with genotype. *J. Med. Genet.* **2021**, *58*, 637–644. [CrossRef] [PubMed]
47. Kaufmann, W.E.; Percy, A.K.; Neul, J.L.; Downs, J.; Leonard, H.; Nues, P.; Sharma, G.D.; Bartolotta, T.E.; Townend, G.S.; Curfs, L.M.G.; et al. Burden of illness in Rett syndrome: Initial evaluation of a disorder-specific caregiver survey. *Orphanet J. Rare Dis.* **2024**, *19*, 296. [CrossRef]
48. Merbler, A.M.; Byiers, B.J.; Garcia, J.J.; Feyma, T.J.; Symons, F.J. The feasibility of using actigraphy to characterize sleep in Rett syndrome. *J. Neurodev. Disord.* **2018**, *10*, 8. [CrossRef]
49. Byiers, B.J.; Merbler, A.M.; Burkitt, C.C.; Symons, F.J. Challenges in Using Parent-Reported Bed and Wake Times for Actigraphy Scoring in Rett-Related Syndromes. *Am. J. Intellect. Dev. Disabil.* **2025**, *130*, 1–12. [CrossRef]
50. Sarber, K.M.; Howard, J.J.M.; Dye, T.J.; Pascoe, J.E.; Simakajornboon, N. Sleep-Disordered Breathing in Pediatric Patients With Rett Syndrome. *J. Clin. Sleep Med.* **2019**, *15*, 1451–1457. [CrossRef]
51. Zhang, X.-Y.; Spruyt, K. Literature Cases Summarized Based on Their Polysomnographic Findings in Rett Syndrome. *Int. J. Environ. Res. Public Health* **2022**, *19*, 3422. [CrossRef]
52. Carotenuto, M.; Esposito, M.; D'aNiello, A.; Rippa, C.D.; Precenzano, F.; Pascotto, A.; Bravaccio, C.; Elia, M. Polysomnographic findings in Rett syndrome: A case–control study. *Sleep Breath.* **2013**, *17*, 93–98. [CrossRef]
53. Ammanuel, S.; Chan, W.C.; Adler, D.A.; Lakshamanan, B.M.; Gupta, S.S.; Ewen, J.B.; Johnston, M.V.; Marcus, C.L.; Naidu, S.; Kadam, S.D.; et al. Heightened Delta Power during Slow-Wave-Sleep in Patients with Rett Syndrome Associated with Poor Sleep Efficiency. *PLoS ONE* **2015**, *10*, e0138113. [CrossRef] [PubMed]
54. Davis, P.; Takach, K.; Maski, K.; Levin, A. A circuit-level biomarker of Rett syndrome based on ectopic phase-amplitude coupling during slow-wave-sleep. *Cereb. Cortex* **2022**, *33*, 2559–2572. [CrossRef] [PubMed]
55. Rodrigues, G.D.; Cordani, R.; Veneruso, M.; Chiarella, L.; Prato, G.; Ferri, R.; Carandina, A.; Tobaldini, E.; Nobili, L.; Montano, N. Predominant cardiac sympathetic modulation during wake and sleep in patients with Rett syndrome. *Sleep Med.* **2024**, *119*, 188–191. [CrossRef] [PubMed]
56. Furqan, M. Trofinetide—A new chapter in rett syndrome's treatment. *Front. Pharmacol.* **2023**, *14*, 1284035. [CrossRef]
57. Lopes, A.G.; Loganathan, S.K.; Caliaperumal, J. Rett Syndrome and the Role of MECP2: Signaling to Clinical Trials. *Brain Sci.* **2024**, *14*, 120. [CrossRef]
58. Percy, A.K.; Ananth, A.; Neul, J.L. Rett Syndrome: The Emerging Landscape of Treatment Strategies. *CNS Drugs* **2024**, *38*, 851–867. [CrossRef]
59. Camillo, L.; Pozzi, M.; Bernardo, P.; Pisano, S.; Nobile, M. Profile of Trofinetide in the Treatment of Rett Syndrome: Design, Development and Potential Place in Therapy. *Drug Des. Dev. Ther.* **2024**, *18*, 5023–5040. [CrossRef]
60. Bricker, K.; Vaughn, B.V. Review of Sleep Disorders and Therapeutic Approaches in Patients With Autism Spectrum Disorder and Rett Syndrome. *Sleep Med. Res.* **2024**, *15*, 228–236. [CrossRef]
61. Fu, C.; Armstrong, D.; Marsh, E.; Lieberman, D.; Motil, K.; Witt, R.; Standridge, S.; Nues, P.; Lane, J.; Dinkel, T.; et al. Consensus guidelines on managing Rett syndrome across the lifespan. *BMJ Paediatr. Open* **2020**, *4*, e000717. [CrossRef]
62. International Rett Syndrome Foundation. Rett Syndrome: Comprehensive Care Guidelines. 2024. Available online: https://www.rettsyndrome.org/wp-content/uploads/2024/12/Comprehensive-Care-Guidelines.pdf (accessed on 1 May 2025).
63. Blackmer, A.B.; Feinstein, J.A. Management of Sleep Disorders in Children With Neurodevelopmental Disorders: A Review. *Pharmacother. J. Hum. Pharmacol. Drug Ther.* **2016**, *36*, 84–98. [CrossRef]
64. Buckley, A.W.; Hirtz, D.; Oskoui, M.; Armstrong, M.J.; Batra, A.; Bridgemohan, C.; Coury, D.; Dawson, G.; Donley, D.; Findling, R.L.; et al. Practice guideline: Treatment for insomnia and disrupted sleep behavior in children and adolescents with autism spectrum disorder: Report of the Guideline Development, Dissemination, and Implementation Subcommittee of the American Academy of Neurology. *Neurology* **2020**, *94*, 392–404. [CrossRef]
65. Grigg-Damberger, M.; Ralls, F. Treatment strategies for complex behavioral insomnia in children with neurodevelopmental disorders. *Curr. Opin. Pulm. Med.* **2013**, *19*, 616–625. [CrossRef]
66. Jan, J.E.; Owens, J.A.; Weiss, M.D.; Johnson, K.P.; Wasdell, M.B.; Freeman, R.D.; Ipsiroglu, O.S. Sleep hygiene for children with neurodevelopmental disabilities. *Pediatrics* **2008**, *122*, 1343–1350. [CrossRef]
67. Epstein, A.; Leonard, H.; Davis, E.; Williams, K.; Reddihough, D.; Murphy, N.; Whitehouse, A.; Downs, J. Conceptualizing a quality of life framework for girls with Rett syndrome using qualitative methods. *Am. J. Med. Genet. Part A* **2016**, *170*, 645–653. [CrossRef]
68. Woodford, E.C.; France, K.G.; Blampied, N.M.; Hanning, U.; Swan, C.E.; McLay, L.K. Behavioral Sleep Interventions for Children with Rare Genetic Neurodevelopmental Conditions: A Retrospective Analysis of Overall Outcomes for 26 Cases. *Adv. Neurodev. Disord.* **2024**, *8*, 1–16. [CrossRef]
69. McArthur, A.J.; Budden, S.S. Sleep dysfunction in Rett syndrome: A trial of exogenous melatonin treatment. *Dev. Med. Child. Neurol.* **1998**, *40*, 186–192. [CrossRef]

70. Cohen, P.A.; Avula, B.; Wang, Y.-H.; Katragunta, K.; Khan, I. Quantity of Melatonin and CBD in Melatonin Gummies Sold in the US. *JAMA* **2023**, *329*, 1401. [CrossRef]
71. Owens, J.A.; Rosen, C.L.; Mindell, J.A.; Kirchner, H.L. Use of pharmacotherapy for insomnia in child psychiatry practice: A national survey. *Sleep Med.* **2010**, *11*, 692–700. [CrossRef]
72. Bruni, O.; Angriman, M.; Calisti, F.; Comandini, A.; Esposito, G.; Cortese, S.; Ferri, R. Practitioner Review: Treatment of chronic insomnia in children and adolescents with neurodevelopmental disabilities. *J. Child. Psychol. Psychiatry* **2018**, *59*, 489–508. [CrossRef]
73. Ellaway, C.J.; Peat, J.; Williams, K.; Leonard, H.; Christodoulou, J. Medium-term open label trial of L-carnitine in Rett syndrome. *Brain Dev.* **2001**, *23*, S85–S89. [CrossRef]
74. Motil, K.J.; Caeg, E.; Barrish, J.O.; Geerts, S.; Lane, J.B.; Percy, A.K.; Annese, F.; McNair, L.; Skinner, S.A.; Lee, H.; et al. Gastrointestinal and nutritional problems occur frequently throughout life in girls and women with rett syndrome. *J. Pediatr. Gastroenterol. Nutr.* **2012**, *55*, 292–298. [CrossRef]
75. Brook, E.; Usman, M. SSRIs in Rett syndrome. *Aust. New Zealand J. Psychiatry* **2015**, *49*, 667–668. [CrossRef]
76. Picchietti, D.L.; Bruni, O.; de Weerd, A.; Durmer, J.S.; Kotagal, S.; Owens, J.A.; Simakajornboon, N. Pediatric restless legs syndrome diagnostic criteria: An update by the International Restless Legs Syndrome Study Group. *Sleep Med.* **2013**, *14*, 1253–1259. [CrossRef]
77. Killian, W.; Riederer, P.; Linkesch, W. Serum iron status in Rett syndrome. *Brain Dev.* **1987**, *9*, 523–524. [CrossRef]
78. Winkelman, J.W.; Berkowski, J.A.; DelRosso, L.M.; Koo, B.B.; Scharf, M.T.; Sharon, D.; Zak, R.S.; Kazmi, U.; Falck-Ytter, Y.; Shelgikar, A.V.; et al. Treatment of restless legs syndrome and periodic limb movement disorder: An American Academy of Sleep Medicine clinical practice guideline. *J. Clin. Sleep Med.* **2025**, *21*, 137–152. [CrossRef]
79. Cherchi, C.; Chiappini, E.; Amaddeo, A.; Testa, M.B.C.; Banfi, P.; Veneselli, E.; Cutrera, R. Management of respiratory issues in patients with Rett syndrome: Italian experts' consensus using a Delphi approach. *Pediatr. Pulmonol.* **2024**, *59*, 1970–1978. [CrossRef]
80. Toward, M.A.; Abdala, A.P.; Knopp, S.J.; Paton, J.F.R.; Bissonnette, J.M. Increasing brain serotonin corrects CO2 chemosensitivity in methyl-CpG-binding protein 2 (Mecp2)-deficient mice. *Exp. Physiol.* **2013**, *98*, 842–849. [CrossRef]
81. Gökben, S.; Ardıç, Ü.A.; Serdaroğlu, G. Use of Buspirone and Fluoxetine for Breathing Problems in Rett Syndrome. *Pediatr. Neurol.* **2012**, *46*, 192–194. [CrossRef]
82. Ohno, K.; Saito, Y.; Ueda, R.; Togawa, M.; Ohmae, T.; Matsuda, E.; Fujiyama, M.; Maegaki, Y. Effect of Serotonin 1A Agonists and Selective Serotonin Reuptake Inhibitors on Behavioral and Nighttime Respiratory Symptoms in Rett Syndrome. *Pediatr. Neurol.* **2016**, *60*, 54–59.e1. [CrossRef]
83. Abdala, A.P.L.; Dutschmann, M.; Bissonnette, J.M.; Paton, J.F.R. Correction of respiratory disorders in a mouse model of Rett syndrome. *Proc. Natl. Acad. Sci. USA* **2010**, *107*, 18208–18213. [CrossRef]
84. Tarquinio, D.C.; Hou, W.; Neul, J.L.; Kaufmann, W.E.; Glaze, D.G.; Motil, K.J.; Skinner, S.A.; Lee, H.-S.; Percy, A.K. The Changing Face of Survival in Rett Syndrome and MECP2-Related Disorders. *Pediatr. Neurol.* **2015**, *53*, 402–411. [CrossRef] [PubMed]
85. Spruyt, K.; Curfs, L.M.G. Non-pharmacological management of problematic sleeping in children with developmental disabilities. *Dev. Med. Child. Neurol.* **2014**, *57*, 120–136. [CrossRef] [PubMed]
86. Hung, P.L.; Wu, K.L.H.; Chen, C.J.; Siu, K.K.; Hsin, Y.J.; Wang, L.J.; Wang, F.S. Music-Based Intervention Ameliorates Mecp2-Loss-Mediated Sociability Repression in Mice through the Prefrontal Cortex FNDC5/BDNF Pathway. *Int. J. Mol. Sci.* **2021**, *22*, 7174. [CrossRef] [PubMed]

children

MDPI

Article

Developmental Patterns in Autism and Other Neurodevelopmental Disorders in Preschool Children

Maria Eugenia Martelli , Federica Gigliotti , Federica Giovannone, Giuliana Lentini, Filippo Manti and Carla Sogos *

Department of Human Neuroscience, Sapienza University of Rome, 00185 Rome, Italy; mariaeugenia.martelli@uniroma1.it (M.E.M.); federica.gig@uniroma1.it (F.G.); federica.giovannone@uniroma1.it (F.G.); giuliana.lentini@uniroma1.it (G.L.); filippo.manti@uniroma1.it (F.M.)
* Correspondence: carla.sogos@uniroma1.it

Abstract: Background: Neurodevelopmental disorders (NDDs) encompass an inclusive group of conditions that appear during the developmental period but continue to persist in adulthood, ranging from particular difficulties to a global impairment of social, cognitive, and emotional functioning. The developmental trajectories associated with these conditions are highly heterogeneous. This study aimed to analyze and compare developmental and adaptive profiles of preschool-aged children with different NDDs to better characterize their developmental trajectories. Methods: We analyzed data from the initial global evaluation of 196 children with NDDs (aged 20 to 71 months), enrolled in three subgroups: 108 with autism spectrum disorder (ASD), 52 with language disorder (LD), and 36 with mixed specific developmental disorder (MSDD). A comprehensive neuropsychiatric evaluation was performed using standardized tools (Griffiths-III, ADOS-2, VABS-II, and ADI-R), and the parents completed the DP-3 and the CBCL $1\frac{1}{2}$-5. Results: Our results showed that all NDDs exhibited poor psychomotor skills, with children with ASD being the most impaired, although their profiles were comparable to those of MSDD in communication and motor areas. CBCL's pervasive developmental problem scale has been shown to provide relevant information for distinguishing children with ASD. Furthermore, DP-3 and VABS-II measure highly differentiated developmental profiles of each diagnostic group. Conclusions: Our results highlighted the importance of including parents'/caregivers' perspectives in defining children's functioning and the possibility of using DP-3 as a screening tool for different neurodevelopmental disorders.

Keywords: developmental profile; adaptive profile; neurodevelopmental disorders; preschool children

1. Introduction

Neurodevelopmental disorders (NDDs) encompass a wide range of conditions that affect brain development, leading to delays or impairments in cognitive, motor, linguistic, and socio-emotional domains [1,2]. These disorders, which can persist throughout life and significantly impact the quality of life, appear early in the child's development, often before school age [3]. However, diagnosing these conditions in preschoolers poses significant challenges due to the complexity and high variability of early development, significant overlap across NDDs [4], and limitations in diagnostic tools that can lead to diagnostic uncertainty, delayed identification, or misdiagnosis.

Over the past 15 years, research has highlighted that developmental profiles in NDDs are highly heterogeneous, not following uniform patterns but instead representing dynamic continua shaped by a complex interplay of genetic, neurobiological, and environmental factors [5,6]. In preschool-aged children, identifying and understanding these trajectories is essential for early diagnosis and implementation of effective interventions tailored to the unique child's needs, which can significantly influence developmental outcomes and quality of life [7].

Differential diagnosis between different NDDs in preschool-aged children is a complex and nuanced process that requires careful assessment of cognitive, linguistic, social, and behavioral domains to reveal strengths and weaknesses in different areas of development [4].

Autism spectrum disorder (ASD) is a disorder characterized by persistent deficits in social communication and interaction, as well as restricted and repetitive patterns of behavior, interests, or activities [3]. In this condition, there is significant variability in developmental trajectories, with early indicators often emerging in social communication and sensory–motor integration. Longitudinal studies suggest that some children exhibit developmental plateaus or regressions, particularly in language and social interaction domains [8].

Cognitive abilities in ASD are heterogeneous; a previous study found that up to 78% of preschool children with ASD had clear or suspected developmental delays and another 20% presented average or above-average cognitive levels, resembling the clinical profile of high-functioning autism [9]. On the other hand, some ASD children may display uneven skill development with strengths in specific areas (such as rote memory or visual–spatial processing) and challenges in executive functioning [10,11].

Verbal skills can vary widely, ranging from nonverbal communication to advanced vocabulary with atypical use. Language delays are quite common in ASD, with challenges in both expressive and receptive language, leading to diagnostic confusion with LD. However, children with ASD often exhibit pragmatic impairments and qualitative differences in language use, such as echolalia or unusual prosody, which are less typical in LD [12]. Nonverbal communication is also frequently affected.

Additionally, impairment in social reciprocity, joint attention (e.g., difficulties in sharing attention with others through pointing or eye contact), and emotional regulation, as well as repetitive behaviors (e.g., hand flapping or fixations on specific objects) and restricted interests, are hallmark features in preschool children with ASD [13], but they can be subtle or transient, particularly in children under the age of three, leading to delayed recognition of the disorder [8].

Language disorder (LD) involves significant and persistent difficulties with language acquisition and use, because of impairments in understanding or producing language, in the absence of intellectual disability, sensory impairments, or other medical conditions [3]. Children with LD had significant difficulties in areas highly dependent on language, such as communication and community participation; the severity of these weaknesses ranges from very mild to substantial enough to qualify as disabilities. On the other hand, these children exhibit strengths in areas less reliant on language, including domestic and personal life activities, play and leisure, coping in social situations, and gross motor skills [14].

While primary language disorder may not involve general cognitive delays, challenges in working memory and processing speed are often noted [15,16].

So, children with LD primarily struggle with the structure and use of language, while their social engagement and nonverbal communication skills are generally within the expected developmental range [17]. However, previous research has shown that language impairments can hinder social interactions, potentially resulting in social withdrawal or behavioral issues due to frustration or misunderstanding [12].

Mixed specific developmental disorder (MSDD), as defined by the International Statistical Classification of Diseases and Related Health Problems 10th Revision (ICD-10), describes a condition characterized by delays or difficulties across multiple developmental domains, including cognition, language, motor skills, social interaction, and behavioral regulation [18], without meeting the full criteria for a specific neurodevelopmental disorder. MSDD is not a distinct diagnostic category in current classifications, such as DSM-5-TR or ICD-11, but is often used clinically to describe heterogeneous developmental profiles in preschool-aged children when there is a significant impairment in the development of several functions without any single developmental domain being predominantly affected.

The main aim of this study was to identify and evaluate the developmental level and the adaptive profile of preschool-aged children with diagnoses of NDDs in order to better understand different developmental trajectories. Furthermore, we compared the profiles of different clinical groups in order to verify any differences between these subpopulations that could have implications for diagnostic and therapeutic strategies.

2. Materials and Methods

2.1. Participants

This study involved 196 preschoolers (M:F = 163:33), ranging from 20 and 71 months (40.7 $\pm$ 10.2), with neurodevelopmental disorders.

Participants were recruited among children referred to the Outpatient Service for Neurodevelopmental Disorders of the Department of Human Neuroscience at Sapienza University of Rome, due to difficulties in interaction, communication, and behavior, between 2021 and 2024.

Inclusion criteria were (a) having an age between 1 and 72 months, (b) having received a clinical diagnosis of NDD, encoded according to the ICD-10 classification (currently adopted in the Italian health care system), (c) being in the care of their parents, and (d) not taking drug treatment or practicing other types of therapy.

Children who had a diagnosis of intellectual disability or associated medical conditions (e.g., neurocutaneous or other genetic syndromes, epilepsy, traumatic brain injury, significant sensory or motor deficits, other chronic diseases, or reactive attachment disorders) were excluded. Further exclusion criteria were the inability to perform a structured evaluation of development, due to severe behavioral problems, and the lack of sufficient knowledge of Italian by parents to complete the entire assessment.

2.2. Procedure

The participants underwent a comprehensive diagnostic evaluation, including medical history, developmental level assessment, and observational behavior analysis, during which the disorder was confirmed. Both parents completed a symptom checklist (Child Behavior Checklist for Ages $1\frac{1}{2}$-5 years—CBCL $1\frac{1}{2}$-5) to jointly assess their child's emotional and behavioral problems, the Vineland Adaptive Behavior Scale, 2nd Edition (VABS-II), to evaluate the child's adaptive functioning, and the Developmental Profile-3 (DP-3) to investigate the child's developmental profile. Specific instruments (Autism Diagnostic Observation Schedule, 2nd Edition—ADOS-2, and Autism Diagnostic Interview-Revised—ADI-R) were used to assess autistic symptoms when clinically indicated.

According to the ICD-10 classification, the total sample was divided into 3 clinical groups: children with LD, MSDD, or ASD.

2.2.1. Developmental Profile

All participants were assessed using the Italian adaptation [19] of the Griffiths Scales of Child Development, 3rd Edition (Griffiths-III) [20], which was developed as an evaluation instrument for children aged up to 72 months of age. The administration takes approximately an hour and a half, depending on the clinician's expertise and the child's physical and emotional disposition.

Griffiths-III provides a detailed profile of child psychomotor development (general developmental quotient—GDQ) and allows the assessment of five domains of development: foundations of learning (subscale A), language and communication (subscale B), eye and hand coordination (subscale C), personal–social–emotional (subscale D), and gross motor (subscale E). Each item is scored as a pass (+1) or a fail (0). Raw scores, obtained from the sum of the items passed in each scale, are calculated to determine the Age Equivalent, Scaled Score, and development quotient (DQ), according to the sex and age of patients. In this study, we considered only DQs.

The DP-3 [21] is a standardized instrument designed to evaluate the development and functioning of children aged up to 12 years old, providing information about strengths and weaknesses. It is the updated and revised version of Developmental Profile-II and consists of either an interview or a parent/caregiver checklist; for this study, we used the second version.

It has 180 items, each describing a particular skill, with yes/no questions, assessing 5 key areas of development: physical (35 items), adaptive behavior (37 items), social–emotional (36 items), cognitive (38 items), and communication (34 items). Each scale provides a raw score which is converted into a standard score; the sum of the standard scores of the five domains is finally converted into the general development score, according to the norm tables. Italian adaptation of the DP-3 showed good reliability, both in terms of internal consistency (with split-half coefficients ranging from 0.64 to 0.96) and test–retest reliability (correlation range: 0.866–0.968) [22].

2.2.2. Adaptive Function Profile

To characterize the adaptive functioning of the participants, the survey interview form of the VABS-II [23] was administered to parents. This semi-structured interview is specifically designed to assess the adaptive level of functioning as a standardized measure in individuals aged up to 90 years old.

The VABS-II measures 11 subdomains grouped into four broad domain composites (communication, daily living skills, socialization, and motor skills). Each item can be scored as 0 (never), 1 (sometimes), or 2 (usually or often). The broad domain raw scores, calculated by summing the raw scores from each subdomain, are converted into standard scores which are then combined to provide an adaptive behavior composite (ABC) score, expressing the individual's global adaptive functioning. The Italian adaptation of the scale showed good/excellent internal consistency reliability for broad domains and ABC (split-half coefficient range: 0.80–0.97) [24].

2.2.3. Emotional and Behavioral Profile

The CBCL $1\frac{1}{2}$-5 [25] is a parent-report screening tool that assesses behavioral, emotional, and social functioning in preschoolers. It consists of 100 items rated on a 3-point scale: 0 = not true, 1 = somewhat true or sometimes true, or 2 = very true or often true. Item raw scores are used to compute T-scores for seven syndromic scales (emotionally reactive, anxious/depressed, somatic complaints, withdrawal, sleep problems, attention problems, and aggressive behavior), five DSM-oriented scales (affective problems, anxiety problems, pervasive developmental problems, attention deficit/hyperactivity problems, and oppositional defiant problems) and three summary scales (internalizing, externalizing, and total). In the present study, we used the Italian version of the scale and considered the T-scores of the DSM-oriented scales and the summary scales.

The CBCL $1\frac{1}{2}$-5 has shown good psychometric properties, including high internal consistency (approximately 75% of scales having a Cronbach's alpha of 0.78 or greater) and strong test–retest reliability (r value range: 0.74–0.90).

2.2.4. Signs and Symptoms of ASD

Specific standardized instruments were administered in the differential diagnosis of patients with autistic features.

The ADOS-2 [26] is a standardized assessment instrument designed to evaluate individuals with a suspected diagnosis of ASD. It consists of a series of semi-structured activities and prompts that allow researchers to observe behaviors related to communication, social interaction, play, and restricted or repetitive behaviors.

This clinical instrument is widely regarded as the "gold standard" for ASD assessment and it is divided into five different 40–60 min modules, each tailored to different age groups and language capabilities (Toddler Module, for children aged 12 to 30 months who have limited or no use of phrase speech; Module 1, for children aged 31 months or older who have limited or no use of phrase speech; Module 2, for children who use phrases but not fluently; Module 3, for children and young adolescents with fluent speech; and Module 4, for older adolescents and adults who are verbally fluent).

The ADOS-2 yields calibrated severity scores (CSSs) for the two domains of social affect and restricted and repetitive behaviors, as well as for the total score.

In this study, either the Toddler Module, Module 1, or Module 2 were used. Furthermore, the severity of the autistic symptoms was measured with the total CSS of the ADOS-2, ranging from 1 to 10. The Toddler Module CSS reported in the current study was computed based on Esler et al. (2015) [27] to allow direct comparison with other modules of the ADOS-2.

The ADI-R [28] is a 93-item standardized structured interview, which explores core symptomatic areas of autism: language development, social interaction, and communication abilities as well as play, interests, and behaviors. The items are split into 4 scales: (A) reciprocal social interaction, (B) communication and language, (C) restricted, repetitive, and stereotyped behaviors, and (D) abnormality of development evident at or before 36 months.

In the present study, we used the Italian version [29], and we took into account the scores of A, B, and C scales.

2.3. *Data Analysis*

All statistical analyses were performed using version 25.0 of the IBM Statistical Package for Social Science software (SPSS, Inc., Chicago, IL, USA, IBM, Somers, NY, USA).

Descriptive statistics were applied to the sociodemographic and clinical data. Continuous variables were presented as mean ± standard deviation (SD). Normality was assessed with the Kolmogorov–Smirnov test. Correlation analyses were performed using Spearman's correlation coefficient. For continuous data, an independent sample t-test and a one-way analysis of variance (ANOVA) with post hoc comparison (Bonferroni) were used.

The dimensional effect of clinical variables on outcome was evaluated by linear regression analysis (step-wise method). A p-value <0.05 represented statistical significance for all tests.

3. Results

3.1. Sociodemographic Data and Clinical Features

The research sample consisted of 196 children, of which 52 (26.5%) met the specified criteria for a diagnosis of LD, 36 (18.4%) for MSDD, and 108 (55.1%) for ASD. The mean age and gender ratio did not differ between the three clinical groups (F = 1.186, $p = 0.308$; F = 0.633, $p = 0.589$).

Developmental level, estimated by Griffiths-III GDQ, was significantly different across the groups (F = 69.146; $p < 0.01$); the post hoc analysis showed that GDQ was significantly higher in the LD group compared to the MSDD group ($p < 0.01$) and the ASD group ($p < 0.01$), while there was no significant difference between the MSDD and the ASD group ($p = 0.061$). A significant difference among groups was also found in all Griffiths-III subscales: foundations of learning (F = 39.087; $p < 0.01$), language and communication (F = 42.148; $p < 0.01$), eye and hand coordination (F = 50.154; $p < 0.01$), personal–social–emotional (F = 57.898; $p < 0.01$), and gross motor (F = 17.050; $p < 0.01$). Significantly higher mean scores were found in the LD group than in the MSDD or the ASD group while there were no statistically significant differences between ASD and MSDD (see Table 1).

Table 1. Between-group comparisons of the Griffiths Scales of Child Development, 3rd Edition.

Griffiths-III Quotients, Mean (SD)	Total Sample (n = 196)	LD Group (n = 52)	MSDD Group (n = 36)	ASD Group (n = 108)	Post Hoc	*p*-Value
FL	65.75 (28.47)	90.36 (15.01)	64.39 (21.96)	54.36 (28.05)	LD vs. ASD LD vs. MSDD MSDD vs. ASD	<0.01 * <0.01 * 0.097
LC	50.89 (27.26)	75.46 (18.97)	47.22 (24.59)	40.28 (23.94)	LD vs. ASD LD vs. MSDD MSDD vs. ASD	<0.01 * <0.01 * 0.348
EHC	66.95 (30.74)	96 (21.83)	64.75 (22.99)	53.69 (27.08)	LD vs. ASD LD vs. MSDD MSDD vs. ASD	<0.01 * <0.01 * 0.069
PSE	56.98 (27.47)	84.33 (19.89)	53.97 (21.27)	44.81 (22.88)	LD vs. ASD LD vs. MSDD MSDD vs. ASD	<0.01 * <0.01 * 0.092
GM	78.67 (22.08)	92.86 (15.32)	73.55 (22.17)	73.53 (21.97)	LD vs. ASD LD vs. MSDD MSDD vs. ASD	<0.01 * <0.01 * 1.000
GDQ	54.67 (26.83)	82.86 (16.01)	51.44 (18.94)	42.17 (22.90)	LD vs. ASD LD vs. MSDD MSDD vs. ASD	<0.01 * <0.01 * 0.061

LD = language disorder; MSDD = mixed specific developmental disorder; ASD = autism spectrum disorder; SD = standard deviation; Griffiths-III = Griffiths Scales of Child Development, 3rd Edition; FL = foundations of learning; LC = language and communication; EHC = eye and hand coordination; PSE = personal–social–emotional; GM = gross motor; GDQ = general development quotient. * $p < 0.05$.

In terms of parent ratings of children's developmental functioning, assessed by the DP-3 checklist, we found significant differences among the three groups in the DP-3 general development quotient (F = 30.111; $p < 0.01$); a significant difference among groups was also found in all mean DP-3 scores (physical: F = 5.387, $p < 0.01$; adaptive behavior: F = 16.117, $p < 0.01$; social–emotional: F = 22.378, $p < 0.01$; cognitive: F = 30.978, $p < 0.01$; and communication: F = 23.606, $p < 0.01$). Post hoc analysis highlighted significantly higher mean scores in the LD group than in the MSDD or ASD group in the cognitive and communication scales. On the physical scale, the LD group obtained significantly higher scores than the ASD group ($p < 0.01$); no statistically significant differences were highlighted between the LD and the MSDD group and between the MSSD and the ASD group. On the adaptive behavior scale, significantly higher scores were found in the LD group compared to ASD ($p < 0.01$); a significant difference was also found between the MSDD and ASD group ($p = 0.023$). On the socio-emotional scale, higher mean scores were highlighted in the LD group than in the MSDD ($p < 0.01$) or the ASD group ($p < 0.01$); no statistically significant differences were found between the MSDD and the ASD group. Regarding the general development quotient, the LD group obtained significantly higher scores than the MSDD ($p < 0.01$) and the ASD group ($p < 0.01$); a statistically significant difference was also highlighted between the MSDD and the ASD group ($p = 0.010$) (see Table 2).

Table 2. Between-group comparisons of the Developmental Profile-3.

DP-3 Scores, Mean (SD)	Total Sample (n = 196)	LD Group (n = 52)	MSDD Group (n = 36)	ASD Group (n = 108)	Post Hoc	*p*-Value
Physical	79.65 (20.37)	87.35 (17.61)	78.25 (22.15)	76.42 (20.20)	LD vs. ASD LD vs. MSDD MSDD vs. ASD	<0.01 * 0.110 1.000
Adaptive behavior	74.66 (20.94)	86.23 (16.15)	78.08 (20.37)	67.95 (20.61)	LD vs. ASD LD vs. MSDD MSDD vs. ASD	<0.01 * 0.166 0.023 *
Social–emotional	62.52 (25.30)	79.79 (23.93)	63.36 (23.53)	53.93 (22.47)	LD vs. ASD LD vs. MSDD MSDD vs. ASD	<0.01 * <0.01 * 0.101
Cognitive	60.77 (28.10)	82.19 (21.11)	63.19 (29.39)	49.66 (24.37)	LD vs. ASD LD vs. MSDD MSDD vs. ASD	<0.01 * <0.01 * 0.014 *
Communication	53.58 (26.21)	70.98 (22.80)	57.42 (27.36)	43.92 (22.66)	LD vs. ASD LD vs. MSDD MSDD vs. ASD	<0.01 * 0.026 * 0.010 *
General development	54.90 (25.69)	74.11 (21.63)	57.61 (26.62)	44.74 (21.49)	LD vs. ASD LD vs. MSDD MSDD vs. ASD	<0.01 * <0.01 * 0.010 *

LD = language disorder; MSDD = mixed specific developmental disorder; ASD = autism spectrum disorder; SD = standard deviation; DP-3 = Developmental Profile-3. * $p < 0.05$.

Analysis of mean VABS-II scores showed significant differences among the three groups in all domains (communication: $F = 29.854$, $p < 0.01$; daily living skills: $F = 45.736$, $p < 0.01$; socialization: $F = 43.111$, $p < 0.01$; and motor skills: $F = 8.869$, $p < 0.01$) and in the adaptive behavior composite score (ABC) ($F = 44.636$; $p < 0.01$). Subsequent post hoc analyses revealed that mean communication, daily living skills, socialization, and ABC scores were higher in the LD group compared to the MSDD group (all $p < 0.01$) or the ASD group (all $p < 0.01$); there was also a significant difference between the MSDD and the ASD group. In the motor skills domain, significantly higher scores were found in the LD group compared to the MSDD ($p = 0.030$) and the ASD group ($p < 0.01$) while there were no statistically significant differences between the MSDD and the ASD group (see Table 3).

Table 3. Between-group comparisons of the Vineland Adaptive Behavior Scale, 2nd Edition.

VABS-II Scores, Mean (SD)	Total Sample (n = 196)	LD Group (n = 52)	MSDD Group (n = 36)	ASD Group (n = 108)	Post Hoc	*p*-Value
Communication	73.86 (15.81)	85.83 (11.16)	74.89 (14.33)	67.75 (14.88)	LD vs. ASD LD vs. MSDD MSDD vs. ASD	<0.01 * <0.01 * 0.025 *
Daily living skills	81.46 (14.39)	94.23 (11.94)	82.33 (11.78)	75.02 (11.95)	LD vs. ASD LD vs. MSDD MSDD vs. ASD	<0.01 * <0.01 * <0.01 *
Socialization	77.98 (12.99)	89.30 (10.54)	78.67 (9.53)	72.30 (11.40)	LD vs. ASD LD vs. MSDD MSDD vs. ASD	<0.01 * <0.01 * <0.01 *
Motor skills	82.89 (14.30)	89.67 (14.23)	81.91 (13.88)	79.95 (13.48)	LD vs. ASD LD vs. MSDD MSDD vs. ASD	<0.01 * 0.030 * 1.000
ABC	76.38 (12.87)	87.94 (9.82)	79.19 (10.32)	70.88 (11.21)	LD vs. ASD LD vs. MSDD MSDD vs. ASD	<0.01 * <0.01 * 0.032 *

LD = language disorder; MSDD = mixed specific developmental disorder; ASD = autism spectrum disorder; SD = standard deviation; VABS-II = Vineland Adaptive Behavior Scale, 2nd Edition; ABC = adaptive behavior composite. * $p < 0.05$.

The Supplementary Materials Figure S1 provides a comparison of developmental patterns among the three clinical groups.

As can be seen in Table 4, on the CBCL 1½-5, a significant difference among groups was found in mean T-scores for all composite scales (internalizing: F = 10.186, $p < 0.01$; externalizing: F = 3.197, $p = 0.043$; and total: F = 5.279, $p < 0.01$) and for three DSM-oriented subscales (affective problems: F = 4.804, $p < 0.01$; pervasive developmental problems: F = 15.539, $p < 0.01$; and attention deficit/hyperactivity problems: F = 3.109, $p = 0.047$). The post hoc analysis highlighted significant differences between the LD group compared to the ASD group. Statistically significant differences were found between the MSDD and the ASD group only in the pervasive developmental problems subscale ($p = 0.011$).

Table 4. Between-group comparisons of the Child Behavior Checklist for Ages 1½-5 years.

CBCL 1½-5 T-Scores, Mean (SD)	Total Sample (n = 196)	LD Group (n = 52)	MSDD Group (n = 36)	ASD Group (n = 108)	Post Hoc	*p*-Value
DSM-oriented scales						
Affective problems	56.92 (7.38)	54.75 (6.41)	55.83 (5.51)	58.33 (8.06)	LD vs. ASD LD vs. MSDD MSDD vs. ASD	0.011 * 1.000 0.223
Anxiety problems	56.83 (8.56)	55.33 (7.73)	56.64 (8.71)	57.62 (8.86)	LD vs. ASD LD vs. MSDD MSDD vs. ASD	0.341 1.000 1.000
Pervasive developmental problems	66.54 (10.14)	61.21 (9.21)	64.47 (9.37)	69.80 (9.61)	LD vs. ASD LD vs. MSDD MSDD vs. ASD	<0.01 * 0.341 0.011 *
Attention deficit/hyperactivity problems	57.61 (7.06)	55.65 (5.95)	57.50 (7.59)	58.59 (7.23)	LD vs. ASD LD vs. MSDD MSDD vs. ASD	0.041 * 0.674 1.000
Oppositional defiant problems	55.28 (6.80)	53.96 (7.80)	54.28 (6.04)	56.25 (6.94)	LD vs. ASD LD vs. MSDD MSDD vs. ASD	0.138 1.000 0.391
Composite scales						
Internalizing	57.63 (10.55)	52.85 (11.12)	56.28 (8.94)	60.38 (9.92)	LD vs. ASD LD vs. MSDD MSDD vs. ASD	<0.01 * 0.355 0.108
Externalizing	55.80 (10.21)	53.13 (10.31)	55 (9.43)	57.35 (10.21)	LD vs. ASD LD vs. MSDD MSDD vs. ASD	0.043 * 1.000 0.684
Total	57.51 (10.82)	53.92 (10.65)	56.42 (9.18)	59.60 (10.99)	LD vs. ASD LD vs. MSDD MSDD vs. ASD	<0.01 * 0.837 0.359

LD = language disorder; MSDD = mixed specific developmental disorder; ASD = autism spectrum disorder; SD = standard deviation; CBCL 1½-5 = Child Behavior Checklist for Ages 1½-5. * $p < 0.05$.

In terms of autistic features, as expected, the mean ADOS-2 CSS in the group with ASD was significantly higher than in the group with MSDD ($p < 0.01$). Similarly, on the ADI-R, all scores were significantly higher in children with ASD (all $p < 0.01$) (see Table 5).

Table 5. T-test comparison between MSDD and ASD group (Autism Diagnostic Observation Schedule, 2nd Edition, and Autism Diagnostic Interview-Revised).

	MSDD Group (n = 36)	ASD Group (n = 108)	*p*-Value
ADOS-2, mean (SD)			
CSS	3.94 (1.45)	6.82 (1.86)	<0.01 *

Table 5. *Cont.*

	MSDD Group (n = 36)	ASD Group (n = 108)	*p*-Value
ADI-R, mean (SD)			
Reciprocal social interaction	6.05 (3.62)	14.70 (6.19)	<0.01 *
Communication and language	6.25 (3.57)	11.09 (3.14)	<0.01 *
Restricted, repetitive, and stereotyped behavior	1.85 (1.53)	4.43 (2.49)	<0.01 *

MSDD = mixed specific developmental disorder; ASD = autism spectrum disorder; SD = standard deviation; ADOS-2 = Autism Diagnostic Observation Schedule, 2nd Edition; CSS = calibrated severity score; ADI-R = Autism Diagnostic Interview-Revised. * $p < 0.05$.

3.2. Correlation Analyses

Bivariate correlational analysis evidenced strong relationships between assessment tools. The Griffiths-III GDQ was negatively correlated with measures of autistic symptoms, such as ADOS-CSS (r = −0.53, p <0.01) and ADI-R (reciprocal social interaction: r = 0.54, $p < 0.01$; communication and language: r = 0.54, $p < 0.01$; and restricted, repetitive, and stereotyped behavior: r = 0.32, $p < 0.01$), and with the CBCL $1\frac{1}{2}$-5 total score (r = −0.19, $p < 0.01$), However, the GDQ was positively correlated with the VABS-II ABC (r = −0.65, $p < 0.01$) and the DP-3 general development score (r = −0.66, $p < 0.01$). Adaptive functioning, measured using VABS-II, showed strong correlations with all assessment tools. Only the motor skills domain did not significantly correlate with the ADOS-2 CSS (r = −0.10, $p = 0.2$). Conversely, CBCL $1\frac{1}{2}$-5 correlational results were less consistent among the scales. Considering the CBCL $1\frac{1}{2}$-5 total score, no significant correlation was observed with the ADOS-2 CSS (r = −0.12, $p = 0.13$), but it was positively correlated with the ADI-R domains (reciprocal social interaction: r = 0.42, $p < 0.01$; communication and language: r = 0.39, $p < 0.01$; and restricted, repetitive, and stereotyped behavior: r = 0.38, $p < 0.01$) and negatively correlated with the Griffiths-III GDQ (r = −0.19, $p < 0.01$), VABS-II ABC (r = −0.44, $p < 0.01$), and the DP-3 general development scores (r = −0.4, $p < 0.01$). Moreover, as expected, we found strong positive relationships between all DP-3 subdomains and measures of psychomotor and adaptive functioning, as well as negative correlations with the ADOS-2 CSS and the ADI-R scales. Only the DP-3 physical domain did not correlate with ADOS-2 CSS (r = −0.09, $p = 0.24$).

3.3. Predictor of Adaptive Functioning and General Developmental Quotient

A first step-wise method was applied with VABS-II ABC scores as the dependent variable and Griffiths-III GDQ, DP-3 general development scores, CBCL $1\frac{1}{2}$-5 externalizing, CBCL $1\frac{1}{2}$-5 internalizing, and CBCL $1\frac{1}{2}$-5 total scores as independent variables across clinical groups. The model was significant, explaining, respectively, 55% of the variance in VABS-II ABC scores in LD children ($R^2 = 0.55$, $p < 0.01$), 54% in the MSDD sample ($R^2 = 0.54$, $p < 0.01$), and 36% in the ASD group ($R^2 = 0.36$, $p < 0.01$).

A second step-wise method was applied with Griffiths-III GDQ as the dependent variable and DP-3 general development scores, ADOS-2 CSS, CBCL $1\frac{1}{2}$-5 externalizing, CBCL $1\frac{1}{2}$-5 internalizing, and CBCL $1\frac{1}{2}$-5 total scores as independent variables. We found a significant effect of the DP-3 general development scores, as well as ADOS-2 CSS on Griffiths-III GDQ in ASD children ($R^2 = 0.50$, $p = 0.02$).

4. Discussion

Neurodevelopmental disorders (NDDs) are highly heterogeneous; however, they share significant overlaps in both primary and secondary symptoms. Especially in early childhood, children exhibit limited verbal abilities, and this may mask distinctive features. This overlap often makes NDDs appear similar, and diagnosing might be more challenging; for example, many early autistic behaviors overlap with those linked to language delays or intellectual disability [4]. This underscores the importance of selecting appropriate clinical instruments or combinations of instruments to identify differences between NDDs and accurately capture their developmental profiles.

In this study, we administered both screening and diagnostic tools to describe the developmental profiles of ASD, LD, and MSDD in children aged from 0 to 72 months, identifying both differences and similarities. The assessment tools were varied in their levels of structuring, ranging from structured performance tests to parent questionnaires, and consisted of direct and reported measures about children's psychomotor development and well-being.

The initial analysis revealed that, on average, LD children's general developmental quotient fell into a lower average range, as was described in the literature [30]. However, they achieved higher scores across all domains of Griffiths-III and in all assessment instruments administered, when compared to other diagnostic groups.

They also exhibited fewer adaptive and socio-emotional problems according to VABS-II and CBCL $1\frac{1}{2}$-5 total scores. These findings partially diverged from the existing literature, which suggests that children with language disorders are at risk for psychosocial difficulties or morbidity [31–35]. We could explain this discrepancy by the fact that many of these works investigated socio-emotional problems in adolescence or late childhood, focusing on the effects of persisting language problems during school age or co-occurrence of low IQ. Conversely, the mean age of our sample was only 40.67 months and there was no significant evidence of strong correlations between language delays and behavioral problems in toddlers, except for withdrawn scores [36]. Indeed, caregivers frequently remain unaware of children's socio-emotional or behavioral difficulties until 36 months of age, when children attend school and parents receive feedback from teachers.

However, considering information from the DP-3, it emerged that LD children had delayed or below-average developmental profiles, with clinical difficulties not only in communication but also in adaptive, socio-emotional, and cognitive functioning.

Therefore, we might assume that DP-3 provided a more detailed and reliable picture of LD children's skills. Indeed, DP-3 proved to also be an effective clinical tool for assessing expressive speech development disorders in preschool children [37].

Children with ASD exhibited the most impaired profile, showing the lowest scores in all domains of Griffiths-III, VABS-II, and DP-3, as well as the highest scores in CBCL $1\frac{1}{2}$-5 domains. However, no significant differences were found in Griffiths-III quotients compared to the MSDD group in communication and motor fields.

The literature reported a prevalence of approximately 50% of global developmental delay or intellectual disability in preschoolers with ASD [38,39], alongside impairments in language, cognitive, and motor fields compared to neurotypical peers [40–43]. Autistic children frequently demonstrate difficulties concerning phonological and visuospatial working memory, executive functions, and Theory of Mind [40,44–47], which significantly impact multiple domains of development and adaptive functioning, as it was confirmed by Griffiths-III, VABS-II, and DP-3 scores. According to VABS-II and DP-3, individuals with ASD showed difficulties mostly in communication and a highly delayed developmental profile. Moreover, the relationship between IQ, language abilities, and adaptive functioning was well documented [48,49]. VABS-II confirmed the results of previous studies [50], revealing the following pattern: motor skills scores > daily living skills scores > socialization scores > communication scores. All domain standard scores positively correlated with Griffiths-III scale scores and negatively with ADOS-2 CSS. The only exception was the Vineland motor domain, which did not correlate with ADOS-2 CSS. When analyzing the adaptive profiles of other clinical groups, we did not observe the same pattern. LD children stood out for their higher daily living skills scores, followed by motor skills scores, social skills scores, and communication scores, though none of these scores fell into the clinical range. Conversely, MSDD children achieved good motor skills, comparable to those of ASD children, followed by daily living skills, social skills, and communication skills. All adaptive profiles significantly differed among diagnoses, except in the motor domain, where no differences were found between ASD and MSDD children. Similarly, the DP-3 physical domain did not significantly differentiate between these groups and no correlations were observed with ADOS-2. The motor skills domain was comparable among ASD and MSDD children, and we hypothesized that our assessment tools might lack the sensitivity needed to detect subtle differences between these profiles, or that motor skills did not characterize their developmental profiles in early childhood.

In ASD impairments, cognitive and social functioning are often combined with disruptive behaviors, such as conduct problems, physical and verbal aggression, and self-injuring [51]. Disruptive behaviors are very common and negatively impact the quality of life [52–54], reducing cooperative attitude, escaping demands, and gaining access to preferred objects or to restricted and repetitive interests [55,56]. We thought that these common conduct problems could interfere with completing tests of Griffiths-III and contribute to lowering scores and adaptive functioning [44].

Regarding the MSDD, we found that their Griffiths-III scores differed significantly from those of LD children and ASD children, except for communication and motor skills.

Interpreting these differences is challenging because of the limited and available literature.

Few studies have explored MSDD functioning and developmental profiles, though interest in their psychiatric comorbidities is increasing [57].

However, we hypothesized that the similarity in developmental profiles might be explained by the frequent application of the MSDD diagnosis to children previously identified as being at risk for autism spectrum disorders. ICD-10, indeed, describes the mixed specific disorder as *"a residual category for disorders in which there is some admixture of specific developmental disorders of speech and language, of academic skills, and motor function, but in which none predominates sufficiently to constitute the principal diagnosis"* [18].

Similar to ASD, mixed specific disorders involve impairments in more than one developmental area, threatening the typical developmental trajectory. However, in these cases, there is not a selective impairment of communication skills or other autistic behavioral anomalies, such as restricted and repetitive interests.

ADOS-2 and ADI-R are rarely administered in case of suspected language disorders but are used when ASD and mixed specific disorders are suspected. These tools are considered highly sensitive in detecting autistic symptoms and our results underscore their crucial role in distinguishing children with ASD and MSDD. As previously reported [44], our study confirmed that ADI-R and ADOS-2 CSS were significantly higher in children with ASD compared to those with mixed developmental disorders. Furthermore, these scores were negatively correlated with Griffiths-III, VABS-II, and DP-3 scores.

From a cross-diagnostic perspective, we found that the Griffiths-III scores efficiently differentiated children with language disorders from those with mixed developmental and ASD. However, it did not fully capture differences between MSDD and ASD profiles across all domains, such as communication and motor skills. Nevertheless, Griffiths-III showed significant correlations with adaptive functioning, developmental profiles, ADOS-2, and ADI-R scales (except for the restricted, repetitive, and stereotyped behavior scale of ADI-R). These findings are consistent with previous studies, further validating its usefulness as an essential tool for neurodevelopmental assessment.

Regarding CBCL $1\frac{1}{2}$-5 scores, we observed consistency across the diagnostic groups, and only the pervasive developmental problem (DSM-PDP) scale detected differences between diagnoses.

This result confirmed findings in the literature, which provided evidence of the utility of CBCL1$\frac{1}{2}$-5 in identifying children with ASD in Level 1 screening. In particular, the DSM-PDP scale effectively distinguished ASD children from neurotypicals, but also from children with other psychiatric disorders [58–61]. We observed significant differences in the DSM-PDP score between ASD children and other NDDs, but not between MSDD and LD children. We hypothesized that the DSM-PDP is more sensitive to ASD compared to other NDDs and that the lack of significant differences between LD and MSDD children could be attributed to the limited sample size.

Then, we found that VABS-II and DP-3 scores were significantly correlated with the scores of each administered instrument. This suggested that adaptive functioning and developmental profiles were closely tied to developmental quotients, socio-emotional well-being, and autistic symptoms. These clinical assessment instruments proved highly sensitive in differentiating the diagnostic group, creating different profiles for each one.

Notably, regression analysis revealed that a significant portion of the variance in adaptive function across neurodevelopmental disorders and, in general, developmental scores of ASD children could be explained by DP-3. We assumed that DP-3 could be an efficient measure of development, bridging the gap between performance tests and clinical settings by providing information about the everyday functioning of patients.

5. Conclusions

The present study provided a descriptive analysis of the most common developmental disorders in early childhood, combining different types of clinical assessment tools: performance-based structured tests, semi-structured observation, semi-structured interviews, and questionnaires. We integrated information from clinical and natural settings to depict reliable, comprehensive, and detailed developmental profiles, highlighting strengths, weaknesses, and specific characterization aspects. We investigated multiple domains of global functioning, including adaptive, psychomotor, and socio-emotional functioning, and we identified overlaps between diagnostic groups to evaluate which clinical instruments were most efficient in distinguishing clinical patterns.

According to our results, all NDDs exhibited low psychomotor skills, with ASD children being the most compromised, although their profiles were comparable with those of MSDD in communication and motor areas. These findings were consistent with other clinical instrument results, which correlated with Griffiths-III scores, except for CBCL 1$\frac{1}{2}$-5 measures, likely due to the early age of the children and the sample size.

Only CBCL's pervasive developmental problem scale provided relevant information in distinguishing ASD children. However, DP-3 and VABS-II measures highly differentiated developmental profiles of each diagnostic group and they were significantly correlated with performance-based tests. These results highlighted the importance of including parents'/caregivers' perspectives in defining children's functioning and the possibility of using DP-3 as a screening tool for different neurodevelopmental disorders. DP-3 could be a very useful assessment tool: its intuitive dichotomous structure allows for the investigation of all development domains, requiring minimal resources.

6. Limitations

Although this study offered a detailed descriptive analysis and valuable insights, certain limitations should be acknowledged. First, while the sample size was sufficient, the diagnostic groups were unbalanced. ASD children were more numerous than those in other groups and females were underrepresented. Future studies could include an equal number of children across all clinical groups and reduce the predominance of males. Second, we did not observe concordance regarding motor differences between children with ASD and MSDD. Although specific assessment instruments are available, their sensitivity and specificity may be reduced in preschool children with NDDs due to peculiar difficulties in behavior, comprehension, and imitation. Moreover, the limited literature on MSDD hindered deep analysis of developmental profiles and restricted comparison with other diagnostic categories. So, it was challenging to draw strong inferences about MSDD children's functioning. Finally, we did not differentiate children based on their cognitive functioning. However, future longitudinal follow-up studies should discern high- and low-functioning children and evaluate the progression of their development profiles.

Supplementary Materials: The following supporting information can be downloaded at https://www.mdpi.com/article/10.3390/children12020125/s1: Figure S1: Developmental patterns in clinical groups.

Author Contributions: M.E.M., F.G. (Federica Gigliotti) and F.G. (Federica Giovannone) conceived the presented idea, developed the theory, and designed the model. F.M. performed the analysis and verified the computations. F.G. (Federica Giovannone) and C.S. enrolled participants and conducted the evaluations. M.E.M., F.G. (Federica Gigliotti) and G.L. built the datasets and calculated their results. C.S., F.G. (Federica Giovannone) and F.M. supervised the procurement of the findings. M.E.M., F.G. (Federica Gigliotti) and F.G. (Federica Giovannone) wrote the draft, while C.S. and F.M. revised it. All authors have read and agreed to the published version of the manuscript.

Funding: This research received no external funding.

Institutional Review Board Statement: The study was conducted in accordance with the Declaration of Helsinki and approved by the Institutional Review Board of the Sapienza University of Rome; session: 7 March 2019 (5365/2019).

Informed Consent Statement: All subjects' parents gave their informed consent for inclusion before participating in the study.

Data Availability Statement: The original contributions presented in the study are included in the article; further inquiries can be directed to the corresponding authors. Additional data are not publicly available due to privacy concerns.

Conflicts of Interest: The authors declare no conflicts of interest.

References

1. Thapar, A.; Cooper, M.; Rutter, M. Neurodevelopmental disorders. *Lancet Psychiatry* **2017**, *4*, 339–346. [CrossRef] [PubMed]
2. Morris-Rosendahl, D.J.; Crocq, M.A. Neurodevelopmental disorders—The history and future of a diagnostic concept. *Dialogues Clin. Neurosci.* **2020**, *22*, 65–72. [CrossRef] [PubMed]
3. American Psychiatric Association. *Diagnostic and Statistical Manual of Mental Disorders*, 5th ed.; American Psychiatric Association: Washington, DC, USA, 2022.
4. De Lima, T.A.; Zuanetti, P.A.; Nunes, M.E.N.; Hamad, A.P.A. Differential diagnosis between autism spectrum disorder and other developmental disorders with emphasis on the preschool period. *World J. Pediatr.* **2023**, *19*, 715–726. [CrossRef] [PubMed]
5. Parenti, I.; Rabaneda, L.G.; Schoen, H.; Novarino, G. Neurodevelopmental disorders: From genetics to functional pathways. *Trends Neurosci.* **2020**, *43*, 608–621. [CrossRef]
6. Scattolin, M.A.A.; Resegue, R.M.; Rosário, M.C.D. The impact of the environment on neurodevelopmental disorders in early childhood. *J. Pediatr.* **2022**, *98*, S66–S72. [CrossRef]
7. Zwaigenbaum, L.; Bauman, M.L.; Stone, W.L.; Yirmiya, N.; Estes, A.; Hansen, R.L.; McPartland, J.C.; Natowicz, M.R.; Choueiri, R.; Fein, D.; et al. Early identification of autism spectrum disorder: Recommendations for practice and research. *Pediatrics* **2015**, *136*, S10–S40. [CrossRef]
8. Landa, R.J.; Gross, A.L.; Stuart, E.A.; Faherty, A. Developmental trajectories in children with and without autism spectrum disorders: The first 3 years. *Child Dev.* **2013**, *84*, 429–442. [CrossRef]
9. Fernell, E.; Hedvall, Å.; Norrelgen, F.; Eriksson, M.; Höglund-Carlsson, L.; Barnevik-Olsson, M.; Svensson, L.; Holm, A.; Westerlund, J.; Gillberg, C. Developmental profiles in preschool children with autism spectrum disorders referred for intervention. *Res. Dev. Disabil.* **2010**, *31*, 790–799. [CrossRef]
10. Charman, T.; Jones, C.R.; Pickles, A.; Simonoff, E.; Baird, G.; Happé, F. Defining the cognitive phenotype of autism. *Brain Res.* **2011**, *1380*, 10–21. [CrossRef]

11. Taddei, M.; Bulgheroni, S.; Toffalini, E.; Pantaleoni, C.; Lanfranchi, S. Developmental profiles of young children with autism spectrum disorder and global developmental delay: A study with the Griffiths III scales. *Autism Res.* **2023**, *16*, 1344–1359. [CrossRef]
12. Georgiou, N.; Spanoudis, G. Developmental language disorder and autism: Commonalities and differences on language. *Brain Sci.* **2021**, *11*, 589. [CrossRef]
13. Mundy, P.; Jarrold, W. Infant joint attention, neural networks and social cognition. *Neural Netw.* **2010**, *23*, 985–997. [CrossRef]
14. McGregor, K.K.; Ohlmann, N.; Eden, N.; Arbisi-Kelm, T.; Young, A. Abilities and disabilities among children with developmental language disorder. *Lang. Speech Hear. Serv. Sch.* **2023**, *54*, 927–951. [CrossRef]
15. Larson, C.; Ellis Weismer, S. Working memory performance in children with developmental language disorder: The role of domain. *J. Speech Lang. Hear. Res.* **2022**, *65*, 1906–1920. [CrossRef]
16. Leonard, L.B.; Weismer, S.E.; Miller, C.A.; Francis, D.J.; Tomblin, J.B.; Kail, R.V. Speed of processing, working memory, and language impairment in children. *J. Speech Lang. Hear. Res.* **2007**, *50*, 408–428. [CrossRef]
17. Bishop, D.V.; Snowling, M.J.; Thompson, P.A.; Greenhalgh, T.; Klee, T.M. CATALISE: A multinational and multidisciplinary Delphi consensus study of problems with language development. Phase 2. *J. Child Psychol. Psychiatry* **2017**, *58*, 1068–1080. [CrossRef]
18. World Health Organization. *The International Statistical Classification of Disease and Related Health Problems*, 10th ed.; World Health Organization: Geneve, Switzerland, 2019.
19. Lanfranchi, S.; Rea, M.; Ferri, R.; Vianello, R. *Studio di Validazione e Standardizzazione Italiana Delle Griffiths III*; Hogrefe Editore: Florence, Italy, 2019.
20. Green, E.; Stroud, L.; O'Connell, R.; Bloomfield, S.; Cronje, J.; Foxcroft, C.; Hurter, K.; Lane, H.; Marais, R.; Marx, C.; et al. *Griffiths Scales of Child Development*, 3rd ed.; Hogrefe: Oxford, UK, 2016.
21. Alpern, G.D. *Developmental Profile 3*; Western Psychological Services: Los Angeles, CA, USA, 2007.
22. Lanfranchi, S.; Vianello, R. *Developmental Profile 3*; Hogrefe: Florence, Italy, 2015.
23. Sparrow, S.S.; Cicchetti, D.V.; Balla, D.A. *Vineland Adaptive Behavior Scales*, 2nd ed.; Pearson Assessments: Livonia, MN, USA, 2005.
24. Balboni, G.; Belacchi, C.; Bonichini, S.; Coscarelli, A. *Vineland Adaptive Behavior Scales, Second Edition (Vineland-II)—Survey Form*; Italian adaptation; Giunti OS: Florence, Italy, 2016.
25. Achenbach, T.M.; Rescorla, L.A. *Manual for the ASEBA Preschool Forms & Profiles: An Integrated System of Multi-Informant Assessment*; Child Behavior Checklist for Ages 1 1/2–5; Language Development Survey; Caregiver-Teacher Report Form; University of Vermont: Burlington, MA, USA, 2000.
26. Lord, C.; Rutter, M.; DiLavore, P.C.; Risi, S.; Gotham, K.; Bishop, S. *Autism Diagnostic Observation Schedule, Second Edition (ADOS-2)*; Western Psychological Services: Torrance, CA, USA, 2012.
27. Esler, A.N.; Bal, V.H.; Guthrie, W.; Wetherby, A.; Ellis Weismer, S.; Lord, C. The autism diagnostic observation schedule, toddler module: Standardized severity scores. *J. Autism Dev. Disord.* **2015**, *45*, 2704–2720. [CrossRef]
28. Le Couteur, A.; Lord, C.; Rutter, M. *Autism Diagnostic Interview-Revised (ADI-R)*; Western Psychological Services: Los Angeles, CA, USA, 2003.
29. Faggioli, R.; Saccani, M.; Persico, A.M.; Tancredi, R.; Parrini, B.; Igliozzi, R. *ADI-R, Autism Diagnostic Interview Revised*; Italian adaptation; Giunti OS: Florence, Italy, 2005.
30. Jin, W.Y.; Wu, L.L.; Hu, L.F.; Li, W.H.; Song, C.; Wang, Y.Y.; Liu, X.L.; Zhu, Z.W. Intelligence profiles and adaptive behaviors of high-functioning autism spectrum disorder and developmental speech and language disorders. *Front. Pediatr.* **2023**, *10*, 972643. [CrossRef]
31. Lloyd-Esenkaya, V.; Russell, A.J.; Clair, M.C.S. What are the peer interaction strengths and difficulties in children with developmental language disorder? A systematic review. *Int. J. Environ. Res. Public Health* **2020**, *17*, 3140. [CrossRef]
32. Jerome, A.C.; Fujiki, M.; Brinton, B.; James, S.L. Self-esteem in children with specific language impairment. *J. Speech Lang. Hear. Res.* **2002**, *45*, 700–714. [CrossRef]
33. Yew, S.G.K.; O'Kearney, R. Emotional and behavioural outcomes later in childhood and adolescence for children with specific language impairments: Meta-analyses of controlled prospective studies. *J. Child Psychol. Psychiatry* **2013**, *54*, 516–524. [CrossRef] [PubMed]
34. Snowling, M.J.; Bishop, D.V.M.; Stothard, S.E.; Chipchase, B.; Kaplan, C. Psychosocial outcomes at 15 years of children with a preschool history of speech-language impairment. *J. Child Psychol. Psychiatry* **2006**, *47*, 759–765. [CrossRef] [PubMed]
35. Hentges, R.F.; Devereux, C.; Graham, S.A.; Madigan, S. Child Language Difficulties and Internalizing and Externalizing Symptoms: A Meta-Analysis. *Child Dev.* **2021**, *92*, e691–e715. [CrossRef]
36. Rescorla, L.; Ross, G.S.; McClure, S. Language delay and behavioral/emotional problems in toddlers: Findings from two developmental clinics. *J. Speech Lang. Hear. Res.* **2007**, *50*, 1063–1078. [CrossRef]

37. Smirnov, I.I.; Popova, E.S.; Serebrovskaya, O.V.; Skipetrova, L.A.; Cheremin, R.A.; Fateeva, V.V. Studying the possibility of using methods for assessing expressive speech developmental disorders in children 3-6 years old. *Zhurnal Nevrol. Psikhiatr. Im. S S Korsakova* **2024**, *124*, 103–109. [CrossRef]
38. Christensen, D.L. Prevalence and characteristics of autism spectrum disorder among children aged 8 years–autism and developmental disabilities monitoring network, 11 sites, United States, 2012. *MMWR Surveill. Summ.* **2016**, *65*, 1–23. [CrossRef]
39. Delehanty, A.D.; Stronach, S.; Guthrie, W.; Slate, E.; Wetherby, A.M. Verbal and nonverbal outcomes of toddlers with and without autism spectrum disorder, language delay, and global developmental delay. *Autism Dev. Lang. Impair.* **2018**, *3*, 2396941518764764. [CrossRef]
40. Cantio, C.; Jepsen, J.R.M.; Madsen, G.F.; Bilenberg, N.; White, S.J. Exploring 'the autisms' at a cognitive level. *Autism Res.* **2016**, *9*, 1328–1339. [CrossRef]
41. Gernsbacher, M.A.; Morson, E.M.; Grace, E.J. Language and speech in autism. *Annu. Rev. Linguist.* **2016**, *2*, 413–425. [CrossRef]
42. Licari, M.K.; Alvares, G.A.; Varcin, K.; Evans, K.L.; Cleary, D.; Reid, S.L.; Glasson, E.J.; Bebbington, K.; Reynolds, J.E.; Wray, J.; et al. Prevalence of motor difficulties in autism spectrum disorder: Analysis of a population-based cohort. *Autism Res.* **2020**, *13*, 298–306. [CrossRef]
43. Schaeffer, J.; Abd El-Raziq, M.; Castroviejo, E.; Durrleman, S.; Ferré, S.; Grama, I.; Hendriks, P.; Kissine, M.; Manenti, M.; Marinis, T. Language in autism: Domains, profiles and co-occurring conditions. *J. Neural Transm.* **2023**, *130*, 433–457. [CrossRef] [PubMed]
44. Davico, C.; Marcotulli, D.; Cudia, V.F.; Arletti, L.; Ghiggia, A.; Svevi, B.; Faraoni, C.; Amianto, F.; Ricci, F.; Vitiello, B. Emotional dysregulation and adaptive functioning in preschoolers with autism spectrum disorder or other neurodevelopmental disorders. *Front. Psychiatry* **2022**, *13*, 846146. [CrossRef] [PubMed]
45. Habib, A.; Harris, L.; Pollick, F.; Melville, C. A meta-analysis of working memory in individuals with autism spectrum disorders. *PLoS ONE* **2019**, *14*, e0216198. [CrossRef]
46. Li, H.H.; Wang, C.X.; Feng, J.Y.; Wang, B.; Li, C.L.; Jia, F.Y. A developmental profile of children with autism spectrum disorder in China using the Griffiths Mental Development Scales. *Front. Psychol.* **2020**, *11*, 570923. [CrossRef] [PubMed]
47. Jansen, J.M.; Green, E.M.; Stroud, L.; Watson, M. Using the Griffiths III and Quartile Charts in Assessing Autism Spectrum Disorder: A Case Study. *JEL* **2019**, *9*, 30–40. [CrossRef]
48. Mayes, S.D.; Calhoun, S.L. Ability profiles in children with autism: Influence of age and IQ. *Autism* **2023**, *7*, 65–80. [CrossRef]
49. Torras-Mañá, M.; Gómez- Morales, A.; González- Gimeno, I.; Fornieles-Deu, A.; Brun-Gasca, C. Assessment of cognition and language in the early diagnosis of autism spectrum disorder: Usefulness of the Bayley Scales of Infant and Toddler Development. *J. Intellect. Disabil. Res.* **2016**, *60*, 502–511. [CrossRef]
50. Ray-Subramanian, C.E.; Huai, N.; Ellis Weismer, S. Brief report: Adaptive behavior and cognitive skills for toddlers on the autism spectrum. *J. Autism Dev. Disord.* **2011**, *41*, 679–684. [CrossRef]
51. Kanne, S.M.; Mazurek, M.O. Aggression in children and adolescents with ASD: Prevalence and risk factors. *J. Autism Dev. Disord.* **2011**, *41*, 926–937. [CrossRef]
52. Kaat, A.J.; Lecavalier, L. Disruptive behavior disorders in children and adolescents with autism spectrum disorders: A review of the prevalence, presentation, and treatment. *Res. Autism Spectr. Disord.* **2013**, *7*, 1579–1594. [CrossRef]
53. Beck, K.B.; Conner, C.M.; Breitenfeldt, K.E.; Northrup, J.B.; White, S.W.; Mazefsky, C.A. Assessment and Treatment of Emotion Regulation Impairment in Autism Spectrum Disorder Across the Life Span: Current State of the Science and Future Directions. *Psychiatr. Clin. N. Am.* **2021**, *44*, 95–110. [CrossRef]
54. Vasa, R.A.; Singh, V.; McDonald, R.G.; Mazefsky, C.; Hong, J.S.; Keefer, A. Dysregulation in Children and Adolescents Presenting to a Multidisciplinary Autism Clinic. *J. Autism Dev. Disord.* **2022**, *52*, 1762–1770. [CrossRef] [PubMed]
55. Reese, R.M.; Richman, D.M.; Zarcone, J.; Zarcone, T. Individualizing functional assessments for children with autism: The contribution of perseverative behavior and sensory disturbances to disruptive behavior. *Focus. Autism Other Dev. Disabil.* **2003**, *18*, 89–94. [CrossRef]
56. Reese, R.M.; Richman, D.M.; Belmont, J.M.; Morse, P. Functional characteristics of disruptive behavior in developmentally disabled children with and without autism. *J. Autism Dev. Disord.* **2005**, *35*, 419–428. [CrossRef]
57. Grimaldi Capitello, T.; Puddu, A.; Piga, S.; Cuttini, M.; Gentile, S. Parental perception of emotional problems in children and adolescents with mixed specific developmental disorder. *J. Child Adolesc. Behav.* **2014**, *2*, 2–9.
58. Levy, S.E.; Rescorla, L.A.; Chittams, J.L.; Kral, T.J.; Moody, E.J.; Pandey, J.; Pinto-Martin, J.A.; Pomykacz, A.T.; Ramirez, A.; Reyes, N.; et al. ASD screening with the Child Behavior Checklist/1.5-5 in the study to explore early development. *J. Autism Dev. Disord.* **2019**, *49*, 2348–2357. [CrossRef]
59. Muratori, F.; Narzisi, A.; Tancredi, R.; Cosenza, A.; Calugi, S.; Saviozzi, I.; Santocchi, E.; Calderoni, S. The CBCL 1.5–5 and the identification of preschoolers with autism in Italy. *Epidemiol. Psychiatr. Sc.* **2011**, *20*, 329–338. [CrossRef]

60. Narzisi, A.; Calderoni, S.; Maestro, S.; Calugi, S.; Mottes, E.; Muratori, F. Child Behavior Check List $1\frac{1}{2}$–5 as a tool to identify toddlers with autism spectrum disorders: A case-control study. *Res. Dev. Disabil.* **2013**, *34*, 1179–1189. [CrossRef]
61. Rescorla, L.A.; Winder-Patel, B.M.; Paterson, S.J.; Pandey, J.; Wolff, J.J.; Schultz, R.T.; Piven, J. Autism spectrum disorder screening with the CBCL/$1\frac{1}{2}$–5: Findings for young children at high risk for autism spectrum disorder. *Autism* **2019**, *23*, 29–38. [CrossRef]

children

MDPI

Article

A Virtual Reality Platform for Evaluating Deficits in Executive Functions in Deaf and Hard of Hearing Children—Relation to Daily Function and to Quality of Life

Shaima Hamed-Daher [1,2], Naomi Josman [3], Evelyne Klinger [4] and Batya Engel-Yeger [3,*]

[1] Department of Special Education, Oranim Academic College, Tiv'on 3600600, Israel; daher.shaima@oranim.ac.il
[2] Department of Early Childhood Education, Beit Berl Academic College, Kfar Sava 4490500, Israel
[3] Department of Occupational Therapy, Faculty of Social Welfare & Health Sciences, University of Haifa, Haifa 3490002, Israel; njosman@univ.haifa.ac.il
[4] Federative Institute for Research on Handicap, University of Bordeaux, 33405 Bordeaux, France; evelyne.klinger@orange.fr
* Correspondence: bengel@univ.haifa.ac.il

Abstract: Background: Childhood hearing loss is a common chronic condition that may have a broad impact on children's communication and motor and cognitive development, resulting in functional challenges and decreased quality of life (QoL). **Objectives:** This pilot study aimed to compare executive functions (EFs) as expressed in daily life and QoL between deaf and hard-of-hearing (D/HH) children and children with typical hearing. Furthermore, we examined the relationship between EFs and QoL in D/HH children. **Methods:** The participants were 76 children aged 7–11 yr: 38 D/HH and 38 with typical hearing. Parents completed the Behavior Rating Inventory of Executive Function (BRIEF) and Pediatric Quality of Life Inventory (PedsQL), while the child performed a shopping task in the virtual action planning supermarket (VAP-S) to reflect the use of EFs in daily activity. **Results:** D/HH children showed significantly poorer EFs (as measured by BRIEF and VAP-S) and reduced QoL. Difficulties in EFs were correlated with lower QoL. BRIEF scores were significant predictors of QoL domains. **Conclusions:** Difficulties in EFs may characterize children with D/HH and reduce their QoL. Therefore, EFs should be screened and treated. VAP-S and BRIEF are feasible tools for evaluating EFs that reflect children's challenges due to EF difficulties in real-life contexts.

Keywords: deaf and hard of hearing children; executive functions; virtual reality; daily activity; quality of life

1. Introduction

Hearing loss is one of the most common chronic conditions in children, impacting about 34 million children worldwide [1]. Hearing loss encompasses both complete and partial loss of hearing ability [2]. Hearing loss is commonly classified as mild, moderate, severe, or profound [3]. In the United States, the majority of hearing loss cases (50–60%) are genetic, including syndromic (15–30%) and non-syndromic (70–85%) varieties [4,5]. Of the remainder, about 35% of cases are associated with infectious disorders or occur as a result of neonatal events [6]. In addition, the etiology of hearing loss is divided into conductive (due to conditions affecting the external or middle ear), sensorineural (caused by damage or diseases related to the inner ear, such as the cochlea with or without auditory nerve involvement), and mixed hearing loss causes [3]. Hearing loss can affect one (unilateral) or both ears (bilateral). In all cases, hearing loss may lead to functional difficulties and delays in children's communication, motor, and cognitive development [3,7,8]. Therefore, the World Health Organization (WHO) highlights the necessity of early identification and appropriate intervention measures to ensure children's optimal development and well-being [9].

When referring to the implications of hearing loss on children's cognitive abilities, a large body of knowledge emphasizes that the difficulty in adequately perceiving auditory sensory information due to hearing loss may affect children's language development, verbal memory, attention, working memory, and behavioral regulation [10–15]. Working memory and behavioral regulation are components of high cognitive abilities called executive functions.

Executive functions (EFs) refer to complex cognitive processes including control, supervisory, and self-regulatory mechanisms. EFs are responsible for organizing and directing all cognitive activities, emotional reactions, and obvious behaviors. EFs are essential for decision-making and performing meaningful, goal-directed actions [16,17]. Therefore, EFs include capacities such as inhibitory control, selection of relevant task goals, working memory activation, planning and organizing information, solving complex problems, shifting, monitoring a course of action, and evaluating success [16,18]. Because EFs are critical for performing and managing almost all activities of daily life and for adaptive responses to environmental demands [16,19], difficulties in EFs may significantly affect each aspect of daily function. EF difficulties become more visible when an individual is asked to function in a new and unexpected situation when performing multiple tasks simultaneously or new patterns of action [18,20,21]. In children, adequate EFs are a crucial part of their development and are essential for academic achievement, proper social interactions, and daily activity performance [22,23].

Hearing loss during childhood may affect EFs [24–26]. Several studies have been conducted on the development of EFs in deaf and hard-of-hearing (D/HH) school-aged children [26–33]. The combined outcomes of these studies show that D/HH children perform significantly lower in all EF tasks compared to their typical hearing peers. Working memory and inhibition are two areas in which differences have been consistently documented [11].

Some authors have explained EF differences by recognizing the complex interrelationships between hearing, language, and EFs [28,30,34–37]. While some authors have suggested that hearing deprivation has a direct impact on EFs and other higher cognitive processes [34,35], others argue that language deprivation can explain the effect of hearing deprivation on EFs [28,30,36,37]. According to the first hypothesis, hearing loss causes an abnormal bias in developmental and neural connectivity, which may impact EFs and other cognitive processes [34]. The second hypothesis argues that the differences in EFs are caused by a deficiency in language development, given that both are closely related and that language is part of cognitive abilities [37]. A third possibility, proposed by Conway et al. [38], suggests that differences in social environments may impact EFs. Additional studies claim that EF difficulties may be a result of vestibular disorders [39,40], which often present in D/HH children [41]. The relationship between vestibular dysfunction and cognitive impairment remains unclear; however, existing research suggests a potential pathway. The increased gaze and postural instability associated with vestibular loss might demand elevated attentional resources for maintaining balance, consequently reducing the cognitive capacity available for other tasks [39]. Hence, there is no scientific consensus regarding the causal nature of decreased EFs in deaf children. Therefore, more scientific research is needed to elucidate the causes or factors associated with poor EFs in deaf children, allowing us to intervene in these differences immediately and successfully.

Difficulties in EFs among D/HH children may reduce their development, social relationships, and emotional status and can explain variance in learning performance and academic achievement [42–49]. For example, Taljaard et al. indicate that lower hearing levels are associated with lower performance across all cognitive domains, including executive functioning [45]. These concerns have long-term implications for educational and occupational development. For example, Qi and Mitchell [44] found that D/HH children performed consistently poorer in reading and mathematics than typical hearing children. Thus, it is essential to screen for executive dysfunction as early as possible, mainly in vulnerable groups such as D/HH children, to ensure optimal development and function [7,23,31,37].

Most existing studies on EFs in D/HH children examine separate EF components, such as inhibition, shifting, and working memory [11,50]. Data are mainly gathered by neuropsychological measures and in laboratory/clinical settings [24,27,51,52], and lack a comprehensive perspective on the implications of EFs on children's daily lives. Ecological valid measures that imitate activities in real-life contexts [16,53–55] may provide knowledge about how EFs affect the daily functioning of D/HH children. This is in line with the International Classification of Functioning, Disability, and Health (ICF) of the World Health Organization [9], which stresses the necessity of health professionals to consider the implications of a health condition (such as hearing loss) and related body dysfunctions (as EF difficulties) on the individuals' ability to carry out everyday activities and participate in daily life contexts (home, school, community).

One standardized evaluation that measures how various executive function (EFs) components affect children's daily lives is the "Behavior Rating Inventory of Executive Function" (BRIEF) [56]. The parents' version of the BRIEF enables gathering information from the children's main caregivers, which aligns with the family-centered approach that encourages gathering information from parents to increase their awareness of the challenges and functional limitations their child encounters. However, there is a need to gather information directly from the child [57]. The use of Virtual Reality (VR) to evaluate EFs in actual life directly from the child, in a friendly manner, could provide a solution. VR is a human–computer interaction platform that allows the creation of realistic temporal and spatial situations or objects by simulating real-world conditions [58]. VR as an ecologically valid EF assessment enables physicians to observe their clients in everyday situations while performing a task in real-time, potentially incorporating conventional neuropsychological evaluation methods and enhancing reliability and psychometric validity [58,59].

In the rehabilitative context, VR offers several beneficial qualities, such as the ability to administer instructions and stimuli through multiple senses (auditory, visual, and tactile), which can be tailored to patients' potential sensory impairments [58]. VR also provides game-like elements that are perceived as interesting and enjoyable by children, enhancing their sense of immersion, motivation, and cooperation [60–62]. Additionally, VR enables individualized treatment based on the abilities and needs of the patients, and has been found to increase independent functioning in real-life scenarios for various clinical populations [54,63–65]. One of the VR platforms used to evaluate executive function (EF) during instrumental activities of daily living (IADL) is the Virtual Action Planning Supermarket (VAP-S) [66,67]. Shopping activities involve the intense use of EFs, such as planning, working memory, and monitoring, making them a relevant task for assessment [53,68]. The VAP-S simulates a medium-sized supermarket with numerous aisles and records the various EFs used by individuals to successfully purchase a list of daily products [66,69]. Previous studies have demonstrated the VAP-S to be a reliable and valid tool for evaluating EF difficulties in neurological and psychiatric populations [54,70–72], with the ability to classify over 70% of participants based on their group and diagnosis [73]. The VAP-S has also shown concurrent validity with other EF assessments, such as the Behavioral Assessment of the Dysexecutive Syndrome (BADS) [74]. However, to the best of our knowledge, this is the first study to apply the VAP-S to children who are deaf or hard of hearing (D/HH).

The present study discusses the importance of quality of life (QoL) in children, particularly for those with chronic conditions such as hearing loss. QoL is defined as an individual's subjective perception of their physical, social, and psychological functioning [9]. Health-Related Quality of Life (HRQoL) is a subcategory that addresses how a chronic condition affects a person's QoL [75]. Therefore, it is a valuable method of assessing psychosocial functioning in children with chronic conditions that impact several aspects of their lives, such as hearing loss. Hearing loss has been reported to affect a child's quality of life [76]. Evidence from previous studies suggests that the consequences of hearing loss extend far beyond audition, negatively affecting components of QoL, such as academic performance [77], emotion and behavior [78], social functioning [79], and psychosocial functioning [80]. Previous studies have found mixed results regarding the impact of hearing loss on children's QoL, with some studies reporting lower QoL [81,82], while others found no significant differences [83–85] or differences only in specific subdomains [80,86]. The inconsistent outcomes may be due to the varying effects of family, peers, and school on children's QoL, as well as their limited capacity to make significant changes to their environment independently [87]. Consequently, special generic tools for measuring QoL in children have been developed, such as the Pediatric Quality of Life Inventory (PedsQL) [88], which evaluates children's QoL from both their parents' and their own perspectives. Since all QoL domains are among those that may be negatively influenced by difficulties in EF, it seems reasonable that children with disorders involving difficulties in EF may be at an increased risk of poor QoL. The most convincing evidence for a link between EF and QoL is provided by conditions such as head injuries and attention-deficit/hyperactivity disorder (ADHD), both of which are related to executive difficulties as primary symptoms [89,90]. Research among these populations indicates that they are more likely to have poor QoL in various areas, such as physical and social functioning, parental emotional well-being, and family related activities [91–93]. Furthermore, additional studies have shown that EF can predict QoL in various populations, including pediatric epilepsy [94], diabetes mellitus [95], and children with congenital heart disease [96].

Since hearing loss and EF may affect the child's physical and psychological health, social interactions, and level of independence, it is important to refer to the interactions between these factors. The present pilot study explored the relationship between EF and QoL among D/HH children. Elaborating knowledge about these interactions may assist in optimizing intervention programs for D/HH children that are focused on improving daily function and QoL.

The present study aimed to (1) compare EF as expressed in daily life (based on parents' reports, using the BRIEF, and in daily activity performance using the VAP-S) and QoL between D/HH and typical hearing children; (2) examine the relationship between VAP-S and BRIEF scores among D/HH children; and (3) examine the relationship between EF and QoL among D/HH children and the ability of EF to predict QoL domains.

Four hypotheses were posited:

Hypothesis 1. *Differences in EF and QoL are expected between D/HH children and their typical hearing peers.*

Hypothesis 2. *Among D/HH children, deficits in EF as measured by the BRIEF are expected to correlate with performance on the VAP-S.*

Hypothesis 3. *Among D/HH children, deficits in EF as measured by the BRIEF and VAP-S are expected to correlate with QoL.*

Hypothesis 4. *Among D/HH children, EF components would predict various QoL domains.*

2. Materials and Methods

2.1. Participants

A total of 76 children aged 7–11 years participated in this pilot study: 38 D/HH and 38 typical hearing children. All participants were recruited from regular education schools north of (BLINDED). Based on assessments performed in their school, a normal cognitive level was found in both groups. In the study group, the severity of hearing loss was determined based on audiologic evaluations and medical records found in the school. Participants' socioeconomic level ranged from low to high based on their parents' reports about their mean monthly income level (according to the criteria published by the Central Bureau for Statistics in Israel, 2020) [97]. Although the groups were supposed to be matched by sociodemographic parameters, according to the final sample, differences were found in mothers' years of education and socioeconomic level, which were higher in the normal group, as shown in Table 1.

Table 1. Participants' socio- demographic information and the study group' hearing impairment characteristics.

	D/HH Children (n = 38)	**Typical Hearing Controls (n = 38)**	***t* (74)**
	$M \pm SD$	$M \pm SD$	
Age	9.09 ± 1.37	9.41 ± 1.43	0.99
Mothers' years of education	11.92 ± 2.48	16.05 ± 3.00	6.54 **
	Number (%)	Number (%)	χ^2
Gender			
Male	20 (52.6%)	16 (42.1%)	0.84
Female	18 (47.7%)	22 (57.9%)	
Socio-economic level			
Low	8 (21.1%)	4 (10.5%)	16.13 **
Average	24 (63.2%)	11 (28.9%)	
High	6 (15.8%)	23 (60.5%)	
The study group' hearing impairment characteristics			
Side of hearing impairment			
Unilateral	11 (28.9%)		
Bilateral	27 (71.1%)		
Severity of hearing impairment			
Mild (20–35 dB)	13 (34.2%)		
Moderate (35–50 dB)	21 (55.3%)		
Moderately- severe (50–65 dB)	2 (5.3%)		
Severe (65–80 dB)	2 (5.3%)		
Type of hearing loss			
Conductive	11 (28.9%)		
Sensorineural	26 (68.4%)		
Mixed	1 (2.6%)		
Device used			
Hearing aid	30 (78.9%)		
Cochlear implant	3 (7.9%)		
Hearing aid + Cochlear implant	5 (13.2%)		
Mode of communication			
Oral	37 (97.4%)		
Signing	0		
Oral + Signing	1 (2.6%)		

** $p \leq 0.01$. M = mean; SD = standard deviation. The socio-economic level was defined according to the criteria published by the Israeli statistical bureau (2020). The severity of hearing impairment was classified according to the World Health Organization criteria [1].

The exclusion criteria for all participants were as follows: severe/chronic physical/mental health conditions (such as cerebral palsy or intellectual developmental deficits). Deficits were identified based on medical records and parents' reports. Furthermore, the inclusion criteria for the typical hearing control group were normal hearing (a normal hearing test where the threshold is lower than 20 dB), as reported by parents in the demographic questionnaire.

2.2. Measures

2.2.1. A Socio-Demographic Questionnaire

This questionnaire included socio-demographic and medical information about the children, such as age, gender, parents' education, developmental difficulties, health status, etc.

2.2.2. The Behavior Rating Inventory of Executive Function—Parents Form (BRIEF) [56]

This standardized parent report, for children aged 5–18 years, characterizes their executive functions in natural, everyday environments [16]. The BRIEF consists of eight subscales: inhibit—resist impulses; shift—adjust allocation of attention and transition between tasks; emotional control—regulate and modulate emotion; initiate—start tasks; working memory—hold information in one's immediate awareness long enough to perform a given task; plan/organize—use future orientation to complete steps in a sequence to meet a goal; organization of materials—effectively manage belongings; and monitor—self-check one's progression with a task and adjust accordingly. The first three subscales combine to form the Behavioral Regulation Index (BRI), and the last five subscales combine to form the Metacognition Index (MI). The BRI and MI are combined into a Global Executive Composite (GEC) score. The BRIEF includes 86 statements describing various behaviors in which the parent rates the behavior frequency in the past six months on a Likert Scale ranging from 1 (never) to 3 (often). Higher scores on sub-scales, indices, and the GEC are indicative of more problems or difficulties with the executive function measured by the respective scale (score > 65). Test–retest reliability r = 0.86 for GEC, r = 0.88 for BRI, r = 0.84 for MI [56].

2.2.3. The Virtual Action Planning Supermarket (VAP-S) [69]

The VAP-S is a shopping task applied in a virtual supermarket and assesses EFs as expressed in an IADL assignment. The individual is asked to purchase seven items from a list of products from various categories, such as milk products, fruits, and vegetables. The child should then proceed to the cashier's desk and pay for the products. A training task that is similar but not identical to the test is also available to enable the user to become acquainted with the virtual environment. To select a product, the participant presses the left mouse button; the item automatically moves to the cart and its icon disappears from the displayed shopping list. When the participant is ready to pay, they must go to a checkout counter where a cashier is present. Otherwise, payment cannot be completed. At the cashier check-out counter, the participant places the items on the conveyor belt by pressing the left mouse button with the cursor pointing to the belt. The participant presses the left mouse button again to return the items to the cart. Payment is achieved by clicking on the wallet icon. The task is completed when the participant proceeds to the supermarket exit with the cart. While performing the task, visual and auditory distractions (such as other shoppers, signs or objects, and background sounds or music) appear to assess EFs, such as attention and inhibition [67,70]. The present study used the upgraded version of the virtual supermarket VAP-S 2 [67], which was visually improved and yielded more outcome measures. The VAP-S versions were modified to resemble an Israeli supermarket: the relevance of the products, the names of the aisles and grocery items, and all elements of the task were translated into Hebrew and Arabic [67,70]. The VAP-S was shown to be an ecologically valid assessment of EF in people with schizophrenia, Parkinson disease, people with mild cognitive impairment (MCI) and people with stroke [71,73].

Outcome Measures: The VAP-S produced a variable report calculated from the recorded data. These included the total distance in meters traversed by the participant (referred to as the trajectory, Figure 1), the total time in seconds it took the user to complete the task, the number of items purchased (the number of items found and successfully moved into the cart), the number of correct actions (i.e., going to a checkout counter with an attending cashier and not to the one with no cashier; placing the items on the conveyor belt; removing the items from the conveyor belt; paying and exiting the supermarket), the number of incorrect actions (i.e., selecting items were not included in the list; selecting same item twice; going to a check-out counter without an attending cashier; exiting the supermarket without paying; staying within the super), the number of pauses, the combined duration of pauses in seconds, and the time to pay (i.e., the time between when the cost was displayed on the screen and when the participant clicked on the purse icon). In addition, The VAP-S automatically recorded the participant's positions to provide an overview of the trajectory, collisions, and stops they made during the virtual shopping task (Figure 1). The eight outcomes can be conceptualized in terms of executive functioning into two categories: (1) variables that evaluate "task completion" as measured by number of purchased products and correct actions (2 variables); and (2) variables that evaluate "efficiency", which is defined as competency in performance or ability to complete work with minimum expenditure of time and effort; efficiency was measured by time, distance, and incorrect actions (6 variables) [71]. To summarize, the main EF components were measured by looking at the participants' planning abilities within the VAP-S and their organization in time and space [71].

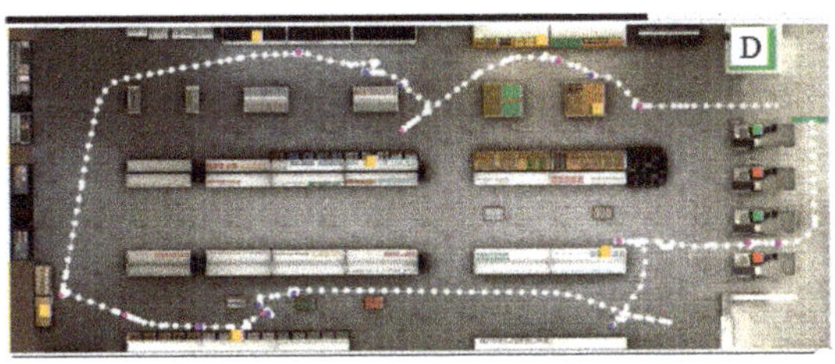

Figure 1. Picture showing the trajectory (path) of a participant during performance of the VAP-S. The departure of the path is indicated with the letter D. White dots correspond to the participant's recorded positions. The orange squares represent the places where products appear on the shopping list. The purple dots represent participants' stops. The blue dots represent collisions made by the participant. The green squares represent checkout counters with a cashier present. The red squares represent checkout counters without a cashier.

2.2.4. The Pediatric Quality of Life Inventory (PedsQL) [88]

The PedsQL assesses QoL in children and adolescents aged between 2 and 18 years. The PedsQL has a self-report version (for children above 5 years) as well as a parent-report version (used in the present study) and consists of 23 items that evaluate four domains of QoL: physical, emotional, social, and school-related QoL. The three domains of emotional, social, and school-related QoL comprise the total score for psychosocial QoL. In addition, the total QoL score is calculated for all the items. The questions are phrased in terms of the frequency of problems experienced over the past month used a 5-point Likert. The scores are converted into a scale of 0 to 100. A higher score indicates a higher QoL.

2.3. Procedure

After receiving permission from the Ethics Committee of the University of Haifa, Ministry of Education, advertisements for participating in the study were published in schools in the north of Israel, calling papers and children to participate in a study on EF and QoL among D/HH children. Parents who agreed to participate with their child in the study contacted the study conductor via phone call, in which they were asked several questions to ensure inclusion criteria. A meeting was set between the study conductor, parents, and children in the child's school. In this meeting, the parents signed a consent form, and the children approved their consent to participate in this study. The parents completed the socio-demographic questionnaire, the BRIEF, and the PedsQL, while their children completed the VAP-S in a quiet room.

2.4. Data Analysis

All statistical analyses were conducted using the SPSS-25 program. Descriptive statistics were calculated for all measures. T test and chi-square tests were performed to examine the differences between the two groups in the relevant demographic variables. Normality tests were applied, and most of the dependent variables showed an abnormal distribution. Hence, the Mann–Whitney test was used to examine whether significant differences existed between the groups in BRIEF, VAP-S, and PedsQL scores. Among D/HH children, the Spearman test was used to examine the correlations between the outcome measures. Based on the correlation results, stepwise linear regression was used to test the contribution of BRIEF and VAP-S scores to the prediction of QoL. As predictors of the emotional, school-related, psychological, and total QoL domains, the following parameters were inserted into the regression: VAP-S: Total distance, total time, and efficiency scores, and BRIEF: MI, BRI, and GEC. To predict the physical QoL domain, the following parameters were inserted into the regression: VAP-S: Total distance score; BRIEF, MI, BRI, and GEC scores. For predictions of the social QOL domain, the BRIEF-MI, BRI, and GEC scores were only inserted into the regression. The correlation between mothers' years of education, socioeconomic level, and the research variables was examined. The results revealed significant findings; thus, this variable was included as a step in the regression analysis. The level of significance was set at $p \leq 0.05$ for all statistical tests.

3. Results

3.1. Hypothesis 1: Comparisons between Groups

When comparing EFs between D/HH and typical hearing children by BRIEF, the D/HH group scored significantly poorer in most BRIEF scales (which are indicated by higher scores)—inhibit, shift, emotional control, initiate, and working memory—in BRIEF-BRI and BRIEF total score (GEC). No significant differences were found in the BRIEF-MI score between the groups (Table 2).

Table 2. The differences between groups in BRIEF scores.

	D/HH Children (n = 38)	Typical Hearing Controls (n = 38)	Z
	Md (IQR)	*Md (IQR)*	
Inhibition	47 (8)	42 (7)	3.79 **
Shift	43 (11.75)	49 (5.25)	2.11 *
Emotional control	45 (7.25)	40 (5.25)	3.19 **
Initiate	43 (11.75)	40 (8)	2.41 *
Working memory	44 (8.75)	40 (6.25)	1.93 *
Plan/Organize	38 (11.25)	38 (3)	0.68
Organization of materials	39 (8.25)	37 (9)	0.17
Monitor	35 (6.5)	35 (5.5)	0.88
BRI	44 (11)	40 (5.25)	3.66 **
MI	38 (10.25)	37 (5.5)	0.81
GEC	45 (12)	43 (5.5)	2.19 *

* $p \leq 0.05$, ** $p \leq 0.01$. Md = Median; IQR = Inter quartile range. BRI = Behavioral Regulation Index; MI = Metacognition Index; GEC = Global Executive Composite.

When comparing EFs between groups, while performing the virtual shopping task (VAP-S), D/HH children scored significantly poorer in all outcome measures, except for 'number of items purchased', 'number of correct actions' and 'time to pay' (Table 3).

Table 3. The differences between groups in VAP-S scores.

	D/HH Children (n = 38)	Typical Hearing Controls (n = 38)	Z
	Md (IQR)	*Md (IQR)*	
Total distance (meters)	190.91 (82.22)	147.78 (32.33)	3.83 **
Total time (seconds)	581.81 (203.17)	420.61 (122.96)	4.57 **
Number of items purchased	7 (0)	7 (0)	0.00
Number of correct actions	13.00 (0)	13.00 (0)	1.00
Number of incorrect actions	6.50 (9.5)	4.00 (4.25)	2.72 **
Number of pauses	14.00 (8.25)	10.50 (4.5)	2.68 **
Duration of pauses (seconds)	196.31 (132.8)	135.22 (80.88)	3.41 **
Time to pay	6.14 (5.91)	5.34 (5.09)	0.88
task completion	20 (0)	20 (0)	1.00
Efficiency	792.09 (269.51)	564.02 (134.12)	4.74 **

** $p \leq 0.01$. Md = Median; IQR = Interquartile range.

When comparing the trajectories of both groups in terms of time, distance, planning, etc., D/HH children showed less efficient performance: difficulties in planning and organization, for example, led to a longer trajectory, with more collisions and stops, and a higher number of incorrect actions (see examples in Figure 2).

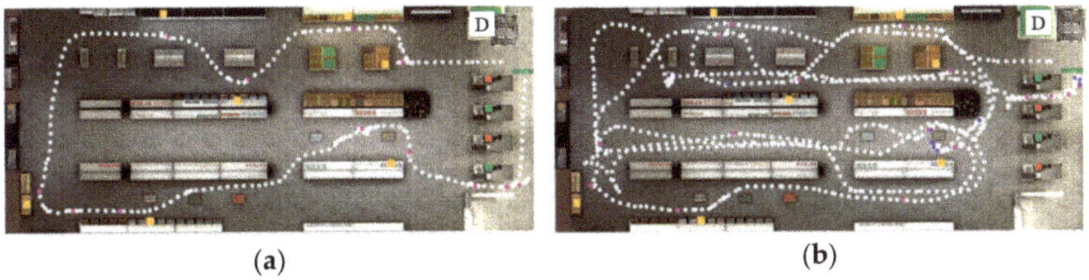

Figure 2. Trajectory (successive white dots) of participants during VAP-S performance. The departure of the path is indicated with the letter D. The orange squares represent the products, blue dots represent the collisions, and purple dots represent the stops. (**a**) Trajectory of a typical hearing child; (**b**) trajectory of a D/HH child. The green squares represent checkout counters with a cashier present. The red squares represent checkout counters without a cashier.

When comparing QoL between groups as assessed by PedsQL, the D/HH group had significantly lower emotional, psychosocial, and school-related QoL, as reflected in the total PedsQL scores as well. No significant differences were found between the groups in physical and social QoL (Table 4).

Table 4. The differences between groups in PedsQL scores.

	D/HH Children (n = 38)	Typical Hearing Controls (n = 38)	Z
	MD (IQR)	*MD (IQR)*	
Physical QoL	100 (12.5)	100 (12.5)	0.06
Emotional QoL	90 (25)	100 (15)	1.96 *
Social QoL	100 (14.06)	100 (1.56)	1.34
School QoL	80 (21.25)	100 (10)	4.02 **
Psychosocial QoL	90 (19.37)	96.67 (8.75)	3.41 **
Total QoL	92.5 (16.09)	96.56 (7.62)	3.43 **

* $p \leq 0.05$, ** $p \leq 0.01$. Md = Median; IQR = Inter quartile range.

3.2. Hypothesis 2: Examining the Correlations between BRIEF and VAP-S Scores, among D/HH Children

Among D/HH children, poorer EF, as measured by BRIEF, was correlated with lower performance in VAP-S. More significant correlations were found between VAP-S scores and BRIEF—emotional control, initiate, working memory, BRI and total score (GEC) (Table 5).

Table 5. The significant correlations between BRIEF and VAP-S scores among D/HH children.

		VAP-S		
		Total Time	Total Distance	Efficiency
BRIEF	Inh	NS	0.31 **	0.20 *
	Sh	NS	0.40 **	0.25 *
	EmC	0.38 **	0.48 **	0.43 *
	Init	0.21 *	0.40 **	0.28 **
	WM	0.25 *	0.36 **	0.30 *
	P/O	NS	0.20 *	NS
	OoM	NS	0.19 *	NS
	Mo	NS	NS	NS
	BRI	0.28 **	0.46 **	0.35 **
	MI	NS	0.32 **	0.20 *
	GEC	0.20 *	0.40 **	0.26 *

NS: not significant; * $p \leq 0.05$, ** $p \leq 0.01$. Only significant correlations are presented in the table. Variables that did not significantly correlate were removed from the table. Inh = Inhibition; Sh = Shift, EmC = Emotional control; Init = Initiate; WM = Working memory; P/O = Plan/Organize; OoM = Organization of materials; Mo = Monitor; BRI = Behavioral Regulation Index; MI = Metacognition Index; GEC = Global Executive Composite.

3.3. Hypothesis 3: Examining the Correlations between EF and QoL, among D/HH Children

Among D/HH children, lower EF, as measured by BRIEF and VAP-S, was correlated with lower QoL. More significant correlations were found with the emotional and school-related QoL (Table 6).

Table 6. The significant correlations between BRIEF, VAP-S and PedsQL scores among D/HH children.

		PedsQL					
		Physical QoL	Emotional QoL	Social QoL	School QoL	Psychosocial QoL	Total QoL
VAP-S	Total distance	−0.30 *	−0.37 *	NS	−0.40 **	−0.30 *	−0.31 *
	Total time	NS	−0.39 **	NS	−0.30 *	−0.31 *	−0.29 *
	Efficiency	NS	−0.44 **	NS	−0.34 *	−0.35 *	−0.34 *
BRIEF	Inh	NS	NS	−0.24 *	−0.38 **	−0.31 **	−0.30 **
	Sh	−0.20 *	−0.59 **	−0.57 **	−0.51 **	−0.63 **	−0.56 **
	EmC	−0.27 **	−0.52 **	−0.47 **	−0.47 **	−0.55 **	−0.52 **
	Init	−0.42 **	−0.44 **	−0.45 **	−0.63 **	−0.60 **	−0.60 **
	WM	−0.34 **	−0.52 **	−0.30 **	−0.63 **	−0.58 **	−0.58 **
	P/O	−0.48 **	−0.47 **	−0.43 **	−0.33 **	−0.39 **	−0.41 **
	OoM	NS	NS	NS	−0.29 **	−0.21 *	−0.21 *
	Mo	−0.42 **	−0.29 **	−0.33 **	−0.24 *	−0.25 *	−0.28 **
	BRI	−0.26 *	−0.48 **	−0.49 **	−0.52 **	−0.56 **	−0.52 **
	MI	−0.44 **	−0.50 **	−0.41 **	−0.52 **	−0.51 **	−0.52 **
	GEC	−0.39 **	−0.51 **	−0.46 **	−0.58 **	−0.56 **	−0.55 **

NS: not significant; * $p \leq 0.05$, ** $p \leq 0.01$. Only significant correlations are presented in the table. Variables that did not significantly correlate were removed from the table. Inh = Inhibition; Sh = Shift, EmC = Emotional control; Init = Initiate; WM = Working memory; P/O = Plan/Organize; OoM = Organization of materials; Mo = Monitor; BRI = Behavioral Regulation Index; MI = Metacognition Index; GEC= Global Executive Composite.

3.4. Hypothesis 4: Predicting QoL of D/HH Children by Their EF

Table 7 presents the results of Stepwise Linear regression analyses of all QoL domains. In general, VAP-S scores were not found to be significant predictors of QoL domains. When referring to QoL domains, the prediction of physical QoL yielded two models: the first included the BRIEF-MI score as a significant predictor, accounting for 44% of the variance (F = 33.3, $p \leq 0.001$), and the second included the BRIEF-BRI score as a significant predictor, accounting for an additional 7% of the variance (F = 22.09, $p \leq 0.001$). Emotional QoL was predicted by the BRIEF-GEC score, which accounted for 54% of the variance (F = 51.11, $p \leq 0.001$). Social QoL was predicted by the BRIEF-BRI score, which accounted for 35% of the variance (F = 23.22, $p \leq 0.001$). School-related QoL was predicted by BRIEF-MI score, accounting for 55% of the variance (F = 51.97, $p \leq 0.001$). The prediction of psychological QoL yielded one model in which the BRIEF-GEC score was a significant predictor, accounting for 65% of the variance (F = 80.81, $p \leq 0.001$). The prediction of the total QoL score yielded one model in which the BRIEF-MI score was a significant predictor, accounting for 73% of the variance (F = 113.63, $p \leq 0.001$).

Table 7. Predicting quality of life among D/HH children by BRIEF scores.

	Model 1			Model 2		
	B	SE *B*	*β*	*B*	SE *B*	*β*
Physical QoL						
BRIEF−MI	−0.82	0.14	−0.66 ***	−1.26	0.22	−1.01 ***
BRIEF−BRI				0.73	0.28	0.45 *
R^2		0.44			0.51	
F for change in R^2		33.3 ***			6.56 *	
Emotional QoL						
BRIEF−GEC	−1.29	0.18	7.74 ***			
R^2		0.54				
F for change in R^2		51.11 ***				
Social QoL						
BRIEF−BRI	−1.17	0.24	−0.59 ***			
R^2		0.35				
F for change in R^2		23.22 ***				
School QoL						
BRIEF−MI	−1.01	0.14	−0.74 ***			
R^2		0.55				
F for change in R^2		51.97 ***				
Psychosocial QoL						
BRIEF−GEC	−1.12	0.13	−0.81 ***			
R^2		0.65				
F for change in R^2		80.81 ***				
Total QoL						
BRIEF−MI	−0.94	0.09	−0.85 ***			
R^2		0.73				
F for change in R^2		113.63 ***				

* $p \leq 0.05$, *** $p \leq 0.001$. BRI = Behavioral Regulation Index; MI = Metacognition Index; GEC = Global Executive Composite.

4. Discussion

This is one of the first studies to examine the EF of D/HH children, as demonstrated by their everyday life settings according to parents' reports and children's daily activity performance in VR. This pilot study examined the differences in EF and QoL between D/HH children and typical hearing controls and explored the relationship between EF and children's QoL among the study group. The main results were that D/HH children had significantly lower EF and QoL. Moreover, greater difficulties with EFs were related to a reduced QoL.

Based on the study results, the first hypothesis was confirmed. The differences in EFs between the groups were manifested in parents' reports and in children's actual activity performance in the virtual supermarket. These results support previous literature on EF difficulties in D/HH children [37,98,99]. Lin et al. [100] suggested that in D/HH children, greater numbers of neural resources are allocated for processing the degraded auditory incoming signals. This may create a cognitive load, limit available resources required for other processes, including EFs, and cause errors, information loss, and slower cognitive processing [101], all of which affect cognitive performance and daily function.

The present pilot study emphasizes the advantages of ecologically valid measures that reflect children's EFs in daily life. According to the BRIEF, D/HH children had lower inhibition, shift, initiation, emotional control, and working memory scores, whereas on the plan/organize and monitor scales, the differences between the groups were not significant. Interestingly, Oberg and Lukomski [102], and Figueras et al. [30] obtained similar results. It is possible that plan/organize and monitor scales are less affected by hearing deprivation in D/HH children. Another possibility is that the timing of the development of various executive skills may place certain skills at greater risk during early school age, whereas others may not be affected until later ages. According to Garon et al. [103], executive skills such as inhibition and working memory may develop earlier than organizational skills, thus making the former more vulnerable than the latter during early school age [104]. Further studies on D/HH children are required to examine this point.

Gathering information from parents, as in BRIEF, is in line with the "family-centered" approach. This approach stresses the importance of including parents' perspectives on their child's challenges in daily life, in order to increase their awareness of the obstacles the child faces in daily life, improve parents' and children's involvement in therapy, and assist them in applying coping strategies and environmental adaptations to improve children's daily function, development, and QoL [105]. However, parents' reports are subjective and rely on their observations. Therefore, it is recommended that a child's performance-based assessment be combined with the evaluation process [106].

The current study found significant differences in VAP-S scores between the groups. This result is supported by earlier studies that used VAP-S to evaluate EF; however, these previous studies were conducted on adult populations [16,54,69,71]. To the best of our knowledge, this is the first study to apply VAP-S in D/HH children. The results showed significant differences in the following VAP-S outcome measures: total distance, total time, number of incorrect actions, number of pauses, duration of pauses, and efficiency (sum of total time, total distance, and number of incorrect actions). These outcomes were found to discriminate between other clinical populations and normal controls with regard to EF as measured by the VAP-S, such as people with Parkinson's disease, stroke, mild cognitive impairment, schizophrenia [16,54,69,71]. Nonetheless, the present pilot study is one of the first to demonstrate the feasibility of VAP-S in measuring EF in D/HH children. The differences in EF between D/HH children and typical hearing controls support VAP-S discriminant validity.

When referring to QoL, as hypothesized, D/HH children had significantly lower QoL than children with typical hearing. Differences were found in emotional QoL (which probably contributed to the difference in psychosocial QoL domains) and school-related QoL. These findings were similar to those reported by Rachakonda et al. [107] and Roland et al. [108]. However, this finding contrasts with that of Alnuhayer et al. [109], who found no significant difference in all PedsQL subscales between D/HH and typical hearing children aged 2–7 years old. In addition, no significant differences in physical QoL were found between the groups. It may be suggested that physical differences between D/HH children and their typical hearing peers at school age are smaller than the differences found in emotional and school-related QoL. The items included in both factors, such as worrying about the future, problems with paying attention in class, and missing school to go to a doctor or hospital, may be more significant in these ages.

The difference in social QoL between groups was close to being significant ($p = 0.06$). Further studies should verify whether this difference is significant by examining a larger sample of children. When referring to the significant differences between both groups in emotional and school-related QoL—psychosocial QoL—indeed, peer relationships and school functioning are increasingly becoming a focus of research investigating D/HH children. The present study supports previous reports highlighting the vulnerability of D/HH children to school and psychosocial functioning [107,108,110]. Parents of D/HH children frequently report their concern and wish that their children, albeit hearing loss, would be included in society, in school settings, and have good academic achievements [111,112], especially when the children study in a regular school system, as in the present study. Studies mention various reasons for the emotional load and its implications on emotional QoL of D/HH children: parents' and teachers' expectations, difficulties with expressive and receptive language development [113], difficulty in converting emotions into abstract concepts and verbal expression, distinguishing between the variety and intensity of emotions [114], as well as the growing social and academic demands and other functional restrictions, may explain the negative emotions such as anger and fear that children with cochlear implants experience [114,115].

Moreover, this pilot study found correlations between the emotional status of children in the study group (as demonstrated by the PedsQL) and their executive functions as measured by BRIEF and VAPS-2. EFs are a worthwhile domain to consider in relation to emotional states as they are also involved in a variety of psychopathologies [116]. From the perspective of developmental cognitive neuroscience, emotion and cognition are closely related and work together to process information and perform actions [117]. Bidirectional influences are likely to occur; cognitive processes play a part in regulating emotions, and emotions can assist people in organizing their thinking, learning, and behavior [118]. As mentioned in the literature, psychological distress may negatively affect executive functions among children in diverse populations like post-traumatic stress disorder (PTSD) [119], depression [120] and anxiety [121]. For instance, a recent systematic review and meta-analysis conducted by Nyvold et al. [119] indicated that children with PTSD have poorer executive functioning overall compared to normal controls. In addition, their findings showed that trauma and PTSD have a negative impact on multiple subdomains of executive function rather than just one or a few subdomains of EF. A similar result was reported in a depressed population, showing that children with higher levels of depressive symptoms had significantly impaired EF performance compared to normal controls [120]. Although not all children with depressive symptoms have an EF impairment, children who present with this comorbidity are at risk for additional cognitive impairments as well as significant psychiatric outcomes, such as longer hospitalizations [122]. Anxiety disorders have also been found to be associated with deficits in EF, as evidenced by studies that found that children with anxiety disorders performed lower than normal controls on some EF tasks [121,123]. Therefore, understanding how EFs are involved in the development of psychopathology may serve therapeutically useful purposes in both prevention and intervention [116].

Accordingly, the relationship between executive functions and emotional status should be further examined in D/HH children to better focus interventions on their specific needs. Researchers and clinicians should note the vicious cycle in which hearing loss leads to functional restrictions that may reduce children's self-efficacy and enhance their emotional load [124,125]. Intervention programs should refer to the emotional profiles of D/HH children, provide help if needed, support children and parents, and enable them to cope better with threats and daily challenges.

When referring to the correlations between VAP-S and BRIEF scores. It is important to note that outcomes from several studies on the use of VR in the rehabilitation of executive functions, particularly VR for shopping, have been encouraging. The current study found significant correlations between the three outcome measures of VAP-S (total time, total distance, and efficiency) and varied BRIEF scores, indicating that these outcome measures appear to be components of EF. This is in line with the literature, which claims that complicated IADL requires the use of executive functions [126]. The significant correlations between the efficiency score of the VAP-S and the BRIEF-MI, BRI, and GEC scores suggest that the VAP-S measure necessitates planning, rule abiding, use of strategy, and organization in time and space, which are main EF components. These findings are consistent with earlier studies that found significant correlations between the VAP-S and the BADS for evaluating EF in people with schizophrenia and people with stroke [54,71].

In summary, the findings of this hypothesis support the use of the VAP-S as an ecologically valid measure of EF in D/HH children, although more studies are needed. Nonetheless, to deeply understand the obstacles and challenges that D/HH children face in their daily lives, it is essential to examine how health condition deficits, such as hearing loss and executive dysfunction, affect their ability to perform daily activities and participate in daily environments. Hence, in line with the ICF model [9], the present pilot study examined the relationship between EF and QoL in D/HH children. The results support the third and fourth hypotheses: greater deficits in EF are correlated with lower QoL, as measured in various domains. Knowledge of the relationship between EF and children's QoL is limited. The existing literature in this regard is mainly focused on children with neurological conditions such as autism [127], epilepsy [128], and cerebral palsy [129], while studies on D/HH children are still lacking. The present study is one of the first to show the significant relationships between EF and physical, social, psychological, and school-related QoL in D/HH children by using ecological measures—parents' report (BRIEF) and children's actual daily activity performance (VAP-S). These results support reports on other clinical pediatric populations, such as children with epilepsy [128], sickle cell disease [130], and attention deficit hyperactivity disorder (ADHD) [131]. The findings highlight how difficulties in various EFs, such as working memory, the ability to regulate emotions, execute goal-directed behavior, and make decisions, may lead to poor coping and negatively affect almost all daily aspects, including academic achievements and social relationships [132,133], leading to cognitive and emotional load and reduced QoL. Given that EF has far-reaching effects on children's cognitive, psychological, and social functions [134,135], EF evaluation should apply measures that reflect these various implications and their expressions in real life.

Interestingly, while correlations existed between the PedsQL domains and all BRIEF scales, only three VAP-S measures (total distance, total time, and efficiency) showed significant correlations with PedsQL domains. As mentioned above, the scores for total distance, total time, and efficiency are the main VAP-S scores derived from various EF components and are affected by low EF abilities. Hence, for example, a low efficiency score may reflect a lower ability to plan, organize, and monitor performance, a higher number of errors, longer time to complete the task, and longer trajectory. The fact that VAP-S successfully differentiated between the EF of D/HH children and typical hearing controls, similar to BRIEF, reflects the parallel validity of these measures.

However, BRIEF scores (MI, BRI, and GEC) were the strongest predictors of low QoL in all the measured domains, whereas VAP-S scores did not significantly predict children's QoL. Therefore, further studies should examine the implications of EF deficits on the daily life of D/HH children, to elucidate functional aspects and reveal feasible measures that reflect them. This approach may assist in optimizing intervention programs for D/HH children and improve not only functions related to comorbidities such as EF but also enable children to better cope with real life in their natural environment. Thus, we may expect optimal development, child inclusion, and well-being.

The results of the present pilot study have important theoretical and practical implications. From a theoretical perspective, the results implement and broaden the ICF model in D/HH children by indicating that an association between body functions (i.e., EFs), activity performance, and QoL exists among these populations. The present study contributes to a deeper understanding of both the concepts of EF and QoL, which in turn contributes to the theoretical foundation of the ecological approach and the establishment of a biopsychosocial model of health. Furthermore, the findings highlight the EF challenges that D/HH children face in their daily life and explore the relationships between EF and QoL, which are still less studied among D/HH children, especially those from regular education.

These findings have practical and clinical implications beyond their theoretical contributions to the existing literature. From a clinical perspective, a deeper and more comprehensive understanding of EF difficulties in D/HH children and their consequences in daily life settings, together with the ability to understand the association between certain EF abilities and specific domains of QoL, may help clinicians implement direct, precise, and effective intervention processes. This helps parents to deal more effectively with the performance difficulties and challenges faced by their D/HH children in daily life. Increased awareness by parents and clinicians, as well as specific knowledge regarding the EF and QoL challenges faced by D/HH children in various settings, may contribute to evaluation and intervention processes that aim to promote their participation and quality of life.

Finally, the research supports receiving knowledge sources that come from both ecological tools based on the child's performance in the context of real life, and from information from standard tools obtained from the parent's point of view, which provides a different perspective on the child's functioning in everyday life. This is undoubtedly an important issue and of great significance in the development of future evaluation and intervention programs.

5. Research Limitations

The current pilot study has several limitations. First, as a pilot study, it has a relatively small sample size, limiting the generalization of the results and conclusions. However, based on the findings of the present study, further studies on larger sample sizes should be performed to strengthen the current results and enable their generalization. Second, the study group included children that study in regular education schools, most of them had mild-moderate hearing loss, and thus may have better participation and inclusion, or better EF as compared to children with severe hearing impairment who study in special education. Hence, this may restrict the generalizability of the study results.

Additionally, in this study, most participants had bilateral hearing loss, but some had unilateral hearing loss; therefore, this study may not adequately represent the experiences of the broader population of D/HH children. It may be assumed that in each group, children may face unique challenges such as sound localization [136], social integration [137] and communication strategies [138]. Future studies should explore the specific experiences and needs of children with unilateral versus bilateral hearing loss to better understand the impact of hearing loss on their development and well-being.

Moreover, the present study relied solely on parent ratings of QoL. Additional studies with larger samples of children with diverse severities of hearing loss are recommended. These studies should apply ecological measures to elucidate deficits in EF, their relationship to hearing impairment severity, and QoL. The diversity of D/HH children will enable a better understanding of how their challenges affect their inclusion and development. These studies should use parents' and children's reports and examine whether any differences exist between them. Interventions should also use frameworks such as the ICF to bridge between hearing impairment, EF, and children's function in real life. Another limitation is that the current study did not address the vestibular function of the study group and did not examine the effect of vestibular deficits on executive functions on EF. This emphasizes the necessity for further research into understanding the complex interaction between vestibular function and cognitive processes.

6. Conclusions

The current pilot study may provide a valuable contribution to the literature by outlining D/HH children's profiles in terms of EF and QoL, as well as emphasizing and elucidating the association between EF and QoL in D/HH children. In this pilot study, several differences were found in the EF and QoL between D/HH and typical hearing controls, highlighting the relevance of screening EF in children with D/HH. The results revealed that EF deficits in D/HH children may be present in their daily lives and affect their activity performance and QoL. In addition, the importance of assessing EF using various tools has been highlighted in the present study. Ecological measures that reflect daily scenarios may help in assessing EF in D/HH children and in creating optimal interventions and training programs for parents and educators, to provide them with practical resources to use when working with D/HH children. These resources could encourage children to participate in more EF-promoting activities at home, in the community, and in school. In line with the ICF model, the children's participation in EF activities may improve and enhance children's daily function, QoL, and optimal development. Finally, investigating the relationship between EF and QoL may contribute significantly to the existing theoretical knowledge of these connections.

Notably, this pilot study is one of the first to examine executive functions through an ecological assessment, integrating both parent reports and the child's performance in a virtual task. Notably, it is the first time that the VAP-S has been utilized with a population of children with hearing impairments. The research introduces professionals to the relevance of using a virtual platform in the assessment and treatment of children with hearing impairments, emphasizing the tool's strengths and its sensitivity in identifying executive function difficulties within this population in a child-friendly manner.

Author Contributions: Conceptualization, formal analysis, investigation, resources, data curation, writing—original draft preparation, writing—review, and supervision, S.H.-D. and B.E.-Y.; methodology and software, N.J.; software, E.K. All authors have read and agreed to the published version of the manuscript.

Funding: This research received no external funding.

Institutional Review Board Statement: The study was approved by the Faculty of Social Welfare and Health Sciences Ethical Committee at University of Haifa (278/17) and the Israeli Ministry of Education's Behavioral Research Ethic Board (9534), ethical date: 13 August 2017.

Informed Consent Statement: Informed consent was obtained from all subjects involved in the study.

Data Availability Statement: Data are unavailable due to privacy and ethical restrictions.

Acknowledgments: We thank Lama Shahbari for collecting the data.

Conflicts of Interest: The authors declare no conflicts of interest.

References

1. World Health Organization. World Report on Hearing. Available online: www.who.int/publications/i/item/9789240020481 (accessed on 20 February 2023).
2. Hotchkiss, J.; Manyisa, N.; Mawuli Adadey, S.; Oluwole, O.G.; Wonkam, E.; Mnika, K.; Yalcouye, A.; Nembaware, V.; Haendel, M.; Vasilevsky, N. The hearing impairment ontology: A tool for unifying hearing impairment knowledge to enhance collaborative research. *Genes* **2019**, *10*, 960. [CrossRef] [PubMed]
3. Graydon, K.; Waterworth, C.; Miller, H.; Gunasekera, H. Global burden of hearing impairment and ear disease. *J. Laryngol. Otol.* **2019**, *133*, 18–25. [CrossRef] [PubMed]
4. Morton, C.C.; Nance, W.E. Newborn hearing screening–a silent revolution. *N. Engl. J. Med.* **2006**, *354*, 2151–2164. [CrossRef]
5. Tanna, R.J.; Lin, J.W.; De Jesus, O. *Sensorineural Hearing Loss*; StatPearls: St. Petersburg, FL, USA, 2021; Available online: https://www.ncbi.nlm.nih.gov/books/NBK565860/ (accessed on 20 March 2023).
6. Prosser, J.D.; Cohen, A.P.; Greinwald, J.H. Diagnostic evaluation of children with sensorineural hearing loss. *Otolaryngol. Clin. N. Am.* **2015**, *48*, 75–982. [CrossRef] [PubMed]
7. Van Wieringen, A.; Boudewyns, A.; Sangen, A.; Wouters, J.; Desloovere, C. Unilateral congenital hearing loss in children: Challenges and potentials. *Hear. Res.* **2018**, *372*, 29–41. [CrossRef]

8. Williams, A.; Pulsifer, M.; Tissera, K.; Mankarious, L.A. Cognitive and behavioral functioning in hearing-impaired children with and without language delay. *J. Otolaryngol. Head. Neck Surg.* **2020**, *163*, 588–590. [CrossRef]
9. World Health Organization. *The International Classification of Functioning, Disability and Health (ICF)*; World Health Organization: Geneva, Switzerland, 2001. Available online: http://apps.who.int/iris/bitstream/handle/10665/42407/9241545429.pdf;jsessionid=EFB5A18701A32C05186DECC5CD1CBEB2?sequence=1 (accessed on 20 February 2023).
10. AuBuchon, A.M.; Pisoni, D.B.; Kronenberger, W.G. Short-term and working memory impairments in early-implanted, long-term cochlear implant users are independent of audibility and speech production. *Ear Hear.* **2015**, *36*, 733–737. [CrossRef] [PubMed]
11. Beer, J.; Kronenberger, W.G.; Pisoni, D.B. Executive function in everyday life: Implications for young cochlear implant users. *Cochlear Implant. Int.* **2011**, *12*, 89–91. [CrossRef]
12. Duncan, A.F.; Matthews, M.A. Neurodevelopmental outcomes in early childhood. *Clin. Perinatol.* **2018**, *45*, 377–392. [CrossRef]
13. Ead, B.; Hale, S.; DeAlwis, D.; Lieu, J.E. Pilot study of cognition in children with unilateral hearing loss. *Int. J. Pediatr. Otorhinolaryngol.* **2013**, *77*, 1856–1860. [CrossRef]
14. Gosselin, P.A.; Ismail, Z.; Faris, P.D.; Benkoczi, C.L.; Fraser, T.L.; Cherry, S.W.; Faulkner, T.I.; Islam, M.S. Effect of hearing ability and mild Behavioural impairment on MoCA and memory index scores. *Can. Geriatr. J.* **2019**, *22*, 165–170. [CrossRef] [PubMed]
15. Moore, D.R.; Zobay, O.; Ferguson, M.A. Minimal and mild hearing loss in children: Association with auditory perception, cognition, and communication problems. *Ear Hear.* **2020**, *41*, 720–732. [CrossRef] [PubMed]
16. Gioia, G.A.; Isquith, P.K. Ecological assessment of executive function in traumatic brain injury. *Dev. Neuropsychol.* **2004**, *25*, 135–158. [CrossRef] [PubMed]
17. Katz, N.; Maeir, A. Higher-level cognitive functions enabling participation: Awareness and executive functions. In *Cognition, Occupation, and Participation across the Life Span: Neuroscience, Neurorehabilitation, and Models of Intervention in Occupational Therapy*, 3rd ed.; Katz, N., Ed.; AOTA Press: Bethesda, MD, USA, 2011; pp. 13–40.
18. Heyl, V.; Hintermair, M. Executive function and behavioral problems in students with visual impairments at mainstream and special schools. *J. Vis. Impair. Blind.* **2015**, *109*, 251–263. [CrossRef]
19. Stuss, D.T.; Levine, B. Adult clinical neuropsychology: Lessons from studies of the frontal lobes. *Annu. Rev. Psychol.* **2002**, *53*, 401–433. [CrossRef]
20. Burgess, P.W.; Veitch, E.; de Lacy Costello, A.; Shallice, T. The cognitive and neuroanatomical correlates of multitasking. *Neuropsychologia* **2000**, *38*, 848–863. [CrossRef]
21. Connor, L.T.; Maeir, A. Putting executive performance in a theoretical context. *OTJR Occup. Particip. Health* **2011**, *31*, 3–7. [CrossRef]
22. Fogel, Y.; Rosenblum, S.; Hirsh, R.; Chevignard, M.; Josman, N. Daily performance of adolescents with executive function deficits: An empirical study using a complex-cooking task. *Occup. Ther. Int.* **2020**, *2020*, 3051809. [CrossRef]
23. Shimoni, M.A.; Engel Yeger, B.; Tirosh, E. Executive dysfunctions among boys with attention deficit hyperactivity disorder (ADHD): Performance-based test and parents report. *Res. Dev. Disabil.* **2012**, *33*, 858–865. [CrossRef]
24. De Giacomo, A.; Murri, A.; Matera, E.; Pompamea, F.; Craig, F.; Giagnotti, F.; Bartoli, R.; Quaranta, N. Executive functions and deafness: Results in a group of cochlear implanted children. *Audiol. Res.* **2021**, *11*, 706–717. [CrossRef]
25. Engel Yeger, B.; Durr, D.H.; Josman, N. Comparison of memory and metamemory abilities of children with cochlear implant and normal hearing peers. *Disabil. Rehabil.* **2011**, *33*, 770–777. [CrossRef] [PubMed]
26. Hall, M.L.; Eigsti, I.M.; Bortfeld, H.; Lillo-Martin, D. Auditory deprivation does not impair executive function, but language deprivation might: Evidence from a parent-report measure in deaf native signing children. *J. Deaf. Stud. Deaf. Educ.* **2017**, *22*, 9–21. [CrossRef] [PubMed]
27. Beer, J.; Kronenberger, W.G.; Castellanos, I. Executive functioning skills in preschool-age children with cochlear implants. *J. Speech Lang. Hear. Res.* **2014**, *57*, 1521–1534. [CrossRef] [PubMed]
28. Botting, N.; Jones, A.M.; Marshall, C.; Denmark, T.; Atkinson, J.; Morgan, G. Nonverbal executive function is mediated by language: A study of deaf and hearing children. *Child Dev.* **2017**, *88*, 1689–1700. [CrossRef] [PubMed]
29. Dye, M.W.G.; Hauser, P. Sustained attention, selective attention and cognitive control in deaf and hearing children. *Hear. Res.* **2014**, *309*, 94–102. [CrossRef]
30. Figueras, B.; Edwards, L.; Langdon, D. Executive function and language in deaf children. *J. Deaf. Stud. Deaf. Educ.* **2008**, *13*, 362–377. [CrossRef]
31. Jones, A.; Atkinson, J.; Marshall, C.; Botting, N.; St Clair, M.C.; Morgan, G. Expressive vocabulary predicts nonverbal executive function: A 2-year longitudinal study of deaf and hearing children. *Child Dev.* **2020**, *91*, e400–e414. [CrossRef]
32. Pisoni, D.B.; Kronenberger, W.G.; Roman, A.S.; Geers, A. Measures of digit span and verbal rehearsal speed in deaf children after more than 10 years of cochlear implantation. *Ear Hear.* **2011**, *32*, 60S–74S. [CrossRef]
33. Vissers, C.; Hermans, D. Social-emotional problems in deaf and hard-of hearing children from an executive and theory and mind perspective. In *Evidence-Based Practices in Deaf Education*; Knoors, H., Marschark, M., Eds.; Oxford University Press: New York, NY, USA, 2018; pp. 455–476.
34. Kral, A.; Kronenberger, W.G.; Pisoni, D.B.; O'Donoghue, G.M. Neurocognitive factors in sensory restoration of early deafness: A connectome model. *Lancet Neurol.* **2016**, *15*, 610–621. [CrossRef]
35. Kronenberger, W.G.; Colson, B.G.; Henning, S.C.; Pisoni, D.B. Executive functioning and speech-language skills following long-term use of cochlear implants. *J. Deaf. Stud. Deaf. Educ.* **2014**, *19*, 456–470. [CrossRef]

36. Nicastri, M.; Giallini, I.; Amicucci, M.; Mariani, L.; De-Vincentiis, M.; Greco, A.; Guerzoni, L.; Cuda, D.; Ruoppolo, G.; Mancini, P. Variables influencing executive functioning in preschool hearing-impaired children implanted within 24 months of age: An observational cohort study. *Eur. Arch. Otorhinolaryngol.* **2021**, *278*, 2733–2743. [CrossRef] [PubMed]
37. Hall, M.L.; Eigsti, I.M.; Bortfeld, H.; Lillo-Martin, D. Executive function in deaf children: Auditory access and language access. *J. Speech Lang. Hear. Res.* **2018**, *61*, 1970–1988. [CrossRef] [PubMed]
38. Conway, C.M.; Pisoni, D.B.; Kronenberger, W.G. The importance of sound for cognitive sequencing abilities: The auditory scaffolding hypothesis. *Curr. Dir. Psychol. Sci.* **2009**, *18*, 274–279. [CrossRef] [PubMed]
39. Bigelow, R.T.; Agrawal, Y. Vestibular involvement in cognition: Visuospatial ability, attention, executive function, and memory. *J. Vestib. Res.* **2015**, *25*, 73–89. [CrossRef] [PubMed]
40. Hanes, D.A.; McCollum, G. Cognitive-vestibular interactions: A review of patient difficulties and possible mechanisms. *J. Vestib. Res.* **2006**, *16*, 75–91. [CrossRef]
41. Kaga, K.; Shinjo, Y.; Jin, Y.; Takegoshi, H. Vestibular failure in children with congenital deafness. *Int. J. Audiol.* **2008**, *47*, 590–599. [CrossRef]
42. Mellon, N.K.; Ouellette, M.; Greer, T.; Gates-Ulanet, P. Achieving developmental synchrony in young children with hearing loss. *Trends Amplif.* **2009**, *13*, 223–240. [CrossRef]
43. Morgan, G.; Curtin, M.; Botting, N. The interplay between early social interaction, language and executive function development in deaf and hearing infants. *Infant. Behav. Dev.* **2021**, *64*, 101591. [CrossRef]
44. Qi, S.; Mitchell, R.E. Large-scale academic achievement testing of deaf and hard-of-hearing students: Past, present, and future. *J. Deaf. Stud. Deaf. Educ.* **2012**, *17*, 1–18. [CrossRef]
45. Taljaard, D.S.; Olaithe, M.; Brennan-Jones, C.G.; Eikelboom, R.H.; Bucks, R.S. The relationship between hearing impairment and cognitive function: A meta-analysis in adults. *Clin. Otolaryngol.* **2016**, *41*, 718–729. [CrossRef]
46. Önal, G.; Huri, M. Relationships between executive functions and occupational performance of children with medulloblastoma. *Br. J. Occup. Ther.* **2021**, *84*, 251–258. [CrossRef]
47. Idstad, M.; Engdahl, B. Childhood sensorineural hearing loss and educational attainment in adulthood: Results from the HUNT study. *Ear Hear.* **2019**, *40*, 1359–1367. [CrossRef] [PubMed]
48. Dammeyer, J.; Marschark, M. Level of educational attainment among deaf adults who attended bilingual-bicultural programs. *J. Deaf Stud. Deaf. Educ.* **2016**, *21*, 394–402. [CrossRef] [PubMed]
49. Rydberg, E.; Gellerstedt, L.C.; Danermark, B. Toward an equal level of educational attainment between deaf and hearing people in Sweden? J. Deaf Stud. *Deaf. Educ.* **2009**, *14*, 312–323. [CrossRef]
50. Pisoni, D.B.; Conway, C.M.; Kronenberger, W.; Henning, S.; Anaya, E. Executive function, cognitive control, and sequence learning in deaf children with cochlear implants. In *The Oxford Handbook of Deaf Studies, Language, and Education*; Marschark, M., Spencer, P.E., Eds.; Oxford University Press: Oxford, UK, 2010; Volume 2, pp. 439–458.
51. Hintermair, M. Executive functions and behavioral problems in deaf and hard-of-hearing students at general and special schools. *J. Deaf. Stud. Deaf. Educ.* **2013**, *18*, 344–359. [CrossRef]
52. Merchán, A.; García, L.F.; Maurno, N.G.; Castañeda, P.R.; González, M.T.D. Executive functions in deaf and hearing children: The mediating role of language skills in inhibitory control. *J. Exp. Child Psychol.* **2022**, *218*, 105374. [CrossRef]
53. Burgess, P.W.; Alderman, N.; Forbes, C. The case for the development and use of "ecologically valid" measures of executive function in experimental and clinical neuropsychology. *J. Int. Neuropsychol. Soc.* **2006**, *12*, 194–209. [CrossRef]
54. Josman, N.; Kizony, R.; Hof, E.; Goldenberg, K.; Weiss, P.L.; Klinger, E. Using the virtual action planning-supermarket for evaluating executive functions in people with stroke. *J. Stroke Cerebrovasc. Dis.* **2014**, *23*, 879–887. [CrossRef]
55. Manchester, D.; Priestly, N.; Jackson, H. The assessment of executive functions: Coming out of the office. *Brain Inj.* **2004**, *18*, 1067–1081. [CrossRef]
56. Gioia, G.A.; Isquith, P.K.; Guy, S.C.; Kenworthy, L. *Behavior Rating Inventory of Executive Function (BRIEF)*; Psychological Assessment Resources: Odessa, FL, USA, 2000.
57. Franck, L.S.; O'Brien, K. The evolution of family-centered care: From supporting parent-delivered interventions to a model of family integrated care. *Birth Defects Res.* **2019**, *111*, 1044–1059. [CrossRef]
58. Pieri, L.; Tosi, G.; Romano, D. Virtual reality technology in neuropsychological testing: A systematic review. *J. Neuropsychol.* **2022**, *17*, 382–399. [CrossRef] [PubMed]
59. Weiss, P.L.; Rand, D.; Katz, N.; Kizony, R. Video capture virtual reality as a flexible and effective rehabilitation tool. *J. Neuroeng. Rehabil.* **2004**, *1*, 1–12. [CrossRef] [PubMed]
60. Ashkenazi, T.; Weiss, P.L.; Orian, D.; Laufer, Y. Low-cost virtual reality intervention program for children with developmental coordination disorder: A pilot feasibility study. *Pediatr. Phys. Ther.* **2013**, *25*, 467–473. [CrossRef] [PubMed]
61. Klinger, E.; Kadri, A.; Sorita, E.; Le Guiet, J.L.; Coignard, P.; Fuchs, P.; Leroy, L.; Du Lac, N.; Servant, F.; Joseph, P.A. AGATHE: A tool for personalized rehabilitation of cognitive functions based on simulated activities of daily living. *IRBM* **2013**, *34*, 113–118. [CrossRef]
62. Mesa-Gresa, P.; Gil-Gómez, H.; Lozano-Quilis, J.A.; Gil-Gómez, J.A. Effectiveness of virtual reality for children and adolescents with autism spectrum disorder: An evidence-based systematic review. *Sensors* **2018**, *18*, 2486. [CrossRef]
63. Gamito, P.; Oliveira, J.; Alves, C.; Santos, N.; Coelho, C.; Brito, R. Virtual reality-based cognitive stimulation to improve cognitive functioning in community elderly: A controlled study. *Cyberpsychol Behav. Soc. Netw.* **2020**, *23*, 150–156. [CrossRef]

64. Lamash, L.; Josman, N.A. metacognitive intervention model to promote independence among individuals with autism spectrum disorder: Implementation on a shopping task in the community. *Neuropsychol. Rehabil.* **2021**, *31*, 189–210. [CrossRef]
65. Liao, Y.Y.; Tseng, H.Y.; Lin, Y.J.; Wang, C.J.; Hsu, W.C. Using virtual reality-based training to improve cognitive function, instrumental activities of daily living and neural efficiency in older adults with mild cognitive impairment: A randomized controlled trial. *Eur. J. Phys. Rehabil. Med.* **2020**, *56*, 47–57. [CrossRef] [PubMed]
66. Klinger, E.; Chemin, I.; Lebreton, S.; Marié, R.M. Virtual action planning in Parkinson's disease: A control study. *Cyberpsychol Behav.* **2006**, *9*, 342–347. [CrossRef]
67. Klinger, E.; Josman, N. Virtual environments to evaluate and treat cognitive deficits in every days function. In Proceedings of the International Conference on Virtual Rehabilitation (ICVR), Tel Aviv, Israel, 22–24 July 2009.
68. Nir-Hadad, S.Y.; Weiss, P.L.; Waizman, A.; Schwartz, N.; Kizony, R. A virtual shopping task for the assessment of executive functions: Validity for people with stroke. *Neuropsychol. Rehabil.* **2017**, *27*, 808–833. [CrossRef]
69. Klinger, E.; Chemin, I.; Lebreton, S.; Marié, R.M. A virtual supermarket to assess cognitive planning. *Cyberpsychol Behav.* **2004**, *7*, 292–293.
70. Josman, N.; Hof, E.; Klinger, E.; Marié, R.M.; Goldenberg, K.; Weiss, P.L.; Kizony, R. Performance within a virtual supermarket and its relationship to executive functions in post-stroke patients. In Proceedings of the International Workshop on Virtual Rehabilitation, New York, NY, USA, 29–30 August 2006.
71. Josman, N.; Schenirderman, A.E.; Klinger, E.; Shevil, E. Using virtual reality to evaluate executive functioning among persons with schizophrenia: A validity study. *Schizophr. Res.* **2009**, *115*, 270–277. [CrossRef] [PubMed]
72. Werner, P.; Rabinowitz, S.; Klinger, E.; Korczyn, A.D.; Josman, N. Use of the virtual action planning supermarket for the diagnosis of mild cognitive impairment: A preliminary study. *Dement. Geriatr. Cogn. Disord.* **2009**, *27*, 301–309. [CrossRef] [PubMed]
73. Josman, N.; Klinger, E.; Kizony, R. Performance within the virtual action planning supermarket (VAP-S): An executive function profile of three different populations suffering from deficits in the central nervous system. In Proceedings of the 7th International Conference on Disability, Virtual Reality and Associated Technologies with ArtAbilitation, Maia, Portugal, 8–11 September 2008.
74. Wilson, B.A.; Alderman, N.; Burgess, P.W.; Emslie, H.; Evans, J. *The Behavioural Assessment of the Dysexecutive Syndrome*; Thames Valley Company: Bury St Edmunds, UK, 1996.
75. McPherson, A.; Webb, G.; Miniscalco, C.; Flynn, T. Language and quality of life in Swedish children with mild hearing loss. *Deaf. Educ. Int.* **2022**, *25*, 309–326. [CrossRef]
76. Aanondsen, C.M.; Jozefiak, T.; Lydersen, S.; Heiling, K.; Rimehaug, T. Deaf and hard-of-hearing children and adolescents' mental health, quality of life and communication. *BMC Psychiatry* **2023**, *23*, 297. [CrossRef] [PubMed]
77. Sharma, R.K.; Chern, A.; Golub, J.S.; Lalwani, A.K. Subclinical hearing loss and educational performance in children: A national study. *Front. Audiol. Otol.* **2023**, *1*, 1214188. [CrossRef]
78. Hameed, N.; Irshad, E.; Mushtaq, R. Emotional and behavioral problems in children with hearing impairment. *Pakistan J. Educ. Res.* **2023**, *6*, 519–531.
79. Bennett, R.J.; Saulsman, L.; Eikelboom, R.H.; Olaithe, M. Coping with the social challenges and emotional distress associated with hearing loss: A qualitative investigation using Leventhal's self-regulation theory. *Int. J. Audiol.* **2022**, *61*, 353–364. [CrossRef]
80. Haukedal, C.L.; Wie, O.B.; Schauber, S.K.; Lyxell, B.; Fitzpatrick, E.M.; Von Koss Torkildsen, J. Social communication and quality of life in children using hearing aids. *Int. J. Pediatr. Otorhinolaryngol.* **2022**, *152*, 111000. [CrossRef]
81. Haukedal, C.L.; Lyxell, B.; Wie, O.B. Health-related quality of life with cochlear implants: The children's perspective. *Ear Hear.* **2020**, *41*, 330–343. [CrossRef]
82. Overgaard, K.R.; Oerbeck, B.; Wagner, K.; Friis, S.; Øhre, B.; Zeiner, P. Youth with hearing loss: Emotional and behavioral problems and quality of life. *Int. J. Pediatr. Otorhinolaryngol.* **2021**, *145*, 110718. [CrossRef] [PubMed]
83. Aanondsen, C.M.; Heiling, K.; Nøvik, T.S.; Jozefiak, T. Quality of Life, family function and mental health of deaf and hard-of-hearing adolescents in mental health services in Norway—A pilot study. *Int. J. Mental Health Deafness* **2018**, *4*, 3–13.
84. Hintermair, M. Quality of life of mainstreamed hearing-impaired children-Results of a study with the Inventory of Life Quality of Children and Youth (ILC). *Z. Kinder Jugendpsychiatr Psychother.* **2010**, *38*, 189–199. [CrossRef]
85. Qi, L.; Zhang, H.; Nie, R.; Xiao, A.; Wang, J.; Du, Y. Quality of life of hearing-impaired middle school students: A cross-sectional study in Hubei province, China. *J. Dev. Phys. Disabil.* **2020**, *32*, 821–837. [CrossRef]
86. Wang, J.; Quach, J.; Sung, V.; Carew, P.; Edwards, B.; Grobler, A.; Gold, L.; Wake, M. Academic, behavioural and quality of life outcomes of slight to mild hearing loss in late childhood: A population-based study. *Arch. Dis. Child* **2019**, *104*, 1056–1063. [CrossRef]
87. Matza, L.S.; Swensen, A.R.; Flood, E.M.; Secnik, K.; Leidy, N.K. Assessment of health related quality of life in children: A review of conceptual, methodological, and regulatory issues. *Value Health* **2004**, *7*, 79–92. [CrossRef]
88. Varni, J.W.; Seid, M.; Kurtin, P.S. PedsQL™ 4.0: Reliability and validity of the pediatric quality of life inventory version 4.0 generic core scales in healthy and patient populations. *Med. Care* **2001**, *39*, 800–812. [CrossRef]
89. Barkley, R.A. *ADHD and the Nature of Self-Control*; Guilford Press: New York, NY, USA, 2005.
90. Baron, I.S. *Neuropsychological Evaluation of the Child: Domains, Methods, and Case Studies*; Oxford University Press: New York, NY, USA, 2018.
91. Klassen, A.F.; Miller, A.; Fine, S. Health-related quality of life in children and adolescents who have a diagnosis of attention-deficit/hyperactivity disorder. *Pediatrics* **2004**, *114*, e541–e547. [CrossRef] [PubMed]

92. Escobar, R.; Soutullo, C.A.; Hervas, A.; Gastaminza, X.; Polavieja, P.; Gilaberte, I. Worse quality of life for children with newly diagnosed attention-deficit/hyperactivity disorder, compared with asthmatic and healthy children. *Pediatrics* **2005**, *116*, e364–e369. [CrossRef]
93. Horneman, G.; Folkesson, P.; Sintonen, H.; von Wendt, L.; Emanuelson, I. Health-related quality of life of adolescents and young adults 10 years after serious traumatic brain injury. *Int. J. Rehabil. Res.* **2005**, *28*, 245–249. [CrossRef]
94. Sherman, E.M.S.; Slick, D.J.; Eyrl, K.L. Executive dysfunction is a significant predictor of poor quality of life in children with epilepsy. *Epilepsia* **2006**, *47*, 1936–1942. [CrossRef] [PubMed]
95. Perez, K.M.; Patel, N.J.; Lord, J.H.; Savin, K.L.; Monzon, A.D.; Whittemore, R.; Jaser, S.S. Executive function in adolescents with type 1 diabetes: Relationship to adherence, glycemic control, and psychosocial outcomes. *J. Pediatr. Psychol.* **2017**, *42*, 636–646. [CrossRef] [PubMed]
96. Gerstle, M.; Beebe, D.W.; Drotar, D.; Cassedy, A.; Marino, B.S. functioning and school performance among pediatric survivors of complex congenital heart disease. *J. Pediatr.* **2016**, *173*, 154–159. [CrossRef]
97. Central Bureau for Statistics in Israel. 2020. Available online: https://www.cbs.gov.il/he/pages/default.aspx (accessed on 1 October 2022).
98. McCreery, R.W.; Walker, E.A. Variation in auditory experience affects language and executive function skills in children who are hard of hearing. *Ear Hear.* **2022**, *43*, 347–360. [CrossRef]
99. Nittrouer, S.; Caldwell-Tarr, A.; Low, K.E.; Lowenstein, J.H. Verbal working memory in children with cochlear implants. *J. Speech Lang. Hear. Res.* **2017**, *60*, 3342–3364. [CrossRef]
100. Lin, F.R.; Ferrucci, L.; Metter, E.J.; An, Y.; Zonderman, A.B.; Resnick, S.M. Hearing loss and cognition in the Baltimore Longitudinal Study of Aging. *Neuropsychology* **2011**, *25*, 763–770. [CrossRef]
101. Campbell, J.; Sharma, A. Compensatory changes in cortical resource allocation in adults with hearing loss. *Front. Syst. Neurosci.* **2013**, *7*, 71. [CrossRef]
102. Oberg, E.; Lukomski, J. Executive functioning and the impact of a hearing loss: Performance-based measures and the Behavior Rating Inventory of Executive Function (BRIEF). *Child Neuropsychol.* **2011**, *17*, 521–545. [CrossRef] [PubMed]
103. Garon, N.; Bryson, S.E.; Smith, I.M. Executive function in preschoolers: A review using an integrative framework. *Psychol. Bull.* **2008**, *134*, 31–60. [CrossRef]
104. Miyake, A.; Friedman, N.P.; Emerson, M.J.; Witzki, A.H.; Howerter, A.; Wager, T.D. The unity and diversity of executive functions and their contributions to complex "frontal lobe" tasks: A latent variable analysis. *Cogn. Psychol.* **2000**, *41*, 49–100. [CrossRef]
105. Pickard, A.S.; Knight, S.J. Proxy evaluation of health-related quality of life: A conceptual framework for understanding multiple proxy perspectives. *Med. Care* **2005**, *43*, 493–499. [CrossRef] [PubMed]
106. Chen, Y.; Fanchiang, H.D.; Howard, A. Effectiveness of virtual reality in children with cerebral palsy: A systematic review and meta-analysis of randomized controlled trials. *Phys. Ther.* **2018**, *98*, 63–77. [CrossRef] [PubMed]
107. Rachakonda, T.; Jeffe, D.B.; Shin, J.J.; Mankarious, L.; Fanning, R.J.; Lesperance, M.M.; Lieu, J.E. Validity, discriminative ability, and reliability of the hearing-related quality of life questionnaire for adolescents. *Laryngoscope* **2014**, *124*, 570–578. [CrossRef] [PubMed]
108. Roland, L.; Fischer, C.; Tran, K.; Rachakonda, T.; Kallogjeri, D.; Lieu, J.E. Quality of life in children with hearing impairment: Systematic review and meta-analysis. *J. Otolaryngol. Head. Neck Surg.* **2016**, *155*, 208–219. [CrossRef]
109. Alnuhayer, O.; Alshawi, Y.; Julaidan, B.; Alromaih, N.; Alakeel, N.; Alballaa, A.; Alromaih, N.I. Quality of life and cochlear implant: Results in Saudi children. *Cureus* **2020**, *12*, e11968. [CrossRef]
110. Fellinger, J.; Holzinger, D.; Sattel, H.; Laucht, M. Mental health and quality of life in deaf pupils. *Eur. Child Adolesc. Psychiatry* **2008**, *17*, 414–423. [CrossRef] [PubMed]
111. Punch, R.; Hyde, M. Social participation of children and adolescents with cochlear implants: A qualitative analysis of parent, teacher, and child interviews. *J. Deaf. Stud. Deaf. Educ.* **2011**, *16*, 474–493. [CrossRef]
112. Wake, M.; Hughes, E.K.; Collins, C.M.; Poulakis, Z. Parent-reported health-related quality of life in children with congenital hearing loss: A population study. *Ambul. Pediatr.* **2004**, *4*, 411–417. [CrossRef]
113. Pimperton, H.; Kennedy, C.R. The impact of early identification of permanent childhood hearing impairment on speech and language outcomes. *Arch. Dis. Child* **2012**, *97*, 648–653. [CrossRef]
114. Stevenson, J.; Pimperton, H.; Kreppner, J.; Worsfold, S.; Terlektsi, E.; Mahon, M.; Kennedy, C. Language and reading comprehension in middle childhood predicts emotional and behaviour difficulties in adolescence for those with permanent childhood hearing loss. *J. Child Psychol. Psychiatry* **2018**, *59*, 180–190. [CrossRef]
115. Stevenson, J.; Kreppner, J.; Pimperton, H.; Worsfold, S.; Kennedy, C. Emotional and behavioural difficulties in children and adolescents with hearing impairment: A systematic review and meta-analysis. *Eur. Child Adolesc. Psychiatry* **2015**, *24*, 477–496. [CrossRef] [PubMed]
116. Lund, J.I.; Boles, K.; Radford, A.; Toombs, E.; Mushquash, C.J. A systematic review of childhood adversity and executive functions outcomes among adults. *Arch. Clin. Neuropsychol.* **2022**, *37*, 1118–1132. [CrossRef] [PubMed]
117. Bell, M.A.; Wolfe, C.D. Emotion and cognition: An intricately bound developmental process. *Child Dev.* **2004**, *75*, 366–370. [CrossRef]
118. Garcia-Andres, E.; Huertas-Martínez, J.A.; Ardura, A.; Fernández-Alcaraz, C. Emotion regulation and executive function profiles of functioning related to the social development of children. *Procedia Soc. Behav. Sci.* **2010**, *5*, 2077–2081. [CrossRef]

119. Nyvold, O.; Nygaard, E.; Augusti, E.M.; Tamnes, C.K. Unity or diversity of executive functioning in children and adolescents with post-traumatic stress symptoms? A systematic review and meta-analysis. *Child Neuropsychol.* **2022**, *28*, 374–393. [CrossRef] [PubMed]
120. Ciuhan, G.C.; Iliescu, D. Depression and learning problems in children: Executive function impairments and inattention as mediators. *Acta Psychol.* **2021**, *220*, 103420. [CrossRef]
121. Dieckhaus, M.F.S.; Hardy, K.K.; Gutermuth-Anthony, L.; Verbalis, A.; Kenworthy, L.; Pugliese, C.E. Anxiety relates to classroom executive function problems in students with ASD, but not ADHD. *Res. Autism Spectr. Disord.* **2021**, *82*, 101739. [CrossRef]
122. Weber, E.B.; Studeny, J.; Kavanaugh, B.C.; Cook, N.E.; Gaudet, C.E.; McCurdy, K.; Holler, K.A. Pediatric depression symptoms, executive functioning weaknesses, and associated neuropsychological and psychiatric outcomes. *J. Child Fam. Stud.* **2018**, *27*, 1661–1670. [CrossRef]
123. O'Rourke, E.J.; Halpern, L.F.; Vaysman, R. Examining the relations among emerging adult coping, executive function, and anxiety. *Emerg. Adulthood* **2020**, *8*, 209–225. [CrossRef]
124. Dammeyer, J. Psychosocial development in a Danish population of children with cochlear implants and deaf and hard-of-hearing children. *J. Deaf. Stud. Deaf. Educ.* **2010**, *15*, 50–58. [CrossRef]
125. Dammeyer, J.; Marschark, M.; Zettler, I. Personality traits, self-efficacy, and cochlear implant use among deaf young adults. *J. Deaf. Stud. Deaf. Educ.* **2018**, *23*, 351–359. [CrossRef]
126. Foster, E.R.; Hershey, T. Everyday executive function is associated with activity participation in Parkinson disease without dementia. *OTJR* **2011**, *31*, 16–22. [CrossRef]
127. De-Vries, M.; Geurts, H. Influence of autism traits and executive functioning on quality of life in children with an autism spectrum disorder. *J. Autism Dev. Disord.* **2015**, *45*, 2734–2743. [CrossRef] [PubMed]
128. Schraegle, W.A.; Titus, J.B. Executive function and health-related quality of life in pediatric epilepsy. *Epilepsy Behav.* **2016**, *62*, 20–26. [CrossRef] [PubMed]
129. Laporta-Hoyos, O.; Ballester-Plané, J.; Póo, P.; Macaya, A.; Meléndez-Plumed, M.; Vázquez, I.; Delgado, E.; Zubiaurre-Elorza, L.; Botellero, V.L.; Narberhaus, A. Proxy-reported quality of life in adolescents and adults with dyskinetic cerebral palsy is associated with executive functions and cortical thickness. *Qual. Life Res.* **2017**, *26*, 1209–1222. [CrossRef] [PubMed]
130. Allen, T.M.; Anderson, L.M.; Rothman, J.A.; Bonner, M.J. Executive functioning and health-related quality of life in pediatric sickle cell disease. *Child Neuropsycho* **2017**, *23*, 889–906. [CrossRef]
131. Gjervan, B.; Torgersen, T.; Nordahl, H.M.; Rasmussen, K. Functional impairment and occupational outcome in adults with ADHD. *J. Atten. Disord.* **2012**, *16*, 544–552. [CrossRef]
132. Best, J.R.; Miller, P.H.; Naglieri, J.A. Relations between executive function and academic achievement from ages 5 to 17 in a large, representative national sample. *Learn. Individ. Differ.* **2011**, *21*, 327–336. [CrossRef]
133. Mendley, S.R.; Matheson, M.B.; Shinnar, S.; Lande, M.B.; Gerson, A.C.; Butler, R.W.; Warady, B.A.; Furth, S.L.; Hooper, S.R. Duration of chronic kidney disease reduces attention and executive function in pediatric patients. *Kidney Int.* **2015**, *87*, 800–806. [CrossRef]
134. Borella, E.; Carretti, B.; Pelegrina, S. The specific role of inhibition in reading comprehension in good and poor comprehenders. *J. Learn. Disabil.* **2010**, *43*, 541–552. [CrossRef]
135. Letkiewicz, A.M.; Miller, G.A.; Crocker, L.D.; Warren, S.L.; Infantolino, Z.P.; Mimnaugh, K.J.; Heller, W. Executive function deficits in daily life prospectively predict increases in depressive symptoms. *Cognit Ther. Res.* **2014**, *38*, 612–620. [CrossRef] [PubMed]
136. Kumpik, D.P.; King, A.J. A review of the effects of unilateral hearing loss on spatial hearing. *Hear. Res.* **2019**, *372*, 17–28. [CrossRef] [PubMed]
137. Laugen, N.J.; Jacobsen, K.H.; Rieffe, C.; Wichstrøm, L. Social skills in preschool children with unilateral and mild bilateral hearing loss. *Deafness Educ. Int.* **2017**, *19*, 54–62. [CrossRef]
138. Lieu, J.E.; Tye-Murray, N.; Fu, Q. Longitudinal study of children with unilateral hearing loss. *Laryngoscope* **2012**, *122*, 2088–2095. [CrossRef] [PubMed]

MDPI AG
Grosspeteranlage 5
4052 Basel
Switzerland
Tel.: +41 61 683 77 34

Children Editorial Office
E-mail: children@mdpi.com
www.mdpi.com/journal/children

www.ingramcontent.com/pod-product-compliance
Lightning Source LLC
Chambersburg PA
CBHW061550210926
51850CB00009B/2062
9783725869749